Promises To Keep

Public Health Policy for American Indians and Alaska Natives in the 21st Century

Edited by
Mim Dixon and Yvette Roubideaux

Foreword by
Michael E. Bird, APHA President, 2000-2001

DEDICATION

To the American Indian and Alaska Native people
Who are entitled to the best possible health care.

To the health care workers
Who sacrifice every day to improve
The health of American Indians and Alaska Natives.

To the warriors of today, the tribal leaders,
Who leave their communities and families
To travel to the halls of Congress to battle
For better health care for all
American Indian and Alaska Native people.

TABLE OF CONTENTS

LIST OF ABBREVIATIONS

AAIP	Association of American Indian Physicians
ADA	American Diabetes Association; also Americans with Disabilities Act
ADM	Alcohol, drug and mental disorders
AFA	Annual Funding Agreement
AFN	Alaska Federation of Natives
AI/AN	American Indian(s) and Alaska Native(s)
AIDLP	American Indian Disability Legislation Project
BCCP	Breast and Cervical Cancer Program (funded by CDC)
BIA	Bureau of Indian Affairs
CCC	Civilian Conservation Corps
CCT	Cancer Care Trials
CDC	Centers for Disease Control and Prevention
CDIB	Certificate of Degree of Indian Blood (issued by the BIA)
CHIP	Child Health Insurance Program
CHR	Community Health Representative
CHN	Community Health Nurse
CHS	Contract Health Services
ESRD	End Stage Renal Disease
FDA	Food and Drug Administration
FDPIR	Food Distribution Program on Indian Reservations
FMAP	Federal Medical Assistance Percentage
FQHC	Federally Qualified Health Center
FTCA	Federal Tort Claims Act
HCBS	Home and Community-Based Services
HCFA	Health Care Financing Administration (renamed Center for Medicaid & Medicare)
HHA	Home Health Agency
IHS	Indian Health Service
IHCIA	Indian Health Care Improvement Act
IPA	Intergovernmental Personnel Act

ISD	Indian Self-Determination
I/T/U	The three components of the Indian health system: 1) the Indian Health Service; 2) Tribally-operated health services; and 3) urban Indian clinics.
JCAHO	Joint Commission on the Accreditation of Healthcare Organizations
MOA	Memorandum of Agreement
NAWWA	Native American Women's Wellness through Awareness
NCAI	National Congress of American Indians
NCHS	National Center for Health Statistics
NCI	National Cancer Institute
NDEP	National Diabetes Education Program
NICOA	National Indian Council on Aging
NIH	National Institutes of Health
NIHB	National Indian Health Board
OAA	Older Americans Act
OMB	Office of Management and Budget
P.L. 93-638 ("638")	Public Law 93-638, The Indian Self-Determination Act
P.L. 93-437 ("437")	Public Law 93-437, The Indian Health Care Improvement Act
QIHP	Qualified Indian Health Program
QMB	Qualified Medicare Beneficiary
RPMS	Resource and Patient Management System
SAIAN	Survey of American Indians and Alaska Natives
SEER	Surveillance, Epidemiology, and End Results (database)
SCSEP	Senior Community Service Employment Program
SLIMB	Selected Low Income Medicare Beneficiary
SNF	Skilled Nursing Facility
TLDC	Tribal Leaders Diabetes Committee
USDA	United States Department of Agriculture
VA	Veterans Administration

ACKNOWLEDGEMENTS

We are delighted with the participation of the extraordinarily knowledgeable authors of the chapters in this volume. For devoting so much energy to this project, we thank Kelly Acton, Dave Baldridge, Linda Burhansstipanov, Ralph Forquera, Yvette Joseph-Fox, Spero M. Manson, David T. Mather and Brett Lee Shelton. This book would not have been possible without the many hours each of these authors shared during their very busy lives, and we are grateful for their efforts and enthusiasm.

The photographs that bring the human face to this story were graciously provided by a number of talented photographers. We thank Alejandro Lopez, Arie Pilz and the National Indian Youth Leadership Project for the photos at the beginning of the introduction and chapters 5, 10, and 11; Rebecca Baca and the National Indian Council on Aging for the photos at the beginning of chapters 3, 6, 8 and 12; Gladys Levis-Pilz and Fieldworks, Inc., for photos at the beginning of chapters 2 and 4; Brett Lee Shelton for permission to use the photo at the beginning of chapter 1; and Walt Hollow for the photo at the beginning of chapter 7.

The American Public Health Association has been enthusiastic in its support for this book from the very beginning; it was Ellen T. Meyer, Director of Publications, who first suggested the concept of a book on American Indian and Alaska Native health. We would like to express our appreciation to Michael Bird, APHA President 2000-2001, for his encouragement and his gracious preface to this volume. Thanks also to Edward A. Tureen, Joseph R. Loehle and the entire APHA production staff.

We would like to thank our families for all the love and support that they have lent to this endeavor. E. James Dixon has been extraordinarily generous in his encouragement, sustenance, patience and humor. Ramon and Cecelia Roubideaux's support, encouragement and intermittent concern over the volume of work involved were greatly appreciated.

As co-editors, we have had the good fortune to work with one another and have grown to appreciate the strengths of our partnership on this project. Our differing styles and backgrounds helped provide balance to the process.

We are grateful for the tireless efforts of the tribal leaders, Indian health professionals, and community health workers as they strive everyday to improve the health of American Indians and Alaska Natives despite the incredible obstacles and challenges placed before them. All of our efforts continue to honor the hopes and dreams of American Indian and Alaska Native people.

Mim Dixon and Yvette Roubideaux
Editors

ABOUT THE AUTHORS

KELLY ACTON, MD, MPH, FACP

Kelly Acton, MD, MPH, is the Director of the Indian Health Service National Diabetes Program. She received her MD degree from Jefferson Medical College in Philadelphia and a Master of Public Health degree from the University of Washington. She is board-certified in internal medicine and a fellow of the American College of Physicians. Dr. Acton has worked in the IHS for almost 17 years, including serving on the Crow and Flathead Indian Reservations in Montana and the Cherokee Indian Reservation in North Carolina. She has published many articles on diabetes in American Indians and successfully led the complex administration of the Special Diabetes Grants for Indians Program.

DAVE BALDRIDGE

Dave Baldridge, a member of Cherokee Nation, has been the Executive Director of the National Indian Council on Aging since 1992. Interpreting Indian aging issues for Congressional subcommittees, federal task forces, state aging organizations, long-term care providers, Indian organizations, tribal- and inter-tribal councils, Mr. Baldridge represents the interests of 230,000 American Indian and Alaska Native elders on a daily basis. A board member of the American Society on Aging, he directs the non-profit NICOA in its dealings within the national aging network, with Indian tribes and organizations, with legislators, and with the elders themselves. He holds a BA in English from the University of New Mexico.

MICHAEL BIRD, MSW, MPH

Michael Bird is the President of the American Public Health Association for 2000–2001. A member of the Santo Domingo and San Juan Pueblos, he is the first American Indian and the first social worker to preside over the American Public Health Association in the 128-year history of the organization. He retired from the Indian Health Service in 1999 after 20 years as a social worker, health care administrator, and innovator of health promotion programs in the Albuquerque Area. He earned his BS in anthropology and his Masters in Social Work from the University of Utah, Salt Lake City. He earned his Masters in Public Health from the University of California, Berkeley. He was a fellow in the U.S. Public Health Service Primary Care Fellowship Program. He served as president of the New Mexico Public Health Association and on the board of Healthnet, New Mexico, a campaign to promote the health of New Mexico people.

LINDA BURHANSSTIPANOV, MPH, DRPH

Linda Burhansstipanov, Western Cherokee, is the Executive Director of Native American Cancer Initiatives (NACI) and the Executive Director of Native American Cancer Research, a Native-owned and operated, non-profit corporation. She earned her MSPH and DrPH from the University of California at Los Angeles (UCLA). She has served on the faculty at California State University Long Beach and UCLA. Dr. Burhansstipanov developed and implemented the Native American Cancer Research Program at the National Cancer Institute of National Institutes of Health. She was the director of the Native American Cancer Research Program of the AMC Cancer Research Center in Denver, CO. Her current research includes several studies and demonstration projects among Native Americans relating to genetics education, increasing mammography screening, developing a breast cancer survivors' support network, increasing participation of women in clinical cancer care trials, and training researchers. She has authored several articles and chapters on cultural issues and cancer control among Native Americans. Dr. Burhansstipanov is a recipient of the National Susan G. Komen Breast Cancer Foundation Award for Community Service by an Individual, the APHA Award for Excellence, and the AVON Breast Health Leadership Award.

MIM DIXON, PHD

Mim Dixon has worked with American Indian and Alaska Native people in the areas of health care, planning and economic development for more than 25 years. She was Health Center Director for Chief Andrew Isaac Health Center (CAIHC), a tribally operated ambulatory care clinic that serves 12,000 Alaska Native people in Fairbanks and 35 villages in Interior Alaska. She was a Policy Analyst for the National Indian Health Board, where she worked on national health policy position papers and was the principal investigator in a number of studies related to the organization and funding of Indian health care. Most recently, she has served as Executive Director of the Division of Health Services for the Cherokee Nation, the second largest tribe in the country. Dr. Dixon earned her BA in economics from Washington University (St. Louis) and her MA and PhD in anthropology from Northwestern University.

RALPH FORQUERA, MPH

Ralph Forquera is Executive Director for the Seattle Indian Health Board, the largest and most comprehensive urban Indian health care delivery system in the nation. He is a member of the Juaneno Band of Mission Indians, Acjachmen Nation. Mr. Forquera has a MPH from California State University, Northridge, and a BS in Health Science & Safety from San Diego State University. He serves on the American Indian Health Commission for Washington State and chairs the Community Health Council of Seattle/King County. He is a co-author of the first population-based study on the health status of urban American Indians and Alaska Natives published in the *Journal of the American Medical Association*, as well as an article entitled, "A Political History of the Indian Health Service," in the December 1999 issue of *The Milbank Quarterly*. Mr. Forquera was the chair of the American Indian, Alaska Native, and Native Hawaiian caucus of the American Public Health Association in 1999–2000.

YVETTE JOSEPH-FOX, MSW

Yvette Joseph-Fox has served as the Executive Director of the National Indian Health Board since 1995. Prior to that she worked as a Professional Staff Member on the U.S. Senate Committee on Indian Affairs for 8 years. She served on President Clinton's Task Force on Health Care Reform Working Group on Indian Health. A member of the Colville Confederated Tribe, she earned her BS in Psychology from Washington State University and a Masters in Social Work from the University of Denver. She is the co-author of a chapter on American Indian and Alaska Native Women in the book *Race, Gender, and Health* edited by Marcia Bayne-Smith. She has produced numerous policy statements on behalf of the 558 federally recognized tribes and advocated on behalf of tribal governments for the passage of federal legislation and appropriations to improve the health of American Indian and Alaska Native people.

SPERO M. MANSON, PHD

Spero M. Manson, Ph.D. is Professor, and Head, Division of American Indian and Alaska Native Programs, Department of Psychiatry, at the University of Colorado Health Sciences Center. Dr. Manson directs several programs, including the National Center for American Indian and Alaska Native Mental Health Research, the Robert Wood Johnson Foundation's Healthy Nations Initiative, the Native Elder Health Care Resource Center, the Native Elder Research Center, the Circles of Care Evaluation Technical Assistance Center, and the Center for Native American TeleHealth and TeleEducation. A member of the Pembina Chippewa tribe, Dr. Manson received his graduate training in medical anthropology at the University of Minnesota. He publishes extensively on the assessment, epidemiology, and prevention of alcohol, drug, and mental disorders across the developmental life span. Dr. Manson is the founding editor of *American Indian and Alaska Native Mental Health Research*. Dr. Manson has received numerous awards for his work, including the Colorado Public Health Association Researcher of the Year, the Indian Health Service's Distinguished Service Award, the prestigious Rema Lapouse Mental Health Epidemiology Award from the American Public Health Association, and the Hammer Award from Vice President Gore (1999).

DAVID T. MATHER, MPH, DRPH

David T. Mather is President of Mather and Associates in Fairbanks, Alaska. He has over 20 years' experience in the direction and management of tribally operated health programs. Dr. Mather was involved in the development and implementation of a Title I Contract for the entire Interior Alaska Service Unit that provides IHS services to the 36 member tribes. He has worked on multiple projects for the Alaska Native Tribal Health Consortium, a multi-tribe organization that provides comprehensive health care services to over 100,000 Alaska Natives & American Indians. Dr. Mather was also the founding lead consultant in the formation of the Alaska Tribal Health Compact, the Title III Agreement that includes 206 Alaska Tribes. Dr. Mather received a MPH from the University of North Carolina at Chapel Hill (1977), and a DrPH from the University of California at Berkeley (1990).

YVETTE ROUBIDEAUX, MD, MPH

Yvette Roubideaux, MD, MPH, is a member of the Rosebud Sioux Tribe and is a Clinical Assistant Professor at the University of Arizona in the College of Public Health and College of Medicine. Her work involves teaching, research and program development in the areas of diabetes and Indian health policy. Dr. Roubideaux is also a consultant for the Division of Diabetes Translation at the Centers for Disease Control and Prevention and the Indian Health Service National Diabetes Program on national projects related to diabetes in American Indians. Dr. Roubideaux is the Chair of the National Diabetes Education Program American Indian Campaign, and she recently completed the Commonwealth Fund/Harvard University Fellowship in Minority Health Policy and the University of Colorado Native Elder Resource Center Native Investigator Program. She is a consultant for the Henry J. Kaiser Family Foundation Native American Health Policy Fellowship Program. Dr. Roubideaux was the President of the Association of American Indian Physicians in 1999–2000.

BRETT LEE SHELTON, MA, JD

Brett Lee Shelton is an enrolled member of the Oglala Lakota Nation who was born in Rapid City, South Dakota, and grew up in South Dakota and Colorado.

He received his BS in Business magna cum laude from Baker University, Baldwin City, Kansas, an MA in Philosophy from the University of Kansas, and his JD from Stanford Law School in California. He has worked as an attorney in private practice and for the Native American Rights Fund, as a policy analyst for the National Indian Health Board, and for the Council of Energy Resources Tribes and Stanford University. He currently operates a private consulting and legal practice in Colorado, and serves as Director of Policy and Research for the Indigenous Peoples Council on Biocolonialism on the Pyramid Lake Reservation in Nevada.

FOREWORD

This book is a first and it is long overdue; it gives us reason to celebrate. Starting this new century with a book on American Indian and Alaska Native health is a powerful statement on behalf of the First Americans: "We still are here. We still exist and have survived. We shall continue in this next century."

The history of Indian health in the Americas predates the history of the United States by centuries, yet American Indian and Alaska Native contributions to this country have been overlooked. Those who first populated the Americas were generally healthy; they had their own systems of health care, and their knowledge of the medicinal use of plants is admirable. American Indians and Alaska Natives developed their own concepts of health, disease and medical practice. A central belief for many of the tribes was the interrelationship of mind, body and spirit. Because they lived close to the land, tribes have always recognized the importance of the environment to health: Earth is our Mother. Today, the validity of these concepts is recognized and acknowledged throughout the world.

I am happy to say that it is a new day. Through the American Public Health Association (APHA), American Indian and Alaska Native people have the opportunity to advance and contribute in partnership with other committed and caring public health professionals. The American Indian/Alaska Native/Native Hawaiian Caucus of the APHA has initiated policy statements that have been embraced by all 30,000 members of the APHA; they address such pressing issues as the devastation caused by diabetes, and the need for adequate funding for services to Native American people.

We must all join hands to lend support to tribes in their efforts to meet the health care needs of their people. Reducing the health disparities that affect American Indian and Alaska Native people will require commitment from politicians and policy makers at the federal and state levels, public health professionals in state and county health departments, private grant-making foundations, universities, researchers, and ordinary people who want to see America keep her promises. This book provides an opportunity for people to increase their base of knowledge on these very complex issues, to find better ways to work cooperatively with tribes, and to reduce the disparities in health for American Indian and Alaska Native people.

Michael Bird
President, APHA
2000–2001

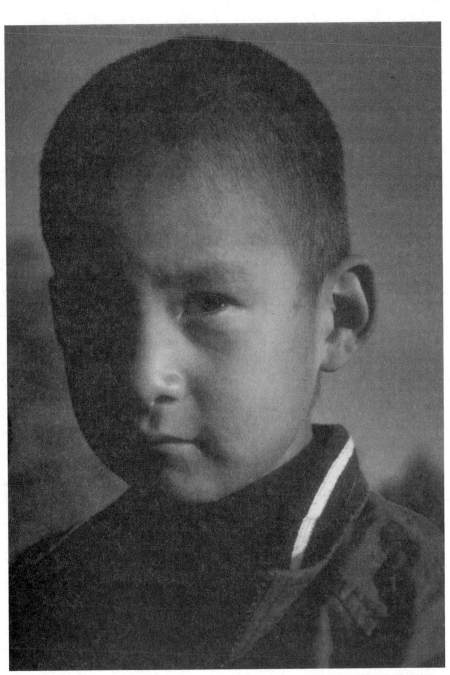

INTRODUCTION
Mim Dixon and Yvette Roubideaux

Raising the health status of American Indians and Alaska Natives to the highest level is one of the most significant public health challenges facing our nation today. While the health status of American Indians and Alaska Natives has improved over the past century, significant disparities still exist in health status, quality of health care, access to health care services, resources and funding for health care, and available services. The Indian health care system has been working to meet these challenges, but there is a clear need for more effective public health efforts and policies to address these disparities. This book examines the most significant issues in the Indian health care system with a focus on current public health practices and recommended changes in policies.

There are more than 2.5 million Americans who are descendents of the original inhabitants of this country. They are members of tribes that have their own distinct languages, cultures and governments. The federal government has recognized 558 of these tribes located in 35 different states. Nearly half of these tribes are located in Alaska, where each Alaska Native village is considered a tribe in itself. Another 100 tribes are located in California. However, the largest American Indian population is in Oklahoma, where many tribes were relocated from their homelands east of the Mississippi River. The largest tribe is the Navajo Nation, which has about 250,000 members in three states, comprising nearly 10 percent of the American Indian population. The smallest tribes have only a few hundred members.

Through law and treaties, the federal government has made a commitment to provide health care free of charge to these American Indians and Alaska Natives (also called "AI/AN" and simply American Indians in this book). Tribes paid for their health care by relinquishing their land to the federal government in the past for the promise of health care in the future. Yet, the federal government has not kept its part of the promise. Congress has never funded Indian health care at a level that would provide health services comparable to that which other Americans receive. As a result, the Indian health care system is struggling to meet the needs of the growing AI/AN population.

With a high birth rate, the population of American Indians and Alaska Natives is growing faster than other minority groups. By 2050 it is estimated that there will be 4.3 million AI/AN in the United States. The AI/AN population is young, with about 1/3 of AI/AN under 15 years old. While educational levels of American Indians have improved significantly, the current data on the number of AI/AN who are high school graduates (65 percent), or have obtained higher education, are still well below that of the general U.S. population. According to the 1990 U.S. Census, the unemployment rate for AI/AN was more than twice that of the U.S. population as a whole and nearly 1/3 of AI/AN were living below the poverty level. Federal policies and high levels of unemployment have resulted in many American Indians leaving their reservations to find jobs and better opportunities for their families. It is estimated that over half the American Indian population lives in urban areas.

Approximately 1.5 million American Indians and Alaska Natives utilize health care facilities and services funded through the Indian Health Service (IHS), a federal program established to provide health care through a system of clinics and hospitals located on or near reservations and other AI/AN communities. The IHS is organized within 12 area offices that oversee 150 service units in Indian communities across the country. The programs and facilities in the Indian health system are jointly administered by the IHS, tribes and urban programs (I/T/U).

Using a public health model, the Indian health programs include community health nursing, community health education, alcohol and substance abuse treatment centers, construction and maintenance of water and sewer systems, and other environmental health services. The IHS also funds a Contract Health Services program to purchase health care services from the private sector where IHS facilities are insufficient or unavailable. The total IHS budget in 2000 was $2.2 billion, which meets less than 60 percent of the health care needs of the AI/AN population.

Despite the availability of free health care, the health status of American Indians and Alaska Natives continues to be worse than any other group in our country. Data collected in 1993 by the Indian Health Service revealed that AI/AN infant mortality rates were higher and life-expectancy was lower than the general population; AI/AN were dying at younger ages compared to other Americans.

Like other Americans, the leading causes of death among AI/AN are heart disease and cancer. While the morbidity and mortality rates from acute health problems such as infectious diseases are declining, the rates of chronic diseases are increasing rapidly as the AI/AN population ages. However, AI/AN still have a tuberculosis rate that is 425 percent greater than the U.S. All Races population. AI/AN also experience significantly greater rates of death due to behavioral health problems, including alcoholism (579 percent greater), accidents (212 percent greater), suicide (70 percent greater), and homicide (41 percent greater). Some of the highest rates of diabetes in the world are now found in Indian communities; regrettably, the death rate from diabetes mellitus is 231 percent greater among AI/AN than the U.S. All Races population.

The good news for chronic diseases, like heart disease, cancer, and diabetes, is that it may be possible to reduce the risk factors for these diseases when people live healthy lifestyles. Addressing the needs of small, isolated, culturally and politically distinct tribes requires special efforts to develop public health solutions and policies. While the general U.S. population is learning the benefits of holistic health and disease prevention, AI/AN communities are recognizing that their own traditional systems of health care were among the first to promote healthy lifestyles, wellness, and community health. AI/AN likely had the first public-health oriented health care system on this continent.

As the poet Robert Frost said, "But I have promises to keep, and miles to go before I sleep." This book reiterates the promises made to American Indians through history and laws. Several complex issues in Indian health are discussed, including the unique role of tribes, organization of health care delivery systems, the changing demography, specific health challenges due to chronic diseases, and unmet health care needs. The concluding chapter outlines the potential of the Indian health care system to provide the highest level of care.

On one hand, the issues related to American Indian and Alaska Native health are very complex. On the other hand, the solutions may be very simple.

As we enter the 21st century, America is experiencing an unprecedented period of economic growth with a surplus in government budgets; it is a time when we have the resources to address the long-neglected health needs of the indigenous people of our country. It is a time when we can honor the commitments that have been made and demonstrate our respect for the venerable Indian nations. It is a time to re-think our policies and funding levels for American Indian and Alaska Native health care. It is a time to act on our highest principles, and to honor the words and promises made by our country.

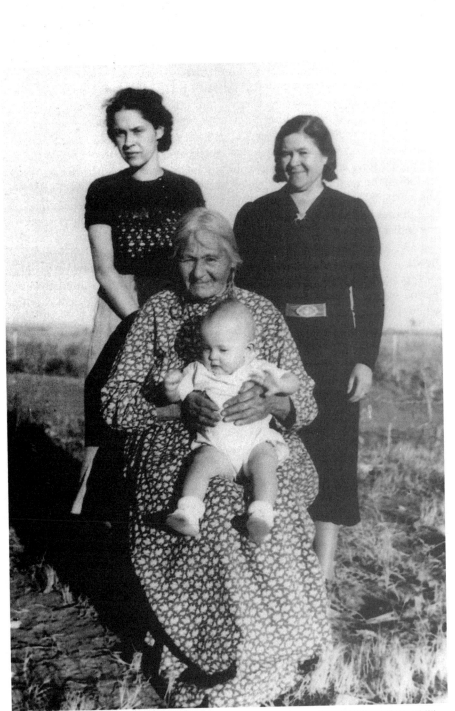

LEGAL AND HISTORICAL BASIS OF INDIAN HEALTH CARE

Brett Lee Shelton

The legal and historical background in which the present health care system for American Indians and Alaska Natives (AI/AN) exists is the result of an ever-changing political landscape. There have been different periods in which different policies dominated, but the threads of each period's politics have remained long after each has passed. From the beginning, tribal self-determination, government-to-government relations between tribes and the United States, and tribal autonomy have existed as common themes beneath federal government—Indian relations. In addition, a federal trust responsibility has grown as a result of the relations between the federal government and the tribes. Both the traditional and the Western Indian health care systems exist within this same complex legal and historical framework; so does the rest of Indian life—the laws, policies, history, and lives of both Indians and non-Indians are all inextricably bound in this story.

OLDEST HEALTH CARE: TRIBAL TRADITIONS

For the tribes of this continent, the beginning of the story is the beginning of time. Prior to European[1] contact, American Indians and Alaska Natives already had their own systems of traditional medicine and health care. These

---

[1] The countries commonly understood as most active in colonizing North America include England, France, Spain, and the Netherlands.

traditional systems survive to this day, although Western systems have been implemented as well. This chapter will review the legal and historical context of the transition from purely traditional systems of health care to the current system. Despite the common conception that contact with Europeans eventually "civilized" the native inhabitants of the Western Hemisphere, in reality many highly-developed societies, with their own systems of health care, already existed. These pre-contact civilizations had extensive knowledge of diseases, medicines, surgery, and health promotion activities (Weatherford 1988). In fact, indigenous knowledge from the Western Hemisphere has contributed much to modern Western medicine (Weatherford 1988).

Mainstream American culture rarely recognizes these contributions, however. Instead, much of the American public's perception of Native American health care has been shaped by misperceptions and distortions. In present times, this influence can be seen in the "new-age" conceptions of "native" practices being available for anyone seeking spiritual and physical health and balance with creation, as just one choice on the spiritual smorgasbord of multiculturalism from which "enlightened" individuals may help themselves (Corbett 1999).

Traditional healing is still practiced among many AI/AN communities today, despite a continuing history of attacks on several fronts, including political attempts to destroy it, demonization by Western religions viewing these practices as "savage" or even "demonic," and distortion by outsiders seeking enlightenment in a form that is virtually unrecognizable to AI/AN people.

It has been no small feat that traditional health care practices have survived, given that American Indians and Alaska Natives have endured an almost constantly changing political and legal landscape, largely imposed on them by a culture that has struggled with how to deal with its "Indian problem." Although anti-Indian policies have pushed for eradication of Indian ways (and, at times, eradication of Indians themselves), there have also been times in which compassion has led to changes that have improved the health of AI/AN people. As a result, a Western health care system has been developed for AI/AN tribes that have been officially recognized as such by the federal government.

EARLY ROOTS OF FEDERAL INDIAN LAW AND POLICY

There are some common themes that run throughout the history of relations between Indian tribes and the United States; there have also been several drastic shifts in certain policies. As the political landscape has changed over the decades, some new laws have developed while others, remnants from earlier times, remain intact or are reinterpreted in light of the prevailing political winds. The result is a very complicated field of law addressing Indian tribes and individual Indians, which is an overlay to laws common to the rest of the country. As the Supreme Court noted as early as 1832, "the relation of the Indians to the United States is marked by peculiarities and cardinal distinctions which exist nowhere else." (*Cherokee Nation v. Georgia*, 30 U.S. (5 Pet.) 1, 16 (1831).)

EUROPEAN ROOTS: DISCOVERY, CONQUEST, AND "INDIAN TITLE"

After they reached the "New" World, the European powers competed to formulate a system to decide who among them got the first opportunity to exploit the resources within any particular area. In other words, they had to decide who could colonize each "newly-discovered" area. Their solutions were the "doctrine of discovery" and the "doctrine of conquest." Put simply, these doctrines provided that the first among them to discover and claim a region and, if necessary, vanquish its inhabitants, had the right to exploit the resources. Among the colonizing nations, the first discoverer had the right to control the land, and the land became that nation's colony.

The doctrines of discovery and conquest were explained clearly in one of the first Supreme Court cases to address the status of Indian tribes in the United States, *Johnson v. McIntosh*. (21 U.S. (8 Wheat.) 543 (1823)). In this 1823 decision, the Court decided that a title to land granted to a non-Indian by the Piankeshaw Nation in Illinois would not be recognized by the United States government and its legal system. The court based its decision on a comparison of "Indian titles" and other titles under the laws of the United States. To explain the differences, the court examined the European predecessors to the law of the United States, particularly the doctrines of discovery and conquest.

Chief Justice John Marshall wrote the opinion for the Court. Marshall's description of European philosophies at the time the colonizing nations "discovered" the Western Hemisphere set in place the foundation upon which the remainder of federal Indian law was built.[2] As the Chief Justice described:

On the discovery of this immense continent, the great nations of Europe were eager to appropriate to themselves so much of it as they could respectively acquire. Its vast extent offered an ample field to the ambition and enterprise of all; and the character and religion of its inhabitants afforded an apology for considering them as a people over whom the superior genius of Europe might claim ascendancy. The potentates of the old world found no difficulty in convincing themselves that they made ample compensation to the inhabitants of the new, by bestowing on them civilization and Christianity, in exchange for unlimited independence. But, as they were all in pursuit of nearly the same object, it was necessary, in order to avoid conflicting settlements, and consequent war with each other, to establish a principle which all should acknowledge as the law by which the right of acquisition, which they all asserted, should be regulated as between themselves. This principle

---

[2] Of course there are other types of law that also affect Indian people. Even before contact, there was tribal "common law"—the day-to-day rules within a group. Today, in addition to their own common law, tribes also have their own enacted laws, consisting of laws that have been legislatively passed by a tribal government and written down.

was that discovery gave title to the government by whose subjects, or by whose authority, it was made, against all other
European governments, which title might be consummated by
possession. (Id. at 572-3.)

So, the doctrine of discovery allowed the European nations, that were eager to
colonize and exploit the resources of the Americas, to decide amongst themselves who would claim particular regions.

The doctrine of discovery required that an area actually be possessed in
order for ownership to be complete. This required dealing with the people
who already lived there when an area was "discovered." Justice Marshall
explained the colonizers' approach to this problem:

> The exclusion of all other Europeans, necessarily gave to the
> nation making the discovery the sole right of acquiring the soil
> from the natives, and establishing settlements upon it. It was
> a right with which no Europeans could interfere. It was a right
> which all asserted for themselves, and to the assertion of
> which, by others, all assented.

> Those relations, which were to exist between the discoverer
> and the natives, were to be regulated by themselves. The
> rights thus acquired being exclusive, no other power could
> interpose between them. (Id. at 573.)

The nations that colonized the Western Hemisphere put in place a system
whereby no nation would be held accountable to others with respect to how it
dealt with the local indigenous people. Morality and justice in dealing with
people who already lived in an area were not required, unless a nation chose to
impose some version of these principles on itself. Each colonizing nation was
free to adopt, or not adopt, any notion of what was right. Marshall gave his
view of what happened next:

> In the establishment of these relations, the rights of the origi-
> nal inhabitants were, in no instance, entirely disregarded; but
> were necessarily, to a considerable extent, impaired. They
> were admitted to be the rightful occupants of the soil, with a
> legal as well as a just claim to retain possession of it, and to use
> it according to their own discretion; but their rights to com-
> plete sovereignty, as independent nations, were necessarily
> diminished, and their power to dispose of the soil at their own
> will, to whomever they pleased, was denied by the original

fundamental principle that discovery gave exclusive title to those who made it. (Id. at 574.)

Thus, the indigenous people of an area were limited by the doctrine of discovery; they could not sell or give their land to any newcomers other than the nation that "discovered" the area in which they lived.

There was a subtle policy shift as more settlers reached the continent. The colonizing nations claimed "dominion," or control, over the land; they claimed the right to the land, whether or not they exercised their exclusive right to make a deal for the land with the local native people. As Marshall explained:

> While the different nations of Europe respected the right of the natives, as occupants, they asserted the ultimate dominion to be in themselves; and claimed and exercised, as a consequence of this ultimate dominion, a power to grant the soil, while yet in the possession of the natives. These grants have been understood by all to convey a title to the grantees, subject only to the Indian right of occupancy. (Id.)

Thus, the notion of land ownership in the United States started with the European doctrine of discovery. The doctrine was originally an arrangement between colonizing nations about whom among them would get first rights to newly "discovered" areas. It was soon transformed into a doctrine whereby the step of actually obtaining the right to the land from the local native people became a mere formality. The local Indians' right was relegated to one of mere occupancy— the right to be on the land and not be found guilty of trespassing.

But land with Indians living on it was not what the colonizers wanted. The right of Indians to occupy the land had to be eliminated before a colonizing nation could make full use of the land. This was accomplished through treaties with the occupying tribes— either treaties of peace or treaties of war.[3] It was usually more cost effective to negotiate a treaty without first having to defeat a tribe in war, therefore treaties of peace were a preferred method for removing tribal rights to land.

Many tribes were understandably unwilling to leave their ancestral lands. The colonizers used the doctrine of conquest as a means to remove Indians who were not willing to give up their lands. Simply put, under the doctrine of conquest, a nation may defeat another nation in war, and subsequently obtain title to the defeated nation's land and control of its people. Because the doctrine of discovery prevented other European nations from speaking out against such an approach, the doctrine of conquest was a readily available means of dealing with tribes that were not willing to move. Justice Marshall described

---

[3] For a thorough collection of treaties and other related documents, as well as a helpful analysis, see Vine C. Deloria Jr. and Raymond J. DeMallie, *Documents of American Indian Diplomacy: Treaties, Agreements, and Conventions, 1775-1979.* Norman, OK; University of Oklahoma Press; 1999.

the implications of conquest:

> The title by conquest is acquired and maintained by force. The conqueror prescribes its limits. . . . When the conquest is complete. . . the conquered inhabitants can be blended with the conquerors, or safely governed as a distinct people. (Id. at 589–90.)

The fledgling United States was born into the established legal tradition that included the doctrines of discovery and conquest. The roots of the remainder of federal Indian law are in these doctrines.

CONSTITUTIONAL BASIS OF UNITED STATES INDIAN POLICY

Upon gaining its independence, the United States assumed the role previously held by England with respect to American Indians. The federal government formalized its primacy in dealing with indigenous peoples in the commerce and treaty clauses of the Constitution. The commerce clause, which includes the "Indian commerce clause" (Article I, § 8, clause 3), authorizes Congress to regulate commerce "with foreign Nations, and among the several States, and with Indian Tribes." The treaty clause (Article II, § 2, clause 2) grants to the federal government the exclusive authority to make treaties on behalf of the United States.

While these clauses in the Constitution are the cornerstones of federal Indian policy, their precise meanings are continually disputed in the courts. Some basic and broad-ranging rules have become fairly well established. These rules form the basis for federal Indian law, a field of law governing Indian peoples' lives, in addition to the laws of the tribes themselves, the states, and general federal law. The tribes, the federal government, and the states are each sovereigns and may make their own laws. However, certain principles of federal Indian law constrain the ability of each sovereign to make laws that affect AI/AN people.

Some of the earliest principles of federal Indian law developed in response to attempts by states to assert their authority over Indian lands within state boundaries. *Cherokee Nation v. Georgia*,[4] an early Supreme Court case, addressed the relations between tribes, states, and the federal government. The Cherokee Nation had asked the United States courts for an injunction to pre-

---

[4] 21 U.S. (5 Pet.) 1 (1831). The case arose when the Cherokee Nation sought an injunction against the State of Georgia enforcing Georgia laws in land the Cherokees had reserved for themselves in several treaties. Justice Marshall commented that: "If the courts were permitted to indulge their sympathies, a case better calculated to excite them can scarcely be imagined. A people once numerous, powerful, and truly independent, found by our ancestors in the quiet and uncontrolled possession of ample domain, gradually sinking beneath our superior policy, our arts and our arms, have yielded their lands by successive treaties, each of which contains a solemn guarantee of the residue, until they retain no more of their formerly extensive territory than is deemed necessary to their comfortable subsistence. To preserve this remnant the present application is made." Id. at 15. Nevertheless, the court decided it could not grant the Cherokees the relief they requested.

vent the State of Georgia from attempting to enforce state laws within lands of the Cherokees reservations. Starting where he left off in *Johnson v. McIntosh*, Justice Marshall took the opportunity to expound upon the status of the Indian nations:

> Though the Indians are acknowledged to have an unquestionable, and, heretofore, unquestioned right to the lands they occupy until that right is extinguished by a voluntary cession to our government, yet it may well be doubted whether those tribes which reside within the acknowledged boundaries of the United States can, with strict accuracy, be denominated foreign nations. They may, more correctly, perhaps, be denominated domestic dependent nations. They occupy a territory to which we assert a title independent of their will, which must take effect in point of possession when their right of possession ceases. Meanwhile they are in a state of pupilage. Their relation to the United States resembles that of a ward to his guardian.
>
> They look to our government for protection; rely upon its kindness and its power; appeal to it for relief to their wants. . . . They and their country are considered by foreign nations, as well as by ourselves, as being so completely under the sovereignty and dominion of the United States, that attempt to acquire their lands, or to form a political connection with them, would be considered by all as an invasion of our territory, and an act of hostility. (Id. at 17-8.)

Because the United States relegated tribes to a "dependent" status, it also assumed the responsibility to look after their well-being; this was the beginning of the trust relationship, the special relationship between tribes and the United States government. The guardian must look after its wards.[5] Yet at the same time, the tribes retained a right to govern themselves, and the United States continued to honor this right. As Justice Marshall explained:

> Though without land that they can call theirs in the sense of property, their right of self-government has never been taken from them; and such a form of government may exist though the land occupied be in fact that of another. The right to expel them may exist in that other, but the alternative of departing and retaining the right of self-government may exist in them.

---

[5] The trust relationship has subsequently been acknowledged repeatedly by all three branches of the United States government in court opinions, executive documents, and Acts of Congress. The trust responsibility applies to all agencies with programs concerning Indians, and it may not be subordinated to other public interests unless specifically authorized by Congress (see *Nevada v. United States*, U.S. Sup. Ct. 1983).

And such they certainly do possess; it has never been questioned, nor any attempt made at subjugating them as a people, or restraining their personal liberty, except as to their land and trade. (Id. at 27.)

However, the court concluded that it could not issue the injunction the Cherokees sought since it lacked jurisdiction to hear the case because the Cherokee Nation was not a foreign nation.

Georgia's extension of its laws into Cherokee territory gave rise to another early Supreme Court case, *Worcester v. Georgia*. (31 U.S. (6 Pet.) 515 (1832)). In this case, a non-Indian missionary was convicted in Georgia courts of violating a state law by living among the Cherokees without first obtaining a license to do so from the state. Georgia law enforcement officials went into Cherokee territory and forcibly removed the missionary, despite the fact that the Cherokees welcomed him there. The Supreme Court held that Georgia could not exert its authority within Cherokee territory, and overturned the conviction. This time Justice Marshall explained that the United States would protect the tribes' sovereignty:

From the commencement of our government Congress has passed acts to regulate trade and intercourse with the Indians; which treat them as nations, respect their rights, and manifest a firm purpose to afford that protection which treaties stipulate. All these acts . . . manifestly consider the several Indian nations as distinct political communities, having territorial boundaries, within which their authority is exclusive, and having a right to all the lands within those boundaries, which is not only acknowledged, but guaranteed by the United States. . . .

The treaties and laws of the United States contemplate the Indian territory as completely separated from that of the States; and provide that all intercourse [trade] with them shall be carried on exclusively by the government of the Union. (Id. at 556-7.)

The case firmly established that the federal government, and not the individual states, has authority over and responsibility for matters relating to members of Indian tribes; because it assumes the authority, it also assumes the responsibility of protecting the tribes (This policy was extended later to Alaska Natives). However, the federal responsibility only applies to those tribes that are in some way recognized by the federal government, by treaty or other methods, and that remain a "distinct" people.[6]

Thus, three of the most basic and earliest principles of federal Indian law were established: (1) tribes retain much of their inherent sovereignty until it is taken away by the federal government; (2) the federal government, and not individual states, is in charge of Indian affairs; and (3) the federal government only deals with tribal organizations or governments that it has recognized. Further, the trust relationship between recognized tribes and the United States government has started to form.

WESTWARD EXPANSION AND INDIAN REMOVAL

As might be expected, given that the power to control Indian affairs arose from the doctrines of discovery and conquest, the federal government initially placed the War Department in charge of Indian affairs (Cohen 1982). Almost as soon as the United States was founded, pressure to expand the frontier mounted and the country's boundary shifted continually westward. The demand for ever more farmland and timber created a need for the United States to obtain by whatever means necessary, the titles of Indian nations and foreign countries. By the middle of the 19th century, the United States had either been at war with virtually all tribes living east of the Mississippi River, entered a land cession treaty with them, or both. With the Louisiana Purchase in 1803, the United States assumed the right, formerly held by France under the doctrine of discovery, to deal with American Indians living west of the Mississippi River.

INDIAN REMOVAL

Treaties with the various tribes were the primary means of clearing the way for westward expansion of the United States. Many early treaties contained cessions by tribes of considerable amounts of their original homelands for smaller tracts of land reserved for the tribes in exchange for protection promised by the United States. However, beginning with President Thomas Jefferson, the United States began to take a new approach to clear the land of Indian inhabitants. Under the new approach, some tribes were removed from their homelands in exchange for lands west of the Mississippi River (Cohen 1982).

The first land exchange treaty was concluded in 1817 (Treaty with the Cherokees, July 8, 1817, 7 Stat. 156.). Under this treaty, the Cherokee Nation was divided into two groups: one remained east of the Mississippi, and the other relocated to land on the Arkansas and White Rivers in "Indian Territory" or what is today Oklahoma.[7] Treaty-making for the following 30 years focused on removing Indian tribes to new territories west of the Mississippi River

---

[6] See, e.g., *United States v. 43 Gallons of Whiskey*, 93 U.S. 188, 195 (1876), where the Supreme Court held that "as long as these Indians remain a distinct people, with an existing tribal organization, recognized by the political department of the government, Congress has the power to say with whom, and on what terms, they shall deal."

[7] Later, most of those Cherokees who remained East of the Mississippi River were removed to Indian Territory through treaties and force.

(Cohen 1982).

The removal policy was formalized in the Indian Removal Act of 1830 (Act of May 28, 1830, 4 Stat. 411.). This Act empowered the President to establish districts for tribes that decided to exchange their ancestral lands for lands farther west. The result of this removal was the creation of a vast open area available for White settlement, reducing the conflict created by the presence of settlers and sovereign Indian nations on the same lands within state boundaries (Cohen 1982).

EARLIEST FEDERAL HEALTH SERVICES

During the 1800s, the U. S. Army took steps to curb infectious diseases among tribes living in the vicinity of military posts, in order to protect its soldiers and neighboring non-Indians. These efforts marked the first time the federal government provided health services to American Indians. Non-Indian settlers brought smallpox, measles, diphtheria, malaria, and other infectious diseases. Because many American Indians had never been exposed to these diseases, they often were particularly susceptible, and epidemics spreading through neighboring tribes increased the risk of infectious disease for non-Indian settlers and military personnel (Cohen 1982).

While the earliest records of federal provision of health services to American Indians are from the early 19th century, the first congressional appropriation specifically for Indian health care was in 1832 (Act of May 5, 1832, ch. 75, 4 Stat. 514.). This appropriation authorized the purchase and administration of smallpox vaccine.

Beginning in 1836, some treaties between tribes and the United States provided for medical supplies and physicians' services, as partial consideration for tribal land cessions. Some additional federal expenditures for Indian health care were made from tribal treaty funds, and some health services were provided with general educational appropriations distributed to religious and philanthropic organizations active in the "civilization" of Indians (Cohen 1982).

FAR WESTERN TRIBES

As more non-Indian settlers moved west of the Mississippi River, the federal government began to abandon its removal policy in favor of another approach. Instead, the U.S. sought to obtain treaties whereby tribes reserved portions of their land and gave up claims to the remainder of their aboriginal territories. A variety of historical circumstances created different legal situations with regard to Western tribes.

PUEBLO INDIANS. One unique situation arose from the U.S. war with Mexico from 1846 to 1848. At the conclusion of this conflict, Mexico ceded New Mexico Territory to the United States under the Treaty of Guadalupe Hidalgo on February 2, 1848 (Treaty of Guadalupe Hidalgo, 9 Stat. 922 (Feb. 2, 1868).). The next year, the United States concluded a peace treaty with the Navajo Nation, which also inhabited this area (Treaty with the Navajoes, 9 Stat.

974 (Sept. 9, 1849)).

The Pueblo Indians held a special status under both Spanish and Mexican rule. They were considered "wards" of the Spanish crown, and royal grants of land were given to each village in the name of the community. The Spanish government also enacted restrictions on alienation of tribal lands and laws to protect Pueblo lands from trespassers (Cohen 1982). The Mexican government recognized the Spanish land grants and granted the Pueblo Indians citizenship. Whether Pueblo Indians retained citizen status when the area was ceded to the United States was unclear (Cohen 1982), but once New Mexico gained statehood in 1912, the Pueblos were treated in a similar fashion as other Indians within the United States (Cohen 1982).[8]

PLAINS INDIANS. Treaties with multiple tribes were the method of choice for relations with tribes that lived on the Great Plains.[9] In 1846, a treaty was made between the United States and the "Comanche, Ioni, Anadaca, Cadoe, Lepan, Longwha, Keechy, Tahwacarro, Wichita, and Wacoe" Nations (9 Stat. 844 (May 15, 1846).). In 1851, the United States entered a treaty with many "Sioux," Cheyenne, Arapaho, Crow, Assiniboine, Gros Ventre, Mandan, and Arikara Indians at Fort Laramie. (Treaty of Fort Laramie of 1851 (Sept. 17, 1851) C. Kappler, ed. 2 _Indian Affairs: Laws and Treaties_, 594 (Washington: Government Printing Office, 1903–1941)[hereinafter Kappler].) Treaties with other tribes in the west were made about this same time, including the Apaches, Kiowas, and Comanches. (See, e.g., Treaty with the Apaches, 10 Stat. 979 (July 1, 1852); Treaty with the Camanches, Kiowas, and Apaches, 10 Stat. 1013 (July 27, 1853).)

CALIFORNIA TRIBES. Discovery of gold in California brought a stampede of prospectors to the area. To make room for new settlers, Congress appropriated funds and dispatched commissioners to obtain the lands of California Indians by treaty. In 1851, many treaties were negotiated with California Indians in which the tribes surrendered their land for small plots elsewhere. These treaties also contained terms subjecting the Indians to state law (Cohen 1982).

The United States Senate rejected the treaties of California in 1852, largely because the California state legislature formally objected to the assignment of any new lands to Indians. The tribes, however, had already started to perform on their end of the agreements, and were on their way to the proposed reservations—they had given up their lands and had no place to go. Eventually several small reservations or "rancherias" were created for California Indians. However, the landlessness created by rejection of the early California treaties has never been completely addressed (Cohen 1982).

---

[8] See also _United States v. Sandoval_, 231 U.S. 28 (1913), confirming federal guardianship over Pueblos in spite of outright tribal ownership of their lands and claims of United States citizenship by the Pueblo Indians. The Court refused to rule on whether the Pueblo Indians were in fact United States citizens.

[9] This policy was also pursued at about the same time with tribes in Oregon Territory, the Puget Sound region, and other tribes of the far Northwest. The first treaty with Oregon Territory tribes was the Treaty with the Rogue River Tribe, 10 Stat. 1018 (Sept. 10, 1853). The Rogue River Indians eventually settled on the Siletz and Grand Ronde Reservations in Oregon.

DEPARTMENT OF INTERIOR ASSUMES RESPONSIBILITY FOR INDIAN HEALTH CARE

Indian health care passed from the military and missionaries to civilian control in 1849, when the Bureau of Indian Affairs (BIA) was transferred from the War Department to the newly formed Department of the Interior (Act of March 3, 1849, ch. 108, § 5, 9 Stat. 395.). The first attempt by the BIA to expand services occurred 24 years later, when a medical and educational division was established. Funding for the new division was inadequate, however, and the medical section of the BIA was terminated in 1877 (Cohen 1982). By 1880, only 77 physicians were serving the entire American Indian population in the United States and it territories (Cohen 1982).

It is unclear why funding for medical services to Indians suffered during this time, but a look at the political climate may be revealing. With the rise of a period of "Indian wars," federal policy necessarily shifted from attempting to integrate Indians into society towards vanquishing them in battles and massacres. The need for protecting citizens from contracting diseases from local American Indians was not as pressing when efforts were focused on eradicating American Indians rather than making them fit into the mainstream.

INDIAN WARS AND THE END OF TREATY MAKING

The formation of the Department of the Interior was not the only event in the last half of the 19th century that influenced Indian policy. The period was a time of significant conflict between the United States and many tribes, as valuable minerals were being discovered across the West. Starting with the discovery of gold in California in 1848, and continuing with each discovery in a new location, the demand mounted for land that was still in Indian control.

Battles and skirmishes arose across the West. Official and unofficial forays resulted in slaughters of innocent and defenseless Indian elders, women, and children at places such as Sand Creek in Colorado and the Washita River in Oklahoma and these will forever mar American history. Indian resistance may have peaked with the defeat of Custer and Reno at the Greasy Grass River in 1876. (Non-Indian historians refer to the battle at the Greasy Grass River as "Custer's Last Stand" or "the Battle of the Little Big Horn.") Fighting continued for several decades, until the death knell of Indian military resistance was sounded at the Massacre at Wounded Knee in 1890. The legacy of this period can be seen in the names of places that honor Indian-killers, continuing to communicate a hostile environment for Indians today.[10]

Treaty making actually ended in 1871. (Act of March 3, 1871, ch. 120, § 1, 16 Stat. 544, 566 (codified at 25 U.S.C. § 71).) After that year, the United States dealt with Indians in agreements, statutes, and executive orders with

---

[10] Countless cities, counties, streets, and businesses in the West bear names like Custer, Reno, and Sheridan. The dominant society would be outraged at the prospect of naming cities or streets after Nazi generals. Yet names of places such as Custer State Park, Sheridan in Wyoming, and Reno in Nevada are constant reminders of the dominant society's denial of the genocide that occurred within its own borders.

legal effect very similar to treaties.

ALASKA

The United States acquired Russia's right to Alaska in 1867, near the end of the treaty-making era. The Treaty of Cession provided that Alaska Natives would be treated the same as aboriginal peoples in the rest of the United States. (Treaty of March 30, 1867, 15 Stat. 539.)Treaties were never negotiated with Alaska Natives, and few reservations were created in Alaska. The federal government eventually pursued its relationship with Alaska Natives on a village-by-village basis through the BIA and the Alaska Native Claims Settlement Act, which was passed in 1971 to clear the title to Alaskan land for oil development.

ASSIMILATION AND ALLOTMENT

Westward expansion by the United States resulted in tribes residing in a portion of their original homelands that was much smaller than the territory the tribe traditionally inhabited; frequently, the reservation was not of sufficient size to provide members of a tribe with the necessities of life. The move to reservations had harmful health effects, in part because it often created a shift away from traditional diets. It became increasingly difficult or impossible to hunt and gather traditional foods. Many of the health problems faced by Indians even today can be traced, at least partially, to dietary factors.

Under the trust responsibility, the United States was obligated to help tribal members subsist. The trust responsibility carried with it a high price—it became increasingly expensive to provide food for an increasing number of people placed on an ever-increasing number of reservations. The policy of assimilation gained favor as the best approach for dealing with the "Indian problem." The goal was to bring Indians into the mainstream society, and have them abandon their former ways of life.[11]

ALLOTMENT

A fundamental goal of assimilation was wresting the notion of group ownership from Indians and replacing it with the "civil" notion of private property. It was thought that, if Indians were made to believe in the virtues of private property and taught how to farm, they would soon be able to feed themselves and the government would be relieved of the cost of supporting them.

One of the primary tools of the assimilation policy was allotment of reservation land. Under the allotment policy, the group title of a tribe to the land on its reservation was abolished and replaced with individual plots, usually from 20 to 80 acres, owned by individual Indians. As the Supreme Court

---

[11] The United States' policy of genocide towards Indian people— the destruction of the race and cultures of Indians— is a common, albeit frequently unspoken, theme throughout American history. When the policy of removal and eradication lost favor because it was expensive and embarrassing, the next logical approach was more subliminal: assimilate the Indians into the mainstream culture. As Richard Henry Pratt, founder of the Carlisle Indian Industrial School (an infamous Indian boarding school) put it, the goal of assimilation was to "kill the Indian and save the man" (Woodhead 1995). Variations on this same theme were repeated later in the forms of relocation and termination policies.

explained, "[w]ithin a generation or two, it was thought, the tribes would dissolve, their reservations would disappear, and individual Indians would be absorbed into the larger community of white settlers." (*South Dakota v. Yankton Sioux Tribe*, 522 U.S. 329, 335 (1998).)

Experiments in allotment had been underway for several decades (Cohen 1982), but this approach peaked with the passage of the General Allotment Act of 1887, commonly known as the Dawes Act. (Ch.119, 24 Stat. 388 (codified as amended at 25 U.S.C. §§ 331-334, 339, 341, 342, 348, 349, 354, 381).) By the early 20th century, Congress shifted to a policy of passing allotment acts on a reservation-by-reservation basis. The Indian Department Appropriation Act in 1901 provided for the Secretary of the Interior to assign Indian Inspectors to negotiate treaties with tribes "for the cession to the United States of portions of their respective reservations or surplus unallotted lands." (Indian Department Appropriations Act, 31 Stat. 1077 (Mar. 3, 1901).)

The theory of allotment was that each head-of-family could farm the allotted land and support his family.[12] Allotment was usually only to male heads of families, despite the fact that matriarchal societies were common in Indian communities. After allotment, "excess land" on the reservation was opened for settlement by non-Indians. Thus, more of the rich resources of the West, unavailable previously because they were within reservation boundaries, were thrown open to non-Indian ownership and development.

The results of allotment were, of course, dismal for Indians. In 1887, Indians held 138 million acres of land on reservations. By the time the Dawes Act was repealed in 1934, Indian landholdings had been reduced to only about 52 million acres (Prucha 1984). Allotment not only caused further loss of natural resources, but it also led to reductions of reservation boundaries and loss of some powers to control affairs within reservation boundaries. As one legal scholar explained:

> Much of the remaining Indian land estate was crippled. . . . The tribal land ownership pattern became checkerboarded, with individual Indian, non-Indian, and corporate ownership interspersed. On allotted lands, scores, even hundreds, of heirs succeeded to the original allottee's ownership as generations passed, creating the fractionated heirship problem. . . .
>
> With the land base slashed back once again and with strange new faces within most reservations, tribal councils and courts went dormant. The BIA moved in as the real government. This was the heyday of the Christian missionaries, who were able on many reservations to drive out traditional religions or at least force them underground. The 1880s marked the

---

[12] The distance between the theory and practice of the policy was great. In many cases, the allotment did not provide enough land or land suitable for farming. Water scarcity in the West is also a factor, and many times there was not sufficient water available to even make farming a viable option.

beginning of half a century of twilight operations by the tribes, a time when the essence of the measured separatism—tribal self rule—was debilitated nearly to the ultimate degree. (Wilkinson 1987, p. 20–21)

Allotment and assimilation had far-reaching effects on many facets of American Indian lives, and the impacts continue to this day.

ASSIMILATION AND TRIBAL HEALTH CARE PRACTICES

One aspect of assimilation policy involved banning tribal spiritual and health care practices. It was thought that if Indians gave up all of their old ways of life, their assimilation into the mainstream would be faster and more complete. In a letter to Commissioner of Indian Affairs Hiram Price, Secretary of the Interior H.M. Teller complained that several traditional practices were "a great hindrance to the civilization of the Indians." In addition to complaints about Indian dances, marriage customs, and probate practices, Teller wrote the following about traditional healers:

> Another great hindrance to the civilization of the Indians is the influence of the medicine men, who are always found with the anti-progressive party. The medicine men resort to various artifices and devices to keep the people under their influence, and are especially active in preventing the attendance of the children at public schools, using their conjurers' arts to prevent the people from abandoning their heathenish rites and customs. While they profess to cure diseases by the administering of a few simple remedies, still they rely mainly on their art of conjuring. Their services are not required even for the administration of the few simple remedies they are competent to recommend, for the Government supplies the several agencies with skillful physicians, who practice among the Indians without charge to them. Steps should be taken to compel these imposters to abandon this deception and discontinue their practice, which are not only without benefit to the Indians but positively injurious to them. (H.M. Teller, Secretary of Interior to Hiram Price, Commissioner of Indian Affairs, December 2, 1882.)

In response to the Secretary's complaints, the Commissioner adopted rules for the Court of Indian Offenses which punished participation in Sun Dances by incarceration and/or withholding of rations for up to 30 days (Rules Governing the Court of Indian Offenses, 4th, Department of Interior (Mar. 30, 1883).), and addressed traditional healing as follows:

The usual practices of so-called "medicine men" shall be considered "Indian offenses" cognizable by the Court of Indian Offenses, and whenever it shall be proven to the satisfaction of the court that the influence or practice of a so-called "medicine man" operates as a hindrance to the civilization of a tribe, or that said "medicine man" resorts to any artifice or device to keep the Indians under his influence, or shall adopt any means to prevent the attendance of children at the agency schools, or shall use any of the arts of a conjurer to prevent the Indians from abandoning their heathenish rites and customs, he shall be adjudged guilty of an Indian offense, and upon conviction of any one or more of these specified practices, or any other, in the opinion of the court, of an equally anti-progressive nature, shall be confined in the agency prison for a term of not less than ten days, or until such time as he shall produce evidence satisfactory to the court, and approved by the agent, that he will forever abandon all practices styled Indian offenses under this rule. (Id., #6.)

Despite being outlawed, traditional healing and medicine are so interwoven in culture that the knowledge, beliefs, and practices have persisted in many tribes.

OTHER ASSIMILATION POLICIES

During the allotment era, policies were designed to bring about the complete assimilation of Indians into the mainstream. Indians were re-named according to Anglo-Saxon family traditions to help them assimilate easier and to make it easier to determine who would inherit an individual Indian's private property. Various statutes extended citizenship to subgroups of Indians, including: Indians judged competent to own their allotments without the federal trust relationship, women who married white men, and members of the Five Civilized Tribes.[13] All Indians were declared citizens in 1924 (Act of June 2, 1924, codified at 8 U.S.C. Sec. 1401 (a)(2)).

During this time Congress passed the first law providing for the exercise of federal jurisdiction over intra-tribal affairs. In an appended section to the Appropriations Act of March 3, 1885 (Ch. 341, 23 Stat. 362, 385), Congress provided for federal court jurisdiction over seven major crimes committed by Indians on reservations against any "Indian or other person." This federal Major Crimes Act has since been amended to cover 16 enumerated crimes (It is codified at 25 U.S.C. § 1153 . . .).

Reformers saw the most hope in the education system for turning Indians away from their tribal cultures, languages, and traditions. By the beginning of the 20th century, federal funds that previously had been given to religious organizations for the education of Indian children were redirected to BIA boarding schools and reservation day schools. There was also increased empha-

---

[13]The Cherokee, Choctaw, Chickasaw, Creeks and Seminoles are known as the Five Civilized Tribes.

sis on sending Indians to public schools, particularly in allotted areas where Whites had organized schools for their children (Prucha 1984).

In the BIA boarding school system, children were not permitted, sometimes for several years, to see their parents, grandparents, or other elder relatives, or friends not attending the school. They were not permitted to speak their native language, even to each other in private time; children who spoke their language were severely punished and degraded. Anything that reflected their native culture—Indian dress and hairstyle, religious practices, philosophies—was prohibited (Bush 1996).

The boarding schools also contributed to the spread of disease among Indians. As one Department of the Interior Indian Inspector's report from Arizona in 1899 described:

> The habit prevails at San Carlos as well as at most of these southern schools of taking in such pupils as can be obtained, some of whom are superficially examined and others not at all. Tuberculosis frequently develops, and apparently for no other reason than to maintain a full attendance, they are kept until the last stage is reached, when to prevent a death occurring at the school, they are carted home . . . where in some instances even a few days suffices to bring the end. In this manner the disease is disseminated among the pupils in the schools, and the few days they occupy the home . . . may be, and no doubt is, frequently the cause of other members of the family becoming affected.[14]

The ripple effects of the boarding school system, like all assimilation policies, can still be seen today. Some of the tragic effects that have only recently come into light were a legacy of physical, emotional, and sexual abuse of children, as well as a lack of parenting, and historical grief from this trauma. These are commonly regarded as contributing factors for high rates of alcoholism, depression, suicide, and domestic abuse.

REFORM AND REORGANIZATION

The deplorable health conditions faced by Indian people at the turn of the century was a major contributing factor to the eventual repeal of the formal assimilation policies. In the early decades of the 20th century, it had become clear that the assimilation and allotment policies were wreaking havoc on Indians in many spheres of life.

AUTHORIZATION OF INDIAN HEALTH PROGRAMS

The BIA attempted to reorganize its health services in 1908, when the

---

[14] William J. McConnell to Secretary of the Interior, July 20, 1899, Office of Indian Affairs, Official letters of W.J. McConnell, U.S. Indian Inspector, entry no. 952, quoted in F.P. Prucha (1984, p. 843).

Chief Medical Supervisor position was created.[15] Congress began appropriating funds for BIA health care services in 1910 (Appropriations Act of April 4, 1910, ch. 140, § 1, 36 Stat. 269, 271.). Yet, despite these early efforts, health care on the reservations remained dismal. In 1912, President Taft sent a special message to Congress summarizing the results of several surveys documenting deplorable health and sanitary conditions on reservations (Cohen 1982). Other contemporary reports revealed similarly distressing conclusions. Eventually, appropriations for health care began to increase.

In 1921 Congress passed the Snyder Act (ch. 115, 42 Stat. 208, (codified as amended at 25 U.S.C. § 13)), providing explicit legislative authorization for federal health programs for Indians by mandating the expenditure of funds for "the relief of distress and conservation of health . . . [and] for the employment of . . . physicians . . . for Indian tribes." This provided the first formal authority for federal provision of health care services to members of all federally recognized tribes. Prior to this Act, provision of health care services to Indians was done piecemeal for a variety of reasons: in the interest of protecting non-Indian settlers, as part of religious "educational" programs designed to "civilize" Indians, in observance of treaty obligations when a particular treaty included terms for health care provision, or in the interest of the trust relationship created when the United States assumed control over Indian affairs. BIA health care services received another boost in 1926 when officers from the Commissioned Corps of the Public Health Service (PHS) were first assigned to Indian health programs.

REORGANIZATION

At the request of the Secretary of the Interior, the non-governmental Institute for Government Research conducted a two-year survey of the condition of Indian affairs. The resulting report published in 1928 is frequently called the *Merriam Report*, after Lewis Merriam, the editor and director of the survey that was formally entitled, *The Problem of Indian Administration*. The report compared the Indian service with agencies serving the general population, with the goal of identifying what factors would help Indians meet a minimum standard of health. The report described the devastation caused by allotment, the failures of Indian education, and the dreadful health status of American Indians. Its recommendations were not radical, and still apply today: more money should be appropriated and the Indian service should be reorganized to run more efficiently. While the report still reflected assimilationist philosophies in many regards, it also defined the goal of Indian policy to be "the development of all that is good in Indian culture 'rather than to crush out all that is Indian'" (Cohen (1982, p. 144-5) quoting Institute for Government Research (1928).).

In 1933, longtime Indian reform activist John Collier was appointed

---

[15] American Medical Assoc., Council on Medical Service. *Health Care of the American Indian* (1973), reprinted in Indian Health Care Improvement Act: Hearings before the Subcommittee on Health and Environment of the House Committee on Interstate and Foreign Commerce, 94th Cong., 2nd Sess. 219, 226 (1976); Cohen at 696–697.

Commissioner of Indian Affairs. Collier was determined to undo the damage done by allotment and assimilation. His 1933 report to Congress addressed the need for consolidation of tribal land bases, the importance of day schools rather than boarding schools, decentralization of the Indian service, and more Indian employment by the BIA (1933 Sec. Int. Ann. Rep. at 68-69.). The next year he issued a report that called for a revival of tribalism and the preservation of Indian heritage (1934 Sec. Int. Ann. Rep. at 90.).

Collier's initiatives met opposition that resulted in compromises in Congress (Cohen 1982). However, during Collier's tenure Congress passed several acts that drastically changed the course of Indian policy. The Johnson–O'Malley Act of 1934 (Ch. 147, 48 Stat. 596 (codified as amended at 25 U.S.C. §§ 453-454)) authorized the Secretary of the Interior to contract with states and territories for provision of services for Indians, if the services met standards established by the Secretary. This allowed the BIA, and later the IHS, to contract for provision of Indian health services.

The Indian Reorganization Act of 1934 ("IRA") (Ch. 576, 48 Stat. 984 (codified as amended at 25 U.S.C. §§ 461, 462, 463, 464, 465, 466–470, 471–473, 474, 475, 476–478. 479). This Act is sometimes referred to as the "Wheeler-Howard Act," after its sponsors in Congress.),created sweeping changes designed to encourage economic development, self-determination, cultural plurality, and the revival of tribalism. The IRA included provisions intended to stop the alienation of tribal lands and provide for recovery of some lands lost due to previous federal policies. Tribes were encouraged to organize in a manner much like modern business corporations.[16] Educational and technical training opportunities were created. Limited tribal autonomy was allowed, but federal supervision was retained.

A major difference between the model used by cities and counties and the IRA model is that the IRA model does not contain a separation of powers. Often, the tribal council serves in both the legislative and executive capacities for a tribe, and it may also supervise the judicial branch.

The IRA–form of government is commonly criticized by Indian people because it has supplanted more traditional tribal forms of government that fostered better relationships within tribal communities (Young Bear and Thiesz 1994). As an example, many tribes traditionally use a consensus-based approach to decision making. IRA governments reach decisions by majority vote, which can lead to a disgruntled minority and cause divisions within a tribe (Young Bear and Thiesz 1994). While majority rule can result in decisions being made faster, consensus assures more broad-based support for the final decision.

---

[16] An almost boilerplate constitution was adopted by many tribes during reorganization. Tribal governments organized under these constitutions are frequently referred to as "IRA governments." The appropriateness of the IRA form of government is sometimes questioned because the boilerplate model didn't necessarily reflect the traditional organizational preferences of a given tribe. The criticism is essentially that the IRA governments are substitutions of Anglo-American government forms for traditional tribal ways (Deloria and Lytle 1983, p. 15).

INDIAN CLAIMS COMMISSION

Under the doctrines of discovery and conquest, and subsequent federal law, the United States is not required to compensate tribes for taking their aboriginal title to land. However, Congress has sometimes allowed tribes to pursue claims for such compensation against the United States. Initially, this was accomplished by piecemeal acts granting jurisdiction to hear the claims of individual tribes. In 1946 Congress enacted the Indian Claims Commission Act. (Indian Claims Commission Act of 1946, ch. 959, 60 Stat. 1049.) The Act created a special commission to hear Indian claims for land that was taken before 1946 and that had been used by a given tribe to the exclusion of others. Compensation was not available for areas that were used by more than one tribe. The Indian Claims Commission was originally given a ten-year life, but it did not disband until 1978 because it had difficulty adjudicating the 375 claims filed. When it disbanded, the Commission transferred 102 uncompleted cases to the Court of Claims (Clinton et al 1991).

TERMINATION AND RELOCATION

While the reorganization era was leading to greater self-determination for Indian tribes, the political pendulum quickly reversed course. Assimilation policy reared its head again, this time as a policy of rapid assimilation through termination of tribes, elimination of their reservations, and relocation of Indians away from their homelands.

Spurred in part by a 1949 Hoover Commission Report (*The Hoover Commission Report On The Organization Of The Executive Branch Of The Government* (1949)) a termination program was implemented in the 1950s. It was promoted as a way to "free" the Indians from the supervision and control of the BIA. Ultimately, Congress passed acts terminating the special federal-tribal trust relationship with 109 tribes and bands. The basic elements of the termination plans included sales of tribal lands, imposition of state legislative and judicial authority, elimination of exemptions from state taxation, and an end to tribal sovereignty (Bush 1996). Treaty-based hunting and fishing rights, however, were not abrogated by termination. (*Menominee Tribe v. United States*, 391 U.S. 404 (1968); *Kimball v. Callahan*, 493 F.2d 564 (9th Cir.) cert. denied, 419 U.S. 1019 (1974) (Klamath Tribe treaty hunting and fishing rights).)

The effects of termination on tribal economies, society, and health were devastating. One example is the case of the Klamath Tribe of Oregon. After termination, the economy of the Klamaths was destroyed, and the culture and social fabric of the people were seriously damaged. Tribal alcoholism and suicide rates soared where almost none existed previously. From the time of their termination in 1961 until restoration in 1986, the once self-sufficient, economically viable, socially and spiritually strong Klamath Nation had been demoralized. By 1980, statistics suggest that 28 percent of the tribe died by age 25, and 52 percent died by age 40. An estimated 40 percent of all deaths were alcohol related. Infant mortality was twice the statewide average. The future looked grim as 70 percent of the adults had less than a high school education and poverty levels were three times that of non-Indians in Klamath County, the poorest county in Oregon.[17]

An active policy of Indian relocation was implemented during the termination era. Reservation Indians were relocated to major urban areas for vocational training and better employment opportunities. The result was a marked increase in the urban Indian population in cities across the country.

Another legacy of the termination era, further eroding tribal sovereignty, was enactment of "Public Law 280." (Act of August 15, 1953, P.L. 83-280, codified as amended at 18 U.S.C. § 1162 (criminal) and 28 U.S.C. § 1360 (civil).) This act granted criminal and limited civil authority over Indian country to the states of Alaska, California, Minnesota, Nebraska, Oregon, and Wisconsin.

INDIAN HEALTH SERVICE

Despite early attempts at improvements, Indian health care was inadequate under the BIA. Many critics, including several Indian organizations, urged that the BIA be relieved of responsibility for Indian health care.[18] In 1954, the Transfer Act (Indian Health Facilities Act of 1954, 68 Stat. 674, codified as amended at 42 U.S.C. §§ 2001-2005f.) moved responsibility for Indian health to the PHS, which was a division of the Department of Health, Education, and Welfare. (The Department of Health, Education, and Welfare has been the Department of Health and Human Services since 1980.) Thus, the Indian Health Service was created as an agency in the U.S. Public Health Service.

As the IHS built hospitals and health centers in or near AI/AN communities, Indian health care began to improve:

> Between 1955 and 1968 the rate of Indian infant deaths was reduced by fifty-one percent, maternal deaths by fifty percent, death from influenza and pneumonia by forty-five percent, tuberculosis by seventy-nine percent and gastroenteric deaths by sixty percent. Indian health problems, however, remain severe in comparison with national averages. (Cohen 1982, p. 699)

---

[17] Chairman Allen Foreman et al, "Termination: An account of the termination of the Klamath Reservation from the Tribe's point of view." *Herald And News*, Klamath Falls, Ore. Oct. 13, 1999; 6–7.

[18] See Transfer of Indian Hospitals and Health Facilities to Public Health Service: Hearings on H.R. 303 Before the Subcommittee on Indian Affairs of the Senate Committee on Interior and Insular Affairs, 83rd Cong., 2nd Sess. (1954).

While it has never been adequately funded, the creation of the IHS is one of the few termination era actions of the federal government that was helpful to Indian people.

SELF-DETERMINATION

Termination was ultimately recognized as a failed detour along the road to self-determination.[19]   An early indictor of the tide turning away from termination was passage of the Indian Civil Rights Act in 1968, (25 U.S.C. § 1301-1303.). A section of this Act required tribal consent to any future extension of state authority over Indian country pursuant to Public Law 280. This ended the possibility of further unilateral extensions of state jurisdiction over tribes.

The most significant provisions of the Indian Civil Rights Act applied ten limitations on the powers of tribal governments and authorized writs of habeus corpus in federal courts for persons detained by an Indian tribe. (A writ of habeus corpus essentially orders the release of an individual from detention.) The Indian Civil Rights Act was designed to implement essentially the same civil rights protections at the tribal-government level that are guaranteed in the United States Bill of Rights. One significant difference is that the prohibition against establishment of religion was not included because it would have interfered with some forms of tribal government.

Eventually, the Supreme Court ruled that suits against an Indian tribe based on the Indian Civil Rights Act must be made first in tribal court (*Santa Clara Pueblo v. Martinez*, 436 U.S. 49 (1978)). The Court noted that the Act served two purposes: to protect individual tribal members from tribal violation of their civil rights, and to promote tribal self-government.

The administration of President Richard M. Nixon set the real foundation for the current federal policy of self-determination. In his 1970 Message to Congress, Nixon called for self-determination without termination. In the early to mid–1970s Congress passed several laws designed to strengthen and restore tribal sovereignty, and restored individual tribes that had been terminated. The stage was also set for two other acts of major importance for tribal sovereignty and health care: the Indian Self-Determination and Education Assistance Act of 1975 (P.L. 93–638, codified as amended at 25 U.S.C. §§ 450a–450n) and the Indian Health Care Improvement Act of 1976 (P.L. 94-437, codified at 25 U.S.C. §§ 1601 et seq., and 42 U.S.C. §§ 1395qq and 1396j.).

"INDIAN COUNTRY" — A JURISDICTIONAL MAZE

One of the results of the pendulum-swings in Indian policy has been a very confusing jurisdictional maze within reservation boundaries. As the Supreme Court described it, "[t]he modern legacy of the [allotment] Acts has been a

---

[19] Congress recognized that the Menominee Tribe of Wisconsin Restoration Act in 1973 "represented the first significant rejection of the termination policy of the 1950s and demonstrated that ... that policy had been a failure." H. Rep. Rept. No. 95-623, Siletz Indian Tribe Restoration Act, (passed as P.L. 95-195) at 3, (1977).

spate of jurisdictional disputes between state and federal officials as to which sovereign has authority over lands that were opened by the Acts and have since passed out of Indian ownership." (*Solem v. Bartlett*, 465 U.S. at 467.) Many of these disputes have arisen in the self-determination era, and the details of jurisdiction on reservations are still being resolved in the courts.[20]

Supreme Court cases have explained that tribes no longer enjoy complete control over their lands, as they did at the time Justice Marshall wrote his two opinions about the Cherokee Nation and Georgia. The intervening federal Indian policies have taken a toll on inherent tribal sovereignty according to United States law. Today, the general rule is a double standard of criminal justice on reservations: generally, tribes have criminal jurisdiction over Indians, but not over non-Indians, within reservation boundaries. (*Oliphant v. Suquamish Indian Tribe*, 435 U.S. 191 (1978).) As for regulatory jurisdiction, tribes retain the authority to regulate tribal lands within a reservation. The Supreme Court has described this authority retained by tribes as follows:

> To be sure, Indian tribes retain inherent sovereign power to exercise some forms of civil jurisdiction over non-Indians on their reservations, even on non-Indian fee lands. A tribe may regulate, through taxation, licensing, or other means, the activities of nonmembers who enter consensual relationships with the tribe or its members, through commercial dealing, contracts, leases, or other arrangements. . . . A tribe may also retain inherent power to exercise civil authority over the conduct of non-Indians on fee lands within its reservation when that conduct threatens or has some direct effect on the political integrity, the economic security, or the health or welfare of the tribe. (*United States v. Montana*, 450 U.S. 544 (1981).)

---

[20] As the previous discussion indicates, just what constitutes "Indian country" has varied and been the subject of debate throughout most of the history of U.S.–tribal relations. However, since 1948, "Indian country" has been statutorily defined by 18 U.S.C. § 1151:

> Except as otherwise provided … "Indian country"… means (a) all land within the limits of any Indian reservation under the jurisdiction of the United States government, notwithstanding the issuance of any patent, and, including rights-of-way running through the reservation, (b) all dependent Indian communities within the borders of the United States whether within the original or subsequently acquired territory thereof, and whether within or without the limits of a state, and (c) all Indian allotments, the Indian titles to which have not been extinguished, including rights of way running through the same.

This definition is contained within the federal criminal jurisdiction statutes, but the Supreme Court has held it to generally apply to civil jurisdiction as well. *DeCoteau v. District County Court*, 420 U.S. 425, 427 n.2 (1975).

Not only do tribes retain authority as sovereigns, but also Congress can delegate to tribes authority for any type of jurisdiction.

ALASKA NATIVE CLAIMS

The land claims of Alaska Natives were finally addressed in 1971, through the Alaska Native Claims Settlement Act ("ANSCA"). (Act of December 18, 1971, Pub. L. No. 92-203, codified as amended at 43 U.S.C. §§ 1601 et seq.) In an unusual mix between assimilationist and self-determination policies, Congress authorized over 200 Alaska Native villages and 13 regional organizations to take lands and share in the financial settlement of their land claims. Native corporations were created to hold the settlement funds and lands. Alaska has a complex mix of village governments, tribal governments, village corporations, regional Native profit-making corporations, and regional Native non-profit corporations. In general, it is the regional Native non-profit corporations that provide health care to Alaska Native people. The maze of jurisdictions and organizations in Alaska has made the identification of "Indian Country" the subject of on-going legal disputes. Meanwhile, the tribes in Alaska are unable to engage in tribal gaming and other activities that have become commonplace elsewhere.

INDIAN SELF-DETERMINATION AND EDUCATION ASSISTANCE ACT

The congruence of the desires of many tribes to provide federal Indian programs to their own people, the historical preference of Congress that tribes become self-sufficient, and the goal of the Nixon administration to turn back the termination policy in favor of tribal self-determination led to the Indian Self-Determination and Education Assistance Act of 1975 ("Self-Determination Act" or "P.L. 93-638"). This law directs the Secretary of the Department of the Interior (DOI) and the Secretary of the Department of Health and Human Services (DHHS), upon the request of any Indian tribe, to enter into self-determination contracts with tribal organizations. These "638 contracts" may be for planning, conducting, and administering programs that are provided by the federal government for the benefit of Indians.

Originally, the Act only applied to the activities and programs of the two agencies with the greatest involvement in Indian affairs: the BIA and the IHS. This original enactment of the federal self-determination policy is now a small portion of a much larger scheme governing the processes by which a tribe may assume responsibility for provision of federal services, and is commonly referred to as "Title I" of the Act. One of the earliest amendments to the Act (P.L. 100-472,102 Stat. 2285) expanded self-determination to cover all bureaus within the DOI. This portion of the Self-Determination Act is commonly referred to as "Title II."

Originally under Title I, the BIA retained ultimate control over programs, made budget allocation decisions, and created a burdensome contracting process. Thus, many tribal leaders were dissatisfied with the implementation of the self-determination policy; other tribal leaders worried that contracting for programs would lead to a hidden type of termination[21], or "termination by appropriation." [22]

In 1998, Congress addressed the need for streamlining the contracting process by amending the Self-Determination Act to increase tribal participation in administering federal Indian programs, and by directing the Secretaries of DOI and DHHS to consult with tribes in drafting regulations to implement the amendments. (Indian Self-Determination and Education Assistance Act Amendments of 1988, P.L. 100-472.)

The next major step in the development of self-determination policy was a proposal by tribes to develop the "Tribal Self Governance Demonstration Project." The Demonstration Project eventually became Title III of the Act. Under Title III, self-governance compacting would be tested within the DOI, with the participation of 20 tribes that were to be selected by the Secretary of the Interior. (Title III of the Indian Self-Determination and Education Assistance Act, as added by the 1988 amendments, P.L. 100-472, 25 U.S.C. Sec. 450f note.) Title III also contains provisions designed to protect the trust and treaty relationship between the United States and tribes.

Title III paved the way for major changes in the manner in which tribes could administer federal programs. Under Title I, a tribe that chooses to assume programs must execute a separate contract for each program, while Title III allows tribes and the federal government to execute just one large compact to cover all programs assumed. Whereas a tribe with multiple Title I contracts cannot move funds from one program to another, Title III permits tribes to shift funds between programs when doing so is justified by need or merit. Further, while self-determination contracts under Title I limit the ability of a tribe to redesign programs, self-governance compacts under Title III allow tribes to redesign programs to better meet the needs of their own tribal members.

The next major developmental steps in the self-determination/self-governance policy came when President Bill Clinton signed the Indian Self-Determination Contract Reform Act (P.L. 103-413) in October 1994. The legislation grew out of Congress' dissatisfaction with the failure of the Departments of Interior and Health and Human Services to develop satisfactory regulations implementing the 1988 amendments intended to increase tribal participation in the management of federal Indian programs. In Title I of the 1994 Act, Congress imposed a negotiated-rulemaking process on the Secretaries of DOI and DHHS. The results of this negotiated rulemaking, which involved 48 tribal representatives, were joint final regulations for the

---

[21] Indian Self-Determination and Education Assistance Act Implementation, Hearings before the United States Senate Select Committee on Indian Affairs, 95th Congress, 1st Session, on Implementation of Public Law 93-638 (1977).

[22] Put roughly, the fear is that when tribes take over responsibility to administer programs and the sole remaining activity of the federal government is funding for the programs, it would be very easy for the federal government to attempt to absolve itself of any further responsibility for the tribes, and to cut funding.

awarding of contracts and grants under the Self-Determination Act published in the Federal Register on June 24, 1996. (61 Fed. Reg. 32482, June 24, 1996.) Title II of P.L. 103-413 was the Self-Governance Permanent Authorization Act. In this Act, Congress expressed its satisfaction with the BIA Self-Governance Demonstration Project, and made self-governance a permanent program within the DOI. The Secretary of the Interior was authorized to select up to 20 new tribes per year for participation in self governance. (25 U.S.C. Sec. 458bb.) Furthermore, the law provides that if it is requested by a majority of self governance tribes, the Secretary will initiate negotiated rulemaking with the affected tribes. (25 U.S.C. Sec. 458gg.) The Act also included a provision stating that there was no intent on the part of Congress to diminish the Federal trust responsibility to Indians or Indian tribes. (25 U.S.C. Sec. 458ff(b).)

Recent developments in P.L. 93-638 policy continue to center around self-governance. Self-governance was made a permanent program in IHS on August 18, 2000 when Congress passed Public Law 106-260.

INDIAN HEALTH CARE IMPROVEMENT ACT

The Indian Health Care Improvement Act of 1976 ("IHCIA" or P.L. 93-437) addressed the continuing lag of Indian health behind that of the general population, setting forth a national goal to provide "the highest possible health status to Indians and to provide existing Indian health services with all resources necessary to effect that policy." (25 U.S.C. § 1602.) The Act contained a vast array of provisions designed to increase the quantity and quality of Indian health services and to improve the participation of Indians in planning and providing those services. IHCIA provides for the consolidation and authorization of funding for existing IHS programs, funding authorization for facilities construction, and authorization for health and medical services for urban Indians. IHCIA also established the IHS Scholarship Program to educate AI/AN health professionals to work in Indian communities. It authorized construction of safe water and sanitary waste disposal facilities in Indian homes and communities and allowed preference to Indian contractors in construction projects. For the first time, IHCIA authorized Medicare and Medicaid reimbursement for services performed in Indian health facilities.[23]

GOVERNMENT-TO-GOVERNMENT RELATIONS

Executive documents on government-to-government relations, issued by President Clinton, are another major policy instrument designed to facilitate tribal involvement in federal Indian affairs. A Presidential Memorandum signed on April 29, 1994, directed the heads of each executive department and agency to operate within a government-to-government relationship with federally-recognized tribal governments, to consult with tribal governments prior to taking actions that affect them, to assess the impacts of federal activities on tribal trust resources, and to take steps to remove barriers that impede working

---

[23] Legislation to reauthorize the IHCIA was introduced in 2000 during the 106th Congress, but the legislation was not finalized by the end of the session. The IHCIA will be re-introduced in the 107th Congress in 2001.

directly and effectively with tribal governments. The Executive Order of May 14, 1998, required agencies to have tribal consultation processes in place, and attempts to reduce the imposition of unfunded mandatory federal requirements. Finally, the Executive Order of November 6, 2000, set out specific requirements for consultation programs, as well as provided specific directions to ensure that tribes' authority over their own affairs was not hindered by federal administrative actions. All of these directives recognize that Indian tribes retain the inherent ability and responsibility to look after the interests of their people. This is a reality that Justice Marshall recognized over 150 years ago.

SUMMARY

The legal framework that history has built retains the distinctive marks of each era. Through European conquest, westward expansion, treaty making, Indian wars, assimilation and allotment, reform and reorganization, and termination, federal policies and contemporaneous court cases have diminished tribal lands and eroded tribal sovereignty. The reality and utility of tribal autonomy has sometimes been ignored as the political pendulum has swung toward assimilative policies. The current policy of self-determination seeks to correct many injustices and restore some tribal authority. Termination and assimilation still find proponents in Congress and mainstream society. Tribal leaders are aware that they must be ever vigilant against the political pendulum swinging back toward regressive policies.

The fundamental concepts that have endured throughout the history of tribal relations with the United States are tribal sovereignty, the federal trust responsibility, and a government-to-government relationship. This is the foundation on which the Indian health system has been built and these are the principles that will guide the future of health care for American Indian and Alaska Native people.

ACKNOWLEDGEMENTS:

I would like to acknowledge Judy and Carrie Shelton and the rest of my family, Stephanie E. Birdwell, Mim Dixon, Jhon Goes In Center, Debra Harry, Sebastian "Bronco" LeBeau, Donald M. Ragona, Yvette Roubideaux, and George "Tink" Tinker, for ideas, assistance, and encouragement. Also, Vine Deloria, Jr., and Justice Raymond Austin, Navajo Nation Supreme Court, for inspiration in approach.

REFERENCES

Bush Judith K. *Legal, Historical and Political Context in which Tribes Make Health Care Decisions*. Denver: National Indian Health Board; 1996.

Clinton R, Newton NJ, Price ME. *American Indian Law: Cases and Materials.* 3rd ed. Charlottesville, VA: Michie Co; 1991.

Cohen Felix S. *Handbook of Federal Indian Law.* Charlottesville, VA: Michie Co; 1982.

Corbett Ben. Would the Real Don Juan Please Step Forward: Plastic Medicine Men and White America's Desperate Search for Native Spirituality. *Boulder Weekly.* October 14, 1999.

Deloria, Jr., V. Jr, Lytle C. *American Indians, American Justice.* Austin: Univ. of Texas Press; 1983.

Institute for Government Research. Meriam L, ed. *The Problem of Indian Administration.* Baltimore, MD: The Johns Hopkins Press; 1928.

Prucha, FP. *The Great Father: The United States Government and the American Indians,* Vol II. Lincoln, NE: Univ. of Nebraska Press; 1984.

Weatherford J. *Indian Givers.* New York, NY: Crown Publishers Inc; 1988.

Wilkinson C. *American Indians, Time and the Law: Native Societies in a Modern Constitutional Democracy.* New Haven, CT: Yale Univ. Press.1987.

Woodhead H. ed. *The American Indians: The Reservations,* 6. Alexandria, VA: Time-Life Books; 1995.

Young Bear S Sr, Theisz RD. *Standing in the Light: A Lakota Way of Seeing.* Lincoln, NE: Univ. of Nebraska Press; 1994.

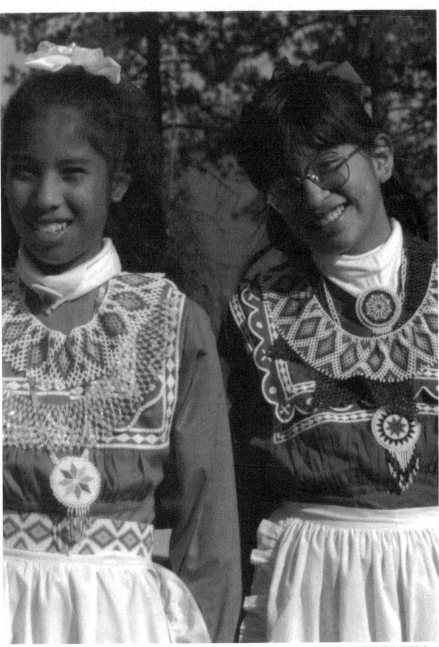

The Unique Role of Tribes
in the Delivery of Health Services
Mim Dixon

Few Americans have had experiences that enable them to understand the concept of a tribe. The Indian nations within our larger nation are invisible to a majority of the American population. Indian health systems are different from the other health systems in the United States because of the unique role of tribes. Understanding how tribes function is important to the development of public policies related to American Indian and Alaska Native (AI/AN) health.

YOU CAN'T BE AN INDIAN WITHOUT A TRIBE

While scientists have rejected the biological concept of race,[1] the popular view of race in America is to categorize people by the color of their skin, eyes, and hair. In the waiting room of an Indian health clinic, there are people with red or blonde hair and those who look like African Americans, as well as people who match the prevailing stereotypes of Native Americans. Any of these individuals may be American Indian or Alaska Native. To know if a person is an American Indian or an Alaska Native, do not look at the color of their skin, hair, or eyes—look in their wallets to see if they have a tribal enrollment card.

Just as the definition of a "European" is being a citizen of a country in

---

[1] The American Anthropological Association Statement on "Race" reviews the literature on the subject and concludes that "the 'racial' worldview was invented to assign some groups to perpetual low status, while others were permitted access to privilege, power, and wealth" (American Anthropological Association 1998).

Europe, people are considered American Indian if they are a citizen of an American Indian nation. Being a member of a tribe means being listed on the membership roll of a specific tribe. A tribal enrollment card is like carrying a passport that identifies an individual as a citizen of a tribe. The H'audenosaunee Nation, also known as the Onondaga Nation of the Six Nations Iroquois Confederacy, actually issues its own passports.

To be an American Indian, a person must be a Crow or Comanche or Jicarilla Apache or Zuni or a member of another tribe. An individual cannot be recognized by the federal government as an Indian without a tribe.[2]

In the year 2000, there were 558 tribes in the United States that are recognized by the federal government. Individual state governments have recognized additional tribes. Some tribes are in the process of trying to secure federal recognition.

FEDERAL RECOGNITION OF TRIBES

To become a federally recognized tribe literally takes an act of Congress. In the past, that act of Congress usually involved approving a treaty, but the treaty-making period ended in 1871. Today, tribes can petition for federal recognition under the Federal Acknowledgment Procedures program that was enacted in 1978, when Congress delegated the authority for tribal recognition to the Executive Branch (Bush 1996). In 1994, Congress passed the Federally Recognized Indian Tribe List Act that requires the Secretary of the Interior to publish an updated list of federally recognized tribes in the *Federal Register* each year. Title II of that Act says that all tribes identified on the list of federally recognized tribes are to be treated the same regardless of how or when they were recognized.

Tribe is a political concept that creates a layer of meaning on top of the ethnological concept of tribe, which relies primarily on shared language and culture. For federal recognition, a tribe is usually considered a group of Native Americans whose existence pre-dates European discovery and which has continued to remain separate and distinct (Bush 1996). However, federal Indian policy has distorted the inherent cultural concept of tribes. For example, the policy of forced removals of Indian people in the 1800s resulted in treaties with those who relocated to reservations, but some members of a tribe may have stayed on their traditional lands and the federal government recognizes the two groups as separate tribes. For example, there is the Cherokee tribe in Oklahoma and the Eastern Band of Cherokee Indians in North Carolina, each with separate political organizations, although they share common origins and cultural traits. Similarly, there is a Seminole Tribe in Florida and the Seminole Tribe of Oklahoma; one Creek tribe is in Oklahoma, but the Poarch Band of Creek

---

[2] While this is true for receiving federal benefits specifically designated for American Indians and Alaska Natives, the federal government also uses the scientifically unjustified concept of "race" in many programs. People can choose whether or not to self-identify as American Indian on birth certificates, in the U.S. Census, or to qualify for some programs designed for "racial minorities." Also, some federal programs require only that the individual be a descendant of a tribal member and not that they be enrolled in a tribe.

Indians is in Alabama; the Mississippi Band of Choctaw Indians is culturally similar to, but politically distinct from, the Choctaw Tribe of Oklahoma.

While a culture may have extended over a vast geographic area prior to European contact, the history of warfare and treaty making may have resulted in divisions that the federal government recognized as tribes. Each of these, in turn, eventually evolved into political units that became responsible for specific reservation lands. The Lakota culture is widespread in North Dakota and South Dakota, but there are many reservations, each recognized as a separate Sioux tribe; similarly, there are many bands of Chippewa in Minnesota, Michigan, and Wisconsin that are recognized as separate tribes. In Alaska, there are different cultures in different geographic areas. For example, the Athabascan Indians inhabit the interior of the state; however, each Athabascan village is regarded as a separate tribe under federal law.

While most federally recognized tribes represent people who share the same language and culture, this is not always the case. Sometimes tribes that were decimated through conflict or disease sought refuge with other tribes and eventually became recognized by the federal government as a single tribe. In some cases, the federal government forced different cultural groups to share the same reservation; they then called this a "confederated" tribe.

TRIBAL ENROLLMENT CRITERIA

Belonging to a tribe is more than just registering for a political party. The tribe sets its requirements for membership and decides who qualifies as a member. Usually, an individual who is a descendent of a tribal member qualifies for membership. In some cases, tribes specify a blood quantum,[3] or a minimum percentage of biological heritage, that must be met to qualify as a tribal member.[4] For example, if an individual is at least one quarter Southern Ute, then he or she can enroll in the Southern Ute Tribe. Other tribes have different requirements for membership.

Belonging to a tribe means more than certifying ethnicity. Some tribes are comprised of clans or other subgroups, so tribal membership can also mean belonging to a clan and carrying out the traditions of that clan, such as rules about kinship and marriage. Even where there is no formal clan structure, extended families may provide an important part of the political and social structure of tribes. Tribal members usually have a place in the social network; they may have responsibilities to others and other tribal members may have responsibilities to them. Decisions are based not on just what is best for the individual, but also what is best for the family, the clan, and the tribe.

Like being a citizen of any country, being a citizen of an Indian nation car-

---

[3] The Bureau of Indian Affairs issues a Certificate of Degree of Indian Blood (CDIB) that is used by some tribes to establish that membership criteria are met. The CDIB also may be used by federal agencies to verify eligibility for federal programs in lieu of tribal enrollment cards.

[4] Tribes that use blood quantum requirements often exclude people whose parents are members of two or more different tribes, or when one parent is not American Indian. This is often a problem for urban Indians who find themselves disenfranchised from their tribal origins and unable to access federal programs for American Indians and Alaska Natives.

ries with it responsibilities as well as benefits—belonging to a tribe means accepting the political and social rules of the tribe. Many tribes have reservations or other lands that are classified as "Indian Country." In Indian Country, tribes have political jurisdiction, much the same as a county government. There are tribal councils that make laws, tribal police that enforce laws, tribal courts that settle disputes, and tribal governments that provide services.

TRIBAL SOVEREIGNTY

Historically, tribes have been considered nations within our larger nation and they have retained their sovereignty to rule over their tribal members and tribal lands. Thus, the laws of the state in which a tribe is located do not necessarily apply in Indian Country. For example, economic enterprises on Indian reservations usually do not have to pay state taxes. Tribes are usually exempt from state licensing laws and can discriminate in employment to give preference to tribal members. At the same time, tribes can pass more restrictive rules than those of the state in which they live, such as prohibiting the sale of alcohol on tribal lands.

Tribal sovereignty is recognized by the federal government. This means that the federal government works with tribes on a government-to-government basis. Relationships between the federal government and tribes are similar to the relationships between the federal government and states. For many federal programs, tribes can receive block grants in the same manner that states receive them. An Executive Order directs federal agencies to consult with tribal leadership before they design programs or make regulations that could affect tribes or tribal members (Clinton 1994).

Sometimes people who are not familiar with tribes are confused about who represents tribes and speaks on their behalf. The elected tribal leaders—often with the titles of Chairman, Governor, or President—are designated by the tribe to represent them in official matters. Also, the elected tribal councils pass resolutions that represent the will of the tribe.

Tribes can use the resolution process to designate another organization to represent them or to act on their behalf. Such is the case for Alaska Natives; in Alaska, the federal government has recognized each Alaska Native village as a separate tribe. Rather than negotiate on their own most of the small tribes have passed resolutions that allow regional non-profit Native corporations to contract with the federal government on their behalf. These regional non-profit Native corporations are considered to be tribal organizations because of these resolutions from the tribes. However, not all organizations that have been formed on a regional or national level to advocate on Indian issues are considered tribal organizations.

Fundamentally, tribes are political organizations with jurisdiction over their members and their lands. If tribes were to lose their sovereignty, they would no longer be tribes. Without tribal sovereignty, American Indians would be just another racial or ethnic group. The future of the tribe is as important as the future of the members of the tribe. While the federal government once engaged in the termination of tribal sovereignty in exchange for cash payments and individual property distributions to tribal members, today most tribes would never willingly enter into this type of arrangement. Most tribal leaders today would put the preservation of tribal sovereignty above all other goals.

TRIBES MAY BE DIFFERENT FROM OTHER TYPES OF GOVERNMENT IN THE U.S.

Tribes can choose any form of government. Some tribes have constitutions, while others do not. In some smaller tribes, all the tribal members participate as a council that makes decisions. Many Pueblos in New Mexico rotate their leadership by having a different person serve as governor each year. Some tribes prohibit women from running for elected office. Many tribes use consensus as a form of decision making, rather than a majority vote. Tribes that have chosen to use the provisions of the Indian Reorganization Act of 1934 (IRA) tend to have governments that look more like the typical city or county governments, but they still differ in two significant ways: (1) there is no separation of powers, and (2) there is no separation of religion and government.

In the federal, state, and local governments of the United States, there is a separation of powers between the legislative and executive branches of government. The congress, legislature, or city council has the power to make laws; while the administrative or executive part of government is charged with carrying out the legislation. In tribal governments, it is not unusual for the tribal council to serve both legislative and administrative functions. The president, chairman, or governor of the tribe may be both the head of the tribal council and the top administrator for the tribe.

Tribes generally do not embrace a "separation of church and state." Spiritual beliefs are an integral part of most Native American cultures, and as such religion is not always a separate formal institution, although Christian missionaries have introduced many formal religions to Indian tribes. In most tribes, there are traditional spiritual leaders. Tribal activities, including tribal council meetings and other governmental activities, often begin and end with prayers. Elected tribal leaders may also be spiritual leaders.

American Indians and Alaska Natives in general tend to look at things in a holistic, integrated way. Most other governments in the United States have rigid categories that identify certain types of responsibilities with specific bodies of government. These clearly defined roles enable people to identify their primary loyalties and to avoid real or potential conflicts of interest, but tribes are relatively small groups of people who are interrelated and they must deal with many potentially conflicting issues. Rather than trying to separate issues into categories, they tend to deal with issues as a whole and to make trade-offs in a more fluid way. For example, decisions about health care delivery systems may also be about increasing employment opportunities for tribal members.

Most tribes have special committees that advise the tribal council on health issues. These may be called a Health Commission, a Health Committee, a Human Services Board, a Health Board, a Health Advisory Board, or some similar name. In some tribes, the health board members are appointed by the tribal council, while in other tribes they may be selected through a general election in which all tribal members vote. The authority and responsibilities of these committees vary from tribe to tribe:

> For some Tribes, the health committee serves as a "clearing house," sifting through lots of information and providing guidance to the health care delivery system. Health committees screen information so that too many details do not go to the Council. Health committees also hear patient complaints and set Tribal health priorities. In some Tribes, the Tribal Council "rubber stamps" all health committee recommendations. In other Tribes, there is duplication at every level, with no clear delineation of roles and responsibilities. (Dixon, Bush, Iron 1997, p. 63)

The roles of tribal councils also vary with regard to health issues:

> Where Indian Health Service (IHS) is providing most of the health services directly, the Tribal Council is asked to advise on program and policy changes. For Tribes that are operating health care programs, Tribal Councils make the final decisions on budgets, changes in rules for eligibility for services, adding or deleting types of services, compacting and contracting, major purchases and facilities construction. Where gaming enterprises have become profitable, Tribal Councils are often asked to use gaming revenues to supplement health budgets, to finance new health programs or to construct new health facilities. Tribal Councils also consider positions on national and State legislation, and adopt Tribal codes and ordinances. Most Tribal Councils hire the top management for Tribal programs. Some Tribal Councils in this study approve all personnel actions, approve contracts requiring the chairperson's signature, and even approve travel to conferences. (Dixon, Bush, Iron 1997, p. 63)

In all of these decisions, the health committees and tribal councils are wearing several hats simultaneously. They must consider the needs of individual tribal members and at the same time protect the interests of the tribe as a whole. They must represent the tribe as an employer, while at the same time representing tribal members who are employees. They may be purchasing health insurance for employees and at the same time billing that insurance for health care services provided at a tribally-operated clinic. Thus, in a single decision they may have to balance the conflicting needs of all parties that they have a duty to represent: consumers, providers, and purchasers of health care.

BASIC BELIEFS THAT GUIDE TRIBAL DECISION-MAKING

Tribes have different cultures and that means different beliefs. Working with a number of tribes over a seven-year period, Americans for Indian Opportunity (AIO) identified four key values which all tribes involved in their work hold in common (Harris and Wasilewski, 1992, p. 7):

- Being a Good Relative

Basing the entire functioning of the community on inclusive relational webs of mutual reciprocal exchange obligations based on kinship principles;

- Inclusive Sharing

Sharing as a mechanism for redistributing "goods" throughout the community;

- Contributing

Setting up the social system so that each person can, not only participate in, but contribute to the community; and

- Non-Coercive Leadership

Leadership (and its associated influence and authority) based on the assumption of responsibility rather than on the ability to coerce others through the exercise of power (or force) over them; leadership based on shared responsibility, not control.

These four values express common ideals that help to shape tribal social relationships and the way people make decisions. HeavyRunner and Morris (1997) have identified additional values that influence the way that American Indian people relate to one another and thus create the context for decision-making. These include cooperation among group members taking precedence over competition; harmony within the group; and attitudes toward time that are inherent in nature rather than imposed by society.

Using intensive interviews with elected tribal leaders from a representative cross-section of tribes, Dixon, Bush, and Iron (1997) identified seven basic beliefs that guide tribal decisions about health care:

- A separate health care delivery system is needed for American Indians.

- Management decisions impact human lives.

- High-quality health care is important.

- Holistic solutions go beyond the health care delivery system.

- Decisions should be made for the long term.

- Information and communications are essential for good decision-making.

- Tribes must act to preserve the federal trust responsibility.

The most fundamental and universal belief expressed by every tribal leader and every tribal health director who participated in the study is the importance for Indian people to have a health care delivery system that is separate from the majority population. One might assume that the federal trust responsibility could be carried out by enrolling tribal members in a managed care plan that was operated by the private sector, and in fact, some tribes have chosen this approach to providing health care for their members. However, most tribal leaders believe that it is important for there to be tribal control over the types of health care provided to tribal members as part of the federal trust responsibility. They explain their reasoning for a separate health care system in the study by Dixon, Bush, and Iron (1997, p. 65):

> One reason they all cited was cultural issues. "From time immemorial, Tribes have taken care of their member's health — it is a traditional function for a Tribe to fill," said one Tribal Chairman. Another leader cited "Tribal feelings of concern for all members' well-being." A Tribal Chair reported that while the members of his Tribe are bilingual, 90 percent speak the Tribal language first and they need interpreters for English. Other cultural issues included the availability of traditional healers and feeling more comfortable in a program that is designed for them. "Understanding by providers that Indian people have different attitudes and beliefs" is important, explained one Tribal Chairperson, because it "means people

are more likely to seek medical care if they believe providers understand them."

Other reasons cited in the study of the need for a separate health care system were more employment opportunities for tribal members; discrimination against Indians in other health care systems; the focus on community health in the present Indian health system, and the ability to address the unique health needs of Indian people that result from their genetic make up, culture, and geographic location. Equally important reasons are ownership, empowerment, sovereignty, and tribal identity.

TRIBAL CHOICES OF HEALTH CARE DELIVERY SYSTEMS

There are two basic choices available to federally-recognized tribes: (1) they can receive their health care through the Indian Health Service, a federal agency in the U.S. Department of Health and Human Services; or (2) they can receive money from the IHS to operate their own health care delivery system. Various combinations of these choices are available, such as tribal management of community health services while relying on the IHS to provide primary care.

If tribes choose to receive their health services through the IHS, they are part of a federal bureaucracy that is organized from the top down. The IHS is a comprehensive primary care system of hospitals and clinics located on or near reservations and AI/AN communities. The headquarters are in Rockville, Maryland, where rules and regulations are promulgated, the budget is decided, and approval must be obtained for any deviation from the basic federal program. The IHS is divided into 12 areas[5], each with an Area Office where administrative functions occur and, in some cases, where there is an IHS tertiary-care hospital. The Areas are further subdivided into Service Units; initially, each Service Unit had a hospital, but today less than one-third of the Service Units have hospitals.[6] Service Units generally provide services to one large tribe or several small tribes. In the Bemidji Area, for example, the Mille Lacs Service Unit serves the Mille Lacs Band of Chippewa in Minnesota, but the Central Wisconsin Service Unit covers four tribes (the Menominee, the Oneida, the Stockbridge-Munsee and the Ho Chunk Nation). However, the Navajo Area has eight Service Units that all provide services to the Navajo Nation, which is the largest tribe in the country with approximately 250,000 members.

If a tribe chooses to manage its own health care system, it has several options under the Indian Self-Determination Act (P.L. 93-638). It can contract with the IHS to take over the management of specific programs. After a good record as a contractor for three years, it is eligible for a compact.[7] A compact

---

[5] The 12 IHS Areas are named: Aberdeen, Alaska, Albuquerque, Bemidji, Billings, California, Nashville, Navajo, Oklahoma City, Phoenix, Portland, and Tucson (Figure 2.1).

[6] There are 150 Service Units and 49 hospitals, of which 37 are operated by IHS and 12 by tribes, according to the IHS report, *Regional Differences in Indian Health*, 1997.

[7] Prior to 2001, when compacting was a demonstration project in the IHS, the number of compacts was limited each year.

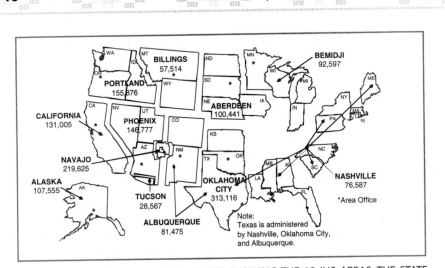

FIGURE 2.1. MAP OF THE UNITED STATES SHOWING THE 12 IHS AREAS, THE STATE BOUNDARIES, AND IHS SERVICE POPULATION BY AREA, FY 2000.
SOURCE: TRENDS IN INDIAN HEALTH, 1998-1999

is more like a treaty or block grant than a contract and allows the tribe considerably more management and administrative authority and more flexibility to move funds between programs and to design new programs. Both contracting and compacting allow tribes the option of taking a portion of the funding from the Service Unit, Area Office, or Headquarters that is intended to provide support services to their tribe.

Neither IHS nor the tribes provide a full range of medical specialty care within their clinics and hospitals, so they must contract with the private sector for some services. The Contract Health Services (CHS) program is used for this purpose. However, congressional appropriations to fund CHS fall far short of the needs. IHS has responded to this limitation by prioritizing services, limiting CHS expenditures to people who live within specified CHS service areas, requiring people who may be eligible for other health care funding to use those alternate resources first, and postponing needed health care when the funds have been fully expended before the end of a fiscal year. Tribes that manage their own health care programs have more latitude to apportion their resources between direct services and contracted services. Some tribes want more access to private health care and put more of their resources into CHS. For some small tribes with limited budgets, the entire health program is provided through CHS. If there are few private sector facilities in a remote area where a tribe is located, tribes are less likely to shift their resources from direct services to CHS.

Not all tribes have the same choices available to them. While the IHS built hospitals and clinics for the larger tribes that were recognized by treaty, the tribes that have been recognized most recently do not have federally-built hospitals. East of the Mississippi River, there is only one IHS hospital, and there are no IHS hospitals in California, Oregon, or Michigan. In states where there are no IHS-built facilities, there is a greater reliance on CHS to pay for services in private and public facilities. Furthermore, many tribes without the bricks-and-mortar of the IHS are virtually required to enter into P.L. 93-638 contracts with the IHS for their health care systems. In California, which has a unique history in the development of Indian health services, there are approximately 100 tribes; these tribes are among the least satisfied with their health care services, because they have fewer choices and lower per capita funding (Dixon et al 1998).

When the Pascua Yaqui Tribe of Arizona was granted federal recognition in 1978, there was no money available to build health facilities for the tribe. The IHS created a Pascua Yaqui Service Unit to receive federal funding and then contracted with a local community health center that was licensed as an HMO to provide services (Dixon 1998). The tribe accepted this unique proposal under protest and began working to find a way to build their own clinic. Over time, as other small tribes have assumed management of their own health care systems, contracting with a managed care plan is an option that has been explored and considered more favorably.

Each tribe has different types and amounts of resources from both the IHS and from their own tribal economic development. Cornell and Kalt (1992) observed that tribes have little control over key factors in economic development, such as market opportunity, distance from markets, and natural resources. Given the limitations of their financial resources and private services available in their geographic area, tribes can make different decisions about how to organize their health services.

Just as Medicaid benefits vary from state to state, individual health care benefits vary from tribe to tribe. However, there is no standard or minimum benefits package for Indian health. Most tribes in California offer only outpatient primary care. While Native non-profit health organizations in Alaska offer both outpatient and inpatient services, most Alaska Native people have to pay for an airline ticket to fly from their village to a regional hospital. In South Dakota, Indian people can obtain both outpatient primary care and inpatient care, but there are few specialized medical services available. While choices are limited for some tribes, the wealthiest tribes, who run gaming casinos, can send their tribal members to the most prestigious private medical facilities in the world.

When a tribal council makes decisions about the organization of their health care services, those decisions affect the choices of tribal members. For example, if a tribe chooses IHS direct services, then tribal members are usually more limited in their ability to access private sector health care, unless they have health insurance through their employer or Medicaid or Medicare. If a tribe chooses to contract or compact a Service Unit and to use that money to enroll all tribal members in a private sector managed care plan, then tribal members usually only have access to that HMO, unless they have alternate resources.

Thus, the tribe in which a person is enrolled determines what types of health benefits that person is eligible to receive. The health care benefits do not accrue to the individual as an American Indian; rather, the health care benefits are vested in the tribe.[8] One of the ways that tribes exercise their sovereignty is to create the rules that allocate health care resources for their tribal members. Another way that a tribe can exercise its sovereignty is to choose to have the Indian Health Service provide direct services to tribal members, recognizing that this choice means that tribal members will be subjected to the rules of the federal bureaucracy that result in the allocation of health care resources.

GOVERNMENT-TO-GOVERNMENT RELATIONSHIP

The federal government has recognized tribal sovereignty since the beginning of the American history. Tribal sovereignty means that the tribe is treated as a nation within a nation. Because the tribe was considered a sovereign nation, the U.S. was able to enter into treaties with tribes. Just as the U.S. government holds meetings with heads of state of foreign nations, the U.S. government is expected to hold meetings with the elected officials that represent tribal nations.

There is a long historic tradition of Indian chiefs traveling to the White House to meet with the president of the United States. As the federal government grew over the years, the government-to-government relationship changed. Most Indian programs were relegated to two federal agencies, the Bureau of Indian Affairs (BIA) and the Indian Health Service. Other federal agencies assumed that the BIA and the IHS were responsible for the tribal consultation component of a government-to-government relationship. However, as Congress has failed to fully fund the BIA and the IHS, tribes have looked to other federal agencies to meet tribal financial needs. Those other agencies have not fully appreciated the legal and historic basis of the government-to-government relationship between the federal government and tribes.

President Bill Clinton issued an Executive Memorandum on Government-to-Government Relationships with Native American Tribal Governments on

---

[8] This situation is actually much more complex. Funding for health care is allotted by tribe and tribes determine who their members are. Prior to 1986, the federal government used eligibility criteria that required the IHS to serve all persons who were descendents of federally recognized tribes, regardless of blood quantum (42CFR). Tribes and the IHS worked together to develop new criteria that would have limited eligibility to enrolled tribal members and those regulations were published in the Federal Register on September 16, 1987. However, Congress placed a moratorium on implementing the new regulations and this language has been added to each annual appropriations bill since 1987. It is anticipated that the reauthorization of the Indian Health Care Improvement Act (P.L. 93-437) will provide another opportunity to develop eligibility criteria. Also, it should be noted that the IHS is an integrated system, so that anyone who is eligible for the IHS can receive the services that are provided at any IHS facility. Urban Indians and members of tribes with less health care funding may travel to other tribal areas to avail themselves of services provided to other tribes that offer more comprehensive health care.

April 29, 1994. It directed each department of the federal government to develop a policy on tribal consultation; a Domestic Policy Council (DPC) Working Group on Indian Affairs guided this effort. The Department of Health and Human Services issued its policy on tribal consultation on August 7, 1997. Since that time, a model has been emerging for tribal consultation that has been used successfully with the allocation of funding under the Diabetes initiative in the Balanced Budget Act of 1997, the fiscal year 2001 federal budget, and the reauthorization of the Indian Health Care Improvement Act.

The federal model for tribal consultation that is emerging has several features. First, a steering committee is formed with elected tribal officials from each of the 12 IHS Areas, as well as representatives from national organizations, such as the National Indian Health Board, the National Congress of American Indians, the Tribal Self-Governance Advisory Committee, and the National Council of Urban Indian Programs. The steering committee is assisted by a technical support staff that is drawn from both government and tribal health programs.

The second feature of the tribal consultation model is a multi-layered process of disseminating information about the issue and gathering comments and suggestions from tribes. Meetings are held with tribes in each Area of the IHS, often with the assistance of Area Health Boards, which are tribally-operated organizations that generally serve the same geographic area as the IHS Area Offices. The purpose of these meetings is to discuss the tribe's options and to explain the process to the tribal leaders in the Area. Then, leaders go back to their tribes to explain the issues and develop tribal recommendations. There may be another meeting in which tribal leaders gather to formulate consensus recommendations on behalf of all the tribes in the Area. The Area Health Board staff may assist in synthesizing these recommendations into a resolution format. These resolutions are taken to each tribal council for approval. After each tribal council has passed the resolution, it becomes an official position of the tribes in the Area. Following this, there will be a national meeting in which each Area presents its resolutions. The steering committee will try to synthesize the recommendations from all the Areas into a unified plan.

The third feature of the federal tribal consultation process is distribution of the unified plan to every federally recognized tribe for review and comment. Based on these comments, the steering committee may make adjustments to the proposed plan, budget, legislation, regulations, or recommendations.

This process requires time, money, and the sharing of power. The results of this approach to tribal consultation have been a high degree of consensus among tribes, as well as a high level of satisfaction that tribal sovereignty has been respected. When the tribes can speak as one voice on an issue, they are better advocates. Furthermore, they can give the federal government clear direction about a tribal position.

TRIBAL/STATE RELATIONSHIPS

Federally recognized tribes are located within 35 of the 50 states. Historically, there has been tension between tribes and state governments since the formation of the United States. The U.S. Constitution gives Congress authority over Indian affairs and limits the rights of states to regulate activities in Indian Country. Federal courts have been asked to settle disputes between states and tribes over a wide range of issues, such as water rights, hunting and fishing rights, land management, child welfare jurisdiction, and gaming. The history of conflict between states and tribes often has resulted in a lack of trust and poor communications.

Some states take the attitude that Indians are a federal responsibility. They reason that the state has no jurisdiction in Indian Country, so the state has no obligation to provide funding or services to the people who live there. Some states do not recognize tribal sovereignty and do not deal directly with tribal governments; while others have developed policies and procedures for tribal consultation that recognize tribal sovereignty—Washington, Oregon and New Mexico have developed official state policy recognizing tribal sovereignty. Some state constitutions say that all state citizens will be treated equally and, therefore, they will not make any special arrangements to respond to the distinct needs of tribes or tribal members.[9] However, these circumstances are changing, in part due to the increased contribution of tribes to the state tax base through gaming.

GOVERNMENT-TO-GOVERNMENT RELATIONSHIP

Most tribes want states to deal with them as they would other governmental agencies and to make funding available to them through state sources and federal block grants. Tribes want to be consulted in the development of legislation and state programs so that the outcomes will be responsive to the needs of Indian people. Tribes want to contract with the state to provide the programs in Indian Country that are being provided elsewhere in the state. Tribal leaders want to sit at the table on an equal basis with state governors.

TRIPLE CITIZENSHIP

Most tribes want states to recognize that American Indians and Alaska Natives have triple citizenship. They are citizens of their tribe, which is a sovereign government; they are citizens of the United States and entitled to all federal programs; and they are citizens of the states in which they reside and therefore entitled to all state programs. In theory, because of this triple citizenship, Indian people should have access to more health resources. For example, an Indian elder who is below the poverty level should have access to health services funded by the Indian Health Service, Medicare, and Medicaid. Ironically,

---

[9] Alaska has taken this approach and has gone to the U.S. Supreme Court to oppose any recognition of Indian Country. Until 1995, Alaska refused to recognize two tribes that had been on the Secretary of the Interior's list of recognized tribes and had approved IRA constitutions dating to the 1940s.

Indian people often have access to fewer resources than other state citizens for a variety of reasons, and have lower health status as a result.

In the health care arena, the motivation for conserving limited public resources for health care has led to arguments over the "payer-of-last-resort" and other techniques associated with cost shifting. In some cases, state programs refuse to pay for services for Indians who had access to the IHS. However, federal regulations require alternate resources, such as state programs, to be used before money can be expended through CHS. As both sides struggle to avoid their responsibility to provide health services, the result is that the Indian consumer receives fewer services rather than more services.

STATE/TRIBAL CONSULTATION

In states where there are few tribes that comprise a very small portion of the population, it is difficult for these tribes to get the attention that they would like from state government. In states where there are many Indian tribes, the state governments have had difficulty consulting with each tribe individually. The state's representatives complain about the turnover in tribal leadership, the poor attendance when they hold meetings, and their confusion over who actually speaks on behalf of tribes (Dixon 1998b). Many small tribes, particularly those that do not manage their own health programs, do not have the technical expertise to interface with the state on health policy issues.

In states where there are predominantly IHS direct services, the state government may find it easier to talk with representatives of the IHS Area Office rather than consulting directly with tribes. However, the IHS Area boundaries do not coincide with state boundaries, except for the Alaska Area and the California Area. Tribes in Arizona are served by three different Area Offices (Navajo, Phoenix, and Tucson), while New Mexico has two Area Offices (Albuquerque and Navajo). The three tribes in Texas are each served by a different Area Office (Nashville, Oklahoma City, and Albuquerque), none of which are located in the state. The other Area Offices serve tribes in several states and are not always staffed to track all the policy developments in each state.

Furthermore, the IHS Area Offices do not actually represent tribes. They are part of a federal bureaucracy, not an extension of tribal government. While the Area Office leadership may need to be at the table to assure that systems work smoothly, this does not preclude the need for tribal consultation.

One way that tribes have found to interface with states is through Area Health Boards. Ideally, the Area Health Boards have representatives from each tribe in the Area. They work through the tribal resolution process to speak collectively on behalf of tribes. The most effective Area Health Boards employ policy analysts with the expertise to track policy issues for the states within their Area. However, there is a huge range in funding and staffing between the Area Health Boards. In some cases, the Area Health Boards receive funding from the IHS Area Offices, but there is no standard funding formula. Membership in some Area Health Boards requires tribes to pay a membership fee and some choose not to do this. Some Area Health Boards do not represent all the tribes in that IHS Area. Furthermore, not all IHS Areas have Area Health Boards.

Within some IHS Areas there are several inter-tribal organizations, sometimes organized to be consistent with state boundaries, but not always. In the Bemidji Area, for example, there is an Inter-Tribal Council of Michigan, as well as a Great Lakes Inter-Tribal Council that represents the tribes in Wisconsin. In some states, there is more than one inter-tribal organization. In New Mexico, for example, there are three inter-tribal organizations: the Albuquerque Area Indian Health Board, the Eight Northern Pueblos, and the All Indian Pueblo Council. None of these represents all the tribes in the state. In states with more than one inter-tribal organization, the organizations may have different political goals and represent different interests.

Regardless of the number of inter-tribal organizations in a state, each of the tribes wants to be acknowledged by the state as a sovereign entity. One tribal leader expressed it this way:

> Although there may be some similarities in the tribes, they are very different and the States need to start learning the differences in these tribes. . . You can't always put one concept of understanding to every tribe in your State. (National Indian Health Board, 1996a, p. 8)

Some states have responded to this need by having an American Indian Liaison, usually located in the department that manages the Medicaid program. The American Indian Liaison makes on-site visits to tribes to better understand their particular health care delivery system and the cultural context in which it operates. This enables the Liaison to provide appropriate technical assistance to the tribes and to participate in the policy development process in a more knowledgeable way. The Liaison provides a point of entry for tribes into the bureaucracy that might otherwise seem faceless and overwhelming. However, the American Indian Liaison position can only be effective if it is empowered to solve problems and if it functions in a department where the leadership is committed to enhancing the Indian health system. Furthermore, the Liaison is not a substitute for tribal consultation.

A study of nine state Medicaid managed care programs identified that the most effective tribal/state relationships occurred where several approaches were used simultaneously:

> The greatest satisfaction on the part of both tribes and states appears to result from using a number of different approach-

es. For example, in Washington there is an official state advisory committee, a tribally organized health committee, and an American Indian Liaison in the Medicaid department. In addition, high-ranking state officials consult personally with people in leadership positions in Indian health. All these efforts appear to be coordinated not only within state government and between tribes, but also with the HCFA American Indian Liaison and the Area Indian health board. Washington has a Centennial Accord that acknowledges tribal sovereignty and establishes a government-to-government relationship. Furthermore, the state has developed a document called the *Native American Health Plan* with the participation of a broad-based Advisory Committee and state-funded staff. (Dixon 1998b, p. 15)

It is significant to note that Washington did not involve the tribes in its initial planning for a statewide Medicaid-managed care waiver. Only after tribal leaders pursued the issues all the way to the governor's office and the federal government also applied pressure, did the state begin to work with the tribes more proactively.

FEDERAL ROLE IN TRIBAL/STATE RELATIONSHIPS

In recent years, the federal Health Care Financing Administration (HCFA) has been asked by tribes to take a greater role in tribal/state relationships in the health care arena. Three developments created the perceived need for this federal role. The first development was that tribes started taking over management of their health services under the Indian Self-Determination Act (P.L. 93-638) in 1975. This put tribes, rather than the IHS, in the position of seeking funding for health services from the state-administered Medicaid programs and other state health financing programs. The second was a push by Congress to give states more control over federal funding through block grants to states. Prior to the block grant approach, the tribes could receive funding directly from the federal government, often through Indian "set-asides" or federal funds that were earmarked for Indian programs. After block grants to states became the *modus operendi*, tribes had to approach states for their share of the federal funding. The third development was the increased use of the Medicaid waiver process to change Medicaid from fee-for-service to managed care programs. Tribes usually were not consulted in the development of state waiver applications and the result was detrimental to Indian health facilities because it reduced their Medicaid income. Therefore, tribes asked HCFA to exercise the federal trust responsibility by reviewing waiver applications from states to assure that Indian health issues were adequately addressed.

The concept of the federal trust responsibility was new to the HCFA, which initially was inclined to regard American Indians and Alaska Natives as one of many ethnic groups that comprised their consumer constituency. The impetus to recognize a special relationship with tribes came from the Executive Memorandum on Government-to-Government Relations with Native American Tribal Governments signed by President Clinton on April 29, 1994.

The leadership of the Department of Health and Human Services initiated a series of regional meetings in 1995 that brought the top leadership of HCFA into Indian Country to learn about the issues and to be part of a problem-solving process. These regional meetings included both tribal leaders and representatives of state governments, as well as federal officials. Although there was no formal process for adopting recommendations, there was a consistent theme about the federal role in promoting tribal/state relations. The following are a sample of the recommendations in the summary reports of these meetings:

- Additional forums are needed to enhance communication between States, tribes, urban Indian programs and the federal government. Issues which require further training, discussion and clarification include tribal sovereignty, multiple citizenship and its implications, and the roles of Native Americans as both consumers and providers of health care. (National Indian Health Board, 1996 b, p. 5)

- The federal government must hold the States accountable in ensuring that there is official concurrence and participation by tribes in changing the health care delivery system, even to the point of getting consent from individual tribes. Particularly when tribes do not have good relationships with the States, the Health Care Financing Administration must negotiate Medicaid waivers with official representatives of the tribes and mediate agreements that are satisfactory to the tribes. (National Indian Health Board, 1996 b, p. 5)

- The Health Care Financing Administration should prohibit granting any State waiver of Medicaid requirements unless the waiver proposal has (1) been reviewed and approved by all affected tribes; (2) been reviewed and approved by the IHS; and (3) been reviewed to assure that the right of Indian people to obtain health services from tribal programs with their Medicaid benefits is not impeded or diminished. (National Indian Health Board, 1996c, p. 19)

- HCFA should review all State Medicaid waiver applications to ensure that the issues of sovereignty and the special federal/tribal relationships for health program funding are addressed, that tribes are involved in all levels of policy development in health care reform, and that the value and importance of traditional medicine in the Indian culture is not overlooked. (National Indian Health Board, 1995, p 6)

While HCFA was under pressure from tribes to protect their interests, the federal agency was also facing the prospect of dissolution as the Congress threatened a revision of the Medicaid program which would turn it into another block grant program for states. Congress and the states were complaining that the Medicaid waiver review process was too slow and too cumbersome. One way to dodge the block grant bullet was to quickly approve the backlog of waiver applications and thus shift power from the federal government to the states. This strategy proved effective as Congress lost interest in block granting Medicaid.

HCFA spent more than three years developing policies on tribal consultation. During that time, statewide managed care waivers were approved for at least eight states with a total of 224 tribes, approximately two-thirds of the tribes located outside of Alaska in California, Michigan, Minnesota, New Mexico, New York, Oklahoma, Oregon and Washington. Interviews with tribal, urban and state representatives from those eight states revealed that people in only half of the eight states felt that the HCFA review made a difference in issues related to Indian health (Dixon 1998b). The study also found that there was a great deal of variation between the regional offices of the HCFA in their handling of state/tribal issues.

IHS/HCFA MEMORANDUM OF AGREEMENT

In addition to the expanded role for HCFA to exercise the federal trust responsibility, federal health care financing policy changed relationships between tribes and states. Prior to 1996, the Medicaid program paid a 100 percent Federal Medical Assistance Percentage (FMAP) for American Indians and Alaska Natives who were served in facilities owned by the IHS. However, when Indians on Medicaid sought care in private facilities or tribally-owned facilities, the federal government would only pay the same matching rate as they paid for other Medicaid recipients in the state. Thus, states were likely to impose the same cost control measures on tribal health programs that they imposed on private providers. While private providers had some latitude to shift costs from Medicaid to private insurers, the Indian health providers had very few non-governmental third party payers to absorb the cost reductions. Congress had recognized this situation and provided for reasonable cost reimbursement to Federally Qualified Health Centers (FQHCs), including both tribal and urban Indian clinics. But, some states sought to phase out FQHC status and reasonable cost reimbursement through their statewide Medicaid managed care waivers.

This was largely resolved for tribes through a Memorandum of Agreement (MOA) between the Indian Health Service and the Health Care Financing

Administration signed December 19, 1996. The MOA stipulated that tribes could be reimbursed for Medicaid services at any one of three rates: at the same rate as IHS facilities; at the FQHC rate; or at the state Medicaid rates. MOA also provided that states would receive the 100 percent FMAP for Medicaid services delivered in tribal facilities. Because the states were not contributing anything to the cost of services to American Indians in tribal clinics, they had no incentive to control costs. In most cases, this resulted in greater flexibility when the states negotiated with tribes in the development of Medicaid managed care programs.

The MOA also resolved a common dispute between tribes and states regarding licensing. Some states had required tribal facilities to be licensed by the state in order to receive Medicaid funding. However, some tribes asserted their sovereignty by refusing to submit to the state for licensing. This often created an impasse in which tribes were unable to collect Medicaid reimbursement for the services they provided to Medicaid recipients. The MOA resolution was to require tribally-owned facilities to meet all state licensing requirements to be eligible for Medicaid funding, but actual licensure was not required for the tribal facilities to receive such funding.

TRIBES AND CULTURAL COMPETENCE

In the rush to convert Medicaid programs from fee-for-service to managed care, the states sought waivers from HCFA that would allow them to deny Medicaid recipients the freedom to choose their own health care providers. These so-called Freedom of Choice Waivers allowed states to enroll Medicaid recipients in managed care plans that restricted their access to providers, limiting them to the panel of providers under contract with the managed care plan. Typically, HCFA requires two consumer protections. First, Medicaid consumers must be able to choose from at least two managed care plans in their area. Second, the states have to assure that "culturally competent care" is provided by the Medicaid managed care plans. However, wording in state Medicaid managed care contracts relating to cultural competence is usually vague, not measurable, and not enforceable.

TRIBAL HEALTH CARE PROVIDES THE GREATEST CULTURAL COMPETENCE

A tribally operated health care delivery system is inherently more culturally competent at providing care to American Indians than a health care delivery system operated by any other organization. A tribe is the political embodiment of a culture. A tribe is the combination of all parts of the culture. Tribal members are the people who live the culture. Elders are responsible for passing their knowledge to younger members of the tribe. Nobody is more knowledgeable about a tribe's culture than its collective membership. Some members of the tribe are acknowledged by others as being the keepers of certain types of specific cultural knowledge. For example, one person may be regarded by tribal members as an authority on healing ceremonies and another may be the keeper of knowledge about the healing properties of plants. In some tribes, there are only a few people left who speak the traditional language— one of the most valuable links to traditional culture.[10]

One might assume that the states and HCFA would develop managed care Medicaid systems that would enhance and preserve the Indian health care delivery system as the best way to deliver culturally competent care. In fact, some states have done this by exempting the American Indian population from being required to use Medicaid managed care plans or by paying Indian health providers for off-plan services delivered to Medicaid beneficiaries.[11]

However, some states have structured Medicaid managed care in such a way that Indian health providers are expected to become providers within the existing networks of managed care plans that receive Medicaid reimbursements.[12] For a variety of reasons, this approach has not been successful and many American Indians are enrolled in Medicaid plans in which there are no Indian health care providers.

Certainly, the managed care plans that do not have Indian health care providers in their networks would be less culturally competent than Medicaid services provided through the Indian health system. The very term "cultural competence" assumes that a person who is not a member of the culture can learn to understand it. The only way they can learn about a different culture is if someone who is a member of that culture shares their knowledge. Even when people are willing to share information about their culture, the outsider will never be fully informed. Some things about the culture can only be understood if one can speak the language and are known only by members of secret societies. Some kinds of knowledge can only be derived from experience.

INCENTIVES FOR STATES TO MINIMIZE CULTURAL COMPETENCE REQUIREMENTS

States that are developing Medicaid managed care contracts generally include some requirement that contractors provide services that are culturally competent. The contractual definition of cultural competence becomes a contractual obligation on the part of the managed care plan that, in turn, results in an expense to the state. Thus, states have a financial incentive to minimize performance standards for cultural competence. Reviews of state contracts with managed care plans indicate that the most common provision relating to cultural competence was to require managed care plans to have interpreter serv-

---

[10] It should be noted that there are some deficiencies in cultural competence within the Indian health care systems. There are not enough tribal members with training as health care professionals, so Indian health systems must employ some people who are not tribal members and try to help them understand the culture of the tribe. Also, the IHS, tribally operated health care delivery systems, and urban Indian programs cannot provide the full range of health services, so individuals may be referred to other provider organizations.

[11] Washington and Oregon are examples of exempting American Indians unless they choose to opt in to managed care plans. Arizona created a special plan for American Indians, which essentially creates a "carve out." Oklahoma pays for off-plan services.

[12] States that have attempted to force Indian health providers into Medicaid managed care networks with limited success are New Mexico, Minnesota, Michigan and California.

ices available (Dixon 1998b, Office of Minority Health 2000); however, this provision rarely applies to American Indians since there is usually a exemption for the managed care plans if a linguistically-distinct population served is less than a specified percentage of the total enrollees in the plan.

States that design programs to enroll American Indian Medicaid beneficiaries in managed care are trying to increase the number of managed care enrollees to the level where it is more attractive and feasible for managed care organizations to bid on Medicaid contracts. States that do this generally have Medicaid administrators who have a very high level of confidence in the ability of managed care to control costs within state government. Furthermore, they believe that managed care is the way of the future and that the Indian health system must adapt to the forces of change. The administrations in these states often take an inflexible position, fearing that there will be no end to special interests and that the entire system will collapse if any group is granted special treatment. However, when states try to force Indian health programs to work through managed care plans to secure Medicaid payments, tribes perceive that the state government does not value them, their sovereignty, or the Indian health care system.

LACK OF STANDARDS RELATING TO CULTURAL COMPETENCE

The reason states are able to skirt the HCFA requirements for cultural competence is related to the huge variety of definitions of cultural competence that have been used. Definitions are developed for cultural groups that do not have their own health care delivery systems and the definitions are intended to improve the existing systems of care that are insensitive to cultural issues.

The most limiting type of definition focuses on the relationship between health care professionals and individual patients. For example, the following definition has been offered by the National Latino Behavioral Health Workgroup (1996, p. 3):

> Cultural competence includes the attainment of knowledge, skills, and attitudes to enable administrators and practitioners within systems of care to provide effective care for diverse populations, i.e., to work within the person's values and reality conditions. Cultural competence acknowledges and incorporates variance in normative acceptable behaviors, beliefs, and values in:
> - determining an individual's mental wellness/illness, and
> - incorporating those variables into assessment and treatment.

The New York State Office of Mental Health convened a Cultural Competence Workgroup that expanded the definition of cultural competence to encompass organizations and systems:

Cultural and Linguistic Competence is a set of con-
gruent behaviors, attitudes, policies and procedures that come
together in a system, agency, or among professionals which
enable that system, agency of those professionals to work
effectively and efficiently in cross-cultural and diverse linguis-
tical situations on a continuous basis. . . .

A culturally and linguistically competent system of
care acknowledges and incorporates, at all levels, the importance of culture and language, the cultural strengths associated with people and communities, the assessment of cross-cultural relations, vigilance towards the dynamics inherent in cultural and linguistic differences; the expansion of cultural and
linguistic knowledge, and the adaptation of services to meet
culturally and linguistically unique needs. (New York State
Office of Mental Health 1996)

The Office of Women and Minority Health at the Bureau of Primary Health
Care in the Health Resources and Services Administration (HRSA) provides an
even broader definition that has also been used by other federal agencies:

'Culture' refers to integrated patterns of human behavior that
include the language, thoughts, communications, actions, customs, beliefs, values and institutions of racial, ethnic, religious
or social groups. 'Competence' implies having the capacity to
function effectively as an individual and an organization within the context of the cultural beliefs, behaviors and needs presented by consumers and their communities. (Office of
Minority Health 1999)

As these definitions indicate, cultural competence is only relevant in cross-cultural situations. None of the definitions considers the possibility that self-governance by a culturally distinct group will maximize cultural competence.

Tribal leaders in Washington State developed a position paper in which
they took a systems approach to dealing with culturally sensitive care. It says
in part:

Lack of understanding by non-Indian providers has resulted
over the years in innumerable instances of inadequate, incomplete, untimely and substandard treatment that has produced
unnecessary pain, suffering, debility and human dignity viola-
tions. . .

To avoid these sorts of situations, many Tribes have instituted
their own clinics where they have direct control over person-

nel and policies. This has worked exceptionally well and many patients who formerly have received less than adequate treatment now have access to culturally sensitive health care services. Most clinics are closely connected to other Tribal health and social services programs. As such, cultural values and intertribal social structure are understood and care plans can be formed to incorporate and maximize all of the support mechanisms that exist. This understanding of American Indian Culture does not exist in the mainstream medical world. (Tribal Leader's Summit on Health Care Reform in Washington State 1994)

The consensus position of tribal leaders and urban Indian clinic administrators is that, if the state wants to assure that Native Americans get culturally competent care, then they should design models that assure access to Indian health facilities (Dixon 1998b).

It was not until 1999 that DHHS first drafted national standards for culturally and linguistically appropriate services (CLAS) in health. The advisory committee to oversee the process of developing draft standards did not include any representatives of tribes or the Indian health system. Furthermore, their review of the literature did not include any documents specific to American Indians, Alaska Natives or the Indian health system. The standards, developed by the DHHS Office of Minority Health, were intended primarily to address the needs of immigrants who did not speak English and who did not have their own health care delivery systems. Nevertheless, this effort would create more specific, measurable, and enforceable approaches to cultural competence. These proposed standards, intended to ensure equal access to quality health care by diverse populations, state that health care organizations and providers should:

1. Promote and support the attitudes, behaviors, knowledge, and skills necessary for staff to work respectfully and effectively with patients and each other in a culturally diverse work environment.

2. Have a comprehensive management strategy to address culturally and linguistically appropriate services, including strategic goals, plans, policies, procedures, and designated staff responsible for implementation.

3. Utilize formal mechanisms for community and consumer involvement in the design and execution of service delivery, including planning, policymaking, operations, evaluation, training and, as appropriate, treatment planning.

4. Develop and implement a strategy to recruit, retain and promote qualified, diverse and culturally compe-

tent administrative, clinical, and support staff that is trained and qualified to address the needs of the racial and ethnic communities being served.

5. Require and arrange for ongoing education and training for administrative, clinical and support staff in culturally and linguistically competent service delivery.

6. Provide all clients with limited English proficiency (LEP) access to bilingual staff or interpretation services.

7. Provide oral and written notices, including translated signage at key points of contact, to clients in their primary language informing them of their right to receive interpreter services free of charge.

8. Translate and make available signage and commonly used written patient educational material and other materials for members of the predominant language groups in service areas.

9. Ensure that interpreters and bilingual staff can demonstrate bilingual proficiency and receive training that includes the skills and ethics of interpreting and knowledge in both languages of the terms and concepts relevant to clinical and non-clinical encounters. Family or friends are not considered adequate substitutes because they usually lack these abilities.

10. Ensure that the clients' primary spoken language and self-identified race/ethnicity are included in the health care organization's management information system as well as any patient records used by provider staff.

11. Use a variety of methods to collect and utilize accurate demographic, cultural, epidemiological and clinical outcome data for racial and ethnic groups in the service area, and become informed about the ethnic/cultural needs, resources, and assets of the surrounding community.

12. Undertake ongoing organizational self-assessment of cultural and linguistic competence and integrate measures of access, satisfaction, quality, and outcomes for CLAS into other organizational internal audits and performance improvement programs.

13. Develop structures and procedures to address cross-cultural ethical and legal conflicts in health care delivery

and complaints or grievances by patients and staff about unfair, culturally insensitive or discriminatory treatment, or difficulty in accessing services, or denial of services.

14. Prepare an annual progress report documenting the organizations' progress with implementing CLAS standards, including information on programs, staffing and resources. (Department of Health and Human Services 1999)

If these standards are actually implemented and incorporated into state Medicaid managed care contracts, they will change the political landscape of managed care. Both state Medicaid agencies and managed care plans will realize that it is most cost effective to meet these standards by serving AI/AN Medicaid consumers in Indian health facilities.

SUMMARY

Tribes have a unique role in the delivery of health services to American Indians and Alaska Natives. Tribes advocate for their tribal members as consumers of health care, while at the same time the tribes also may be providers and purchasers of health care. Unlike other ethnic groups in the United States, American Indians are enrolled in tribes that have political jurisdiction and sovereignty similar to state governments.

When a tribal council makes decisions about the organization of their health care services, those decisions affect the choices of tribal members. There is no minimum benefit package, and the level of funding and types of services provided differ from tribe to tribe. Each tribe has different types and amounts of resources from both the IHS and from their own tribal economic development. The processes and outcomes of tribal decisions are influenced by cultural values.

Federally recognized tribes enjoy a government-to-government relationship with the federal government. Recently, however, federal policies have moved more programs to state control, forcing tribes to negotiate with the states in which they are located. Tribes are asking the federal government to exercise its trust responsibility by providing oversight in tribal/state relationships regarding federally funding programs, such as Medicaid. As Medicaid changes from fee-for-service to managed care, in some states tribes are subject to contractual relationships with managed care organizations that are far removed from the federal trust responsibility. Tribes are not just another provider in Medicaid managed care networks; they have a role that cannot be subsumed by other providers regardless of any standards related to cultural competency.

By understanding the unique role of tribes, federal and state agencies can develop policies to promote and enhance the Indian health system. These policies need to recognize tribal sovereignty, involve tribes in meaningful consultation, empower tribes to design health care systems that best meet the needs of tribal members, and fund those health care systems at a level that assures access to care that meets national standards of quality.

ACKNOWLEDGEMENTS:

I am especially indebted to Judith K. Bush for helping to shape my thoughts on this subject and to Yvette Roubideaux, MD, MPH, for helping me to express those thoughts more clearly.

REFERENCES

American Anthropological Association. Position Paper on "Race." Adopted May 17, 1998, and published on the AAA website http://www.aaanet.org. 1998.

Bazron B, Cross T, Dennis K, Isaacs M. *Towards a Culturally Competent System of Care, Volume I: A Monograph on Effective Services for Minority Children Who Are Severely Emotionally Disturbed*, CASSP Technical Assistance Center, as cited in New York State Office of Mental Health, *New York State Cultural Competence Standards*; 1996.

Bush JK. *Legal, Historical and Political Context in which Tribes Make Health Care Decisions.* Denver, CO: National Indian Health Board; 1996.

Clinton WJ. Executive Memorandum on Government-to-Government Relations with Native American Tribal Governments. April 29, 1994.

Cornell S, Kalt JP. Reloading the Dice: Improving the Chances for Economic Development on American Indian Reservation. In: Cornell S, Kalt JP, eds. *What Can Tribes Do? Strategies and Institutions in American Indian Economic Development.* Los Angeles: American Indian Studies Center, University of California; 1992.

Department of Health and Human Services. Call for Comments on Draft Standards on Culturally and Linguistically Appropriate Health Care and Announcement of Regional Informational Meetings on Draft Standards. *Federal Register* 64: no. 240: (December 15, 1999) p. 70042—70044.

Dixon M. *Managed Care in American Indian and Alaska Native Communities.* Washington, DC: American Public Health Association; 1998a.

Dixon M. *Indian Health in Nine State Medicaid Managed Care Programs.* Denver, CO: National Indian Health Board; 1998b.

Dixon M, Bush JK, Iron PE. Factors Affecting Tribal Choice of Health Care Organizations. In: *A Forum on the Implications of Changes in the Health Care Environment for Native American Health Care*. Washington, D.C.: The Henry J. Kaiser Family Foundation; 1997.

Dixon M, Shelton BL, Roubideaux Y, Mather D, Smith CM. *Tribal Perspectives on Indian Self-Determination and Self-Governance in Health Care Management*. Vol. 2. Denver, CO: National Indian Health Board; 1998.

Harris L, Wasilewski J. *This is What We Want to Share: CORE CULTURAL VALUES*. Bernalillo, NM: Americans for Indian Opportunity; 1992.

Health Care Financing Administration. Department Policy on Consultation with American Indian/Alaska Native Tribes and Indian Organizations. August 7, 1997.

HeavyRunner I, Morris JS. *Traditional Native Culture and Resilience. Research/Practice*. Minneapolis, MN: The College of Education & Human Development, University of Minnesota. Spring 1997.

Indian Health Service, U.S. Department of Health and Human Services. *Regional Differences in Indian Health 1997*. Rockville, MD: Indian Health Service; 1997.

Indian Health Service and the Health Care Financing Administration. Memorandum of Agreement (MOA) signed December 19, 1996.

National Latino Behavioral Health Workgroup. *Cultural Competence Guidelines in Managed Care Mental Health Services for Latino Populations*. Publication 3B85. Boulder, CO: Western Interstate Commission for High Education; 1996

National Indian Health Board. *Regional Forum on Indian Health Care: Alaska, California and Portland Areas*, Clackamas, Oregon, March 22-24, 1995. National Indian Health Board; 1995.

National Indian Health Board. *Regional Forum on Indian Health Care: Aberdeen Area*, Bismarck, North Dakota, July 19-21, 1995. National Indian Health Board; 1996a.

National Indian Health Board. *Regional Forum on Health Care: Bemidji/Billings Areas*, Bloomington, Minnesota, May 31-June 2, 1995, National Indian Health

Board; 1996b.

National Indian Health Board. *Southwest Regional Forum on Indian Health Care: Albuquerque, Navajo, Phoenix, and Tucson Areas*, Scottsdale, Arizona. June 14-16, 1995, National Indian Health Board. 1996c.

Office of Minority Health, Department of Health and Human Services. *Assuring Cultural Competence in Health Care: Recommendations for National Standards and an Outcomes-Focused Research Agenda.* Available at http://www.omhrc.gov. accessed March 16, 2000.

Tribal Leader's Summit on Health Care Reform in Washington State. Position Paper No. 3, Tribal Health Service Delivery Systems. Adopted August 2-4, 1994, and appended to Letter to Governor Mike Lowry from Henry Cagey, Chairman, Lummi Nation, regarding implementation of the Health Services Act of 1993, dated August 29, 1994.

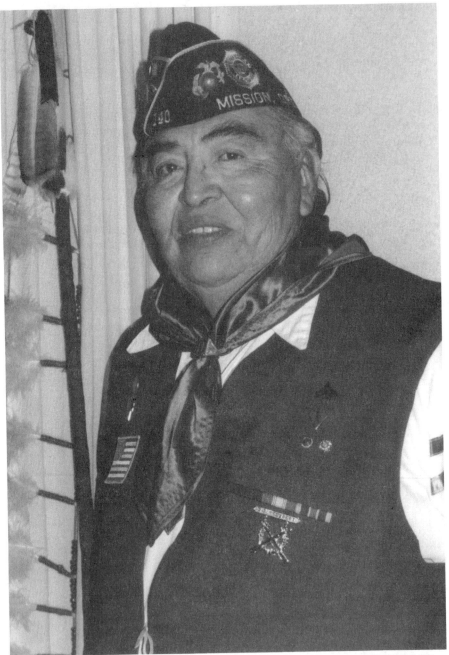

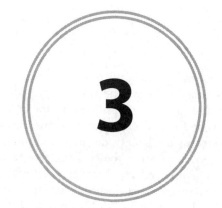

ACCESS TO CARE FOR AMERICAN INDIANS AND ALASKA NATIVES

Mim Dixon

Issues related to access to care for American Indians and Alaska Natives (AI/AN) are often thought to be different than those for many other Americans, however there are some similarities. AI/AN communities have many of the same factors that affect access to care as other rural communities that are characterized by poverty and low employment. While the Indian Health Service (IHS) was designed to make health care more accessible for AI/AN, the IHS is significantly under-funded and does not provide access to all types of health care. AI/AN have greater access to care and greater choices when they have alternate resources, such as Medicaid, Medicare, and private insurance. However, the growing trend toward managed care is limiting access for both those with and without alternate resources.

GEOGRAPHY, POVERTY, AND EDUCATION

American Indians and Alaska Natives live in some of the most remote geographic areas and these circumstances result in some of the same access problems that affect other Americans who live in rural areas. In their review of contemporary American health care systems, Scutchfield and Williams (1998) state:

> Rural health care has required unique and innovative solutions in many communities, especially in the absence of adequate supplies of physicians and facilities, and remains a challenging test of the ingenuity and resourcefulness of the health services system. (Scutchfield and Williams 1998, p. 1121)

Low population density means that it is not economically feasible for private sector physicians, hospitals, and other health care providers to locate in most rural areas. Private sector health care facilities in rural areas tend to be limited in scope and concentrated in regional centers. Thus, access to private sector medical care is impacted by availability, distance, and transportation.

Cost of services can be a barrier to accessing private medical services for any American who is unemployed, employed in a job without health benefits, or living with an income so low that health insurance is unaffordable. Poverty and unemployment are high in many AI/AN communities, creating even less access to health insurance than for the U.S. population as a whole. The 1990 U.S. Census found that unemployment rates among American Indians were more than double that of the U.S. population as whole and the median household income of AI/AN was one-third less than the rest of the U.S. (Indian Health Service 1997). As a result, 32 percent of AI/AN were living below the poverty level, compared to only 13 percent of the total U.S. population (Indian Health Service 1997).

With more people living below the poverty level, one might assume that AI/AN are more likely to be covered by Medicaid, the federal–state program that provides health care coverage to the poor. However, Rosenbaum (1997) found this to be untrue:

> One of the great paradoxes of Medicaid is that despite its vital role in American health care financing, the program remains elusive to millions of individuals in great need of assistance. Nowhere is the paradoxical nature of Medicaid more in evidence than in the case of the 2.3 million American Indians and Alaska Natives, one of the poorest and most pervasively uninsured groups of individuals. All of the traditional reasons that help explain Medicaid's failure to reach poor Americans generally (e.g., restrictive categorical and financial eligibility standards; locational, procedural and administrative barriers to enrollment) apply to coverage of Indians. In addition, there is reason to believe that Medicaid participation among Indians may be lower than that of other low income populations and that their disproportionately low rate of enrollments arises from certain aspects of the program which fall with greater force on Indians, particularly those who live on reservations. (Rosenbaum 1997, p. 151)

Thus, while the 1990 Census found 32 percent of AI/AN living below the poverty level, a 1987 Survey of American Indians and Alaska Natives (SAIAN) by the Agency for Health Care Policy and Research (AHCPR) found that only 11.4 percent of AI/AN were receiving Medicaid benefits (Kauffman et al 1997).

Furthermore, many AI/AN elders are not eligible for Medicare because they have lived subsistence lifestyles and have not worked the required number of quarters in a job that is covered by Social Security. Many of those who are eligible for Medicare cannot afford the Part B supplemental coverage for outpatient services, or elect not to pay the premiums for Part B because they believe that they are entitled to these services at no charge through the Indian Health Service.

Education can also affect access to care, as people with less education may have a difficult time navigating the health care bureaucracies, reading directions, and filling out necessary paperwork. These problems are further compounded by the fact that English is a second language for many rural and elderly AI/AN. People with less education also may be less likely to understand the need for prevention and early treatment. According to the 1990 Census, only 65 percent of AI/AN over 25 years old had graduated from high school (IHS 1997), and only 9 percent of AI/AN were college graduates, compared to 20 percent of the U.S. population as a whole (IHS 1997).

Geographic location, unemployment, poverty and education are interrelated. Remote locations with low population density have a more difficult time attracting employers. Low education levels also affect employment opportunities, and subsequently, high unemployment leads to high rates of poverty. Poverty can mean substandard housing conditions, no telephones, and lack of transportation. All of these factors work together to create barriers to accessing the private health care delivery system in our country.

Low socioeconomic status is more prevalent among ethnic minorities in the United States. However, when researchers adjust for income and parental education, ethnic minorities still have lower utilization of health services than the majority population (Flores et al 1999). Non-financial factors that have been related to ethnic disparities in health and use of services include cultural differences, language problems, folk illness belief, parental beliefs, and provider practices (Flores et al 1999). While the health status of ethnic minorities is generally worse than that of the White population in the United States, research has also shown that rural minorities experience disproportionately high rates of certain kinds of illnesses and experience substantially greater barriers to accessing health care (Mueller et al 1999).

It is not clear whether socioeconomic status affects health directly or indirectly through discrimination and racial segregation, environmental factors such as nutrition and exposure to carcinogens, or barriers in accessing health care. However, research has shown that lower community socioeconomic status is related to higher mortality from all causes, cardiovascular mortality, infant mortality, suicide, birth weight, neural tube defects, cardiovascular diseases, long-term limiting illness, chronic conditions, disability, depression, child health outcomes, pediatric injury, chronic disease symptoms, smoking and physical activity (Yen and Syme 1999).

INDIAN HEALTH SERVICE

Access to care issues for AI/AN are different from other low income Americans living in rural areas due to the Indian Health Service (IHS), a federal agency in the U.S. Department of Health and Human Services. The IHS was founded on the idea that meeting the federal trust responsibility for the AI/AN people would require a government health program. Because of the geographic problems of access, this government program was conceived as a direct service organization, rather than as a form of health insurance like Medicaid or Medicare.

It was understood from the beginning that AI/AN communities had insufficient numbers of patients with commercial health insurance and that living conditions were so harsh that it would be difficult to attract private health care professionals to locate there. Originally, the IHS was designed as a series of federally constructed and operated hospitals that were staffed by health professionals from the U.S. Commissioned Corps. The Commissioned Corps is a uniformed service, similar to the Navy, that staffs federal health programs, including the IHS, federal prisons, the National Institutes of Health (NIH), and the Centers for Disease Control and Prevention(CDC).

IHS[1] clinics and hospitals provide services free of charge to AI/AN who are members or descendents of federally recognized tribes. Because of the federal trust responsibility, they cannot deny services to eligible people. At the present time, there is no means test for eligibility. By providing free services, the IHS has removed the cost-of-services barrier. However, the scope of services provided by the IHS is defined differently from most forms of health insurance and is generally limited by the level of funding appropriated by Congress.

Since the IHS was first organized under the Transfer Act of 1954, the Indian health system has changed to encompass more tribally operated programs, more health workers who are tribal members, and fewer Commissioned Corps health professionals. Also, government policies and programs, as well as economic conditions, resulted in the relocation of many AI/AN to urban areas (See Chapter 5). Title 5 of the Indian Health Care Improvement Act of 1974 created minimal funding for urban Indian clinics to help provide health care for the growing numbers of AI/AN in urban areas. However, urban Indian clinics

---

[1] To make this chapter more readable, the term "IHS" is used for both IHS programs and programs that are operated by tribes that contract or compact IHS programs under P.L. 93-638, the Indian Self-Determination Act. Because urban Indian programs have different factors relating to access, urban Indian clinics are discussed specifically in this chapter and not included in the term "IHS." The term "Indian health system" is used to encompass IHS, tribally-operated programs and urban Indian clinics, also known as the "I/T/U."

are located in only a few cities and some provide very limited services. Indians who require more extensive services and do not have other resources often return to their tribal reservation or community to obtain health or dental care. Currently, the Indian health system has evolved into a tripartite service called the "I/T/U," representing the IHS, tribally operated programs, and urban Indian clinics.

While the overall organization of the Indian health system has evolved, the basic constraints of geography, low population density, and inadequate funding have remained the same. Although the IHS was intended to solve the problems of access to care for AI/AN people, access to care remains a problem and the health of AI/AN is generally worse than other groups in the United States.

ACCESS TO PRIMARY CARE AND PREVENTION SERVICES

Generally, the IHS has done a very good job of making primary care available to AI/AN communities. To address the problems of economies of scale and the difficulty of recruiting health professionals to rural areas, the IHS has pioneered models of primary care that use mid-level practitioners, paraprofessionals, and local individuals as community health practitioners.

In Alaska, the Community Health Aide Program trains and hires indigenous people to provide primary care and emergency care in the villages with supervision via telephone from physicians and mid-level practitioners in larger communities. There is also a system of sub-regional centers in Alaska with physician assistants and nurse practitioners who provide primary care. These mid-level practitioners are supervised by physicians located in regional centers. Improved digital imagery, combined with new funding for telemedicine, is creating new opportunities to provide medical support for village-based practitioners.

In nearly every primary care discipline, the IHS has developed positions and training programs that extend the reach of the limited number of health care professionals and at the same time create employment opportunities for local tribal members. For example, tribal members are trained to be eye care providers supervised by optometrists, mental health workers supervised by clinical psychologists, and medical social work associates supervised by social workers. Also, the Indian health system delegates a wider range of functions and responsibilities to health workers than is usually found in the job descriptions for these positions. For example, dental assistants in the IHS system have been trained for expanded practice. Another strategy is to create positions that can function with a supervisor who is not a licensed health care professional. An example is Community Health Representatives (CHRs), who have served as outreach workers since the program was established in 1968. CHRs make home visits, take vital signs, teach about health issues, provide transportation to appointments, and often assist in case finding and case management.

In the Indian health system, access to care is addressed by taking services to people in the community, rather than waiting for them to come to a clinic to seek care. Unlike the private sector model of health care, the Indian health system has a Community Health Nursing (CHN) program. CHNs are instrumental in maternal and child health, immunizations, elder care, and patient education. CHNs do home visits, as well as clinic work. Often CHNs are nurse practitioners.

While the CHNs and CHRs often work in the community outside the clinical setting, they still interact with people who are diagnosed with illnesses. Another category of community health workers, the Community Health Educators, provides more broad-spectrum community health education and prevention programs. To reduce the high incidence of death due to injury, unique programs have been developed to get smoke and carbon monoxide detectors in homes, ensure access to life jackets, and provide training in firearm safety.

The emphasis on community approaches to primary care and prevention makes it impossible to compare the costs and benefits of IHS to the medically oriented benefit packages offered by health insurance. For example, the IHS has funded hostels where pregnant women can stay near hospitals as they await delivery, thus reducing the chances of an unattended home birth in a remote Alaska Native village. The IHS also constructs community water and sanitation projects, gives rabies vaccinations to dogs, and provides other broad public health programs.

The primary care and preventive services unique to the IHS have helped close the gap between AI/AN and other Americans in their rates of neonatal mortality and communicable diseases. The infant mortality rate dropped by 61 percent from 1972–1974 to 1992–1994. The neonatal mortality rate for AI/AN in 1992–1994 was lower than the U.S. All Races rate (Indian Health Service 1997).[2] Since 1973, maternal mortality decreased by 50 percent, tuberculosis mortality declined by 74 percent and gastrointestinal mortality dropped by 81 percent (Indian Health Service n.d.).

While access to primary care is generally good, there are some deficiencies. First, there is high turnover among physicians and other health professionals in the Indian health system. This not only creates discontinuity of care, but also there are times when positions are not filled and there are long waiting times to get medical care. One solution is to train more AI/AN people in the health professions. Title 1 of the Indian Health Care Improvement Act (P.L. 93-437) authorizes a scholarship program for AI/AN for pre-professional and professional training for health careers. But, funding for health professional training scholarships is not sufficient and training facilities generally are not accessible. A second problem with accessibility of primary care is that Congress has not provided funding for health care for some recently recognized tribes or increased funding to accommodate population growth among tribes. Thus, pri-

---

[2] According to IHS (1997) *Trends*, the neonatal mortality rate for AI/AN in 1992-1994 (5.2 deaths per 1,000 live births) was one-tenth lower than the U.S. All Races rate of 5.3 and 21 percent higher than the U.S. White rate of 6.3. Postneonatal mortality is much higher for AI/AN (5.8 compared to 3.1 for U.S. All Races and 2.5 for Whites), thereby driving up the infant mortality rate. In 1993, the AI/AN infant mortality rate was 30 percent higher than U.S. All Races.

mary care services are insufficient or nonexistent for some tribes.

Perhaps an even bigger issue is access to primary care services that require expensive technology, such as mammograms. While it is generally accepted that the IHS performs Pap tests on women at rates that are higher that the population as a whole (this cannot be verified, however, as quality assurance data are not aggregated for the Indian health system), this test is relatively inexpensive, portable, and can be administered by a variety of types of health care providers located in or traveling to AI/AN communities. Other types of diagnostic tests that are considered essential to quality primary care, such as mammograms and flexible sigmoidoscopy, require equipment that is not portable, is more expensive to purchase and maintain, and must be used by skilled health professionals. It is not feasible to locate a mammography unit, for example, in every Alaska Native village. The Indian health system does not have sufficient travel funds for Alaska Native people who live in villages not connected to the limited highway system to fly to regional hospitals for primary care screening services.

ACCESS TO SPECIALTY CARE

IHS and tribally operated hospitals have a limited range of medical specialists on staff. The AI/AN population is too small to support large teams of medical specialists and the salaries are too low to recruit physicians in most subspecialties. Recognizing these economic factors, the IHS often contracts with the private sector to provide specialty medical services to AI/AN. This program is called "Contract Health Services" or "CHS." CHS has different rules and procedures for accessing care than the primary care direct service portion of the IHS. These rules often impede access to specialty medical care.

While anybody who is AI/AN can present themselves to an IHS clinic and receive primary care, there are restrictions on who can receive specialty care through the CHS system. Generally, a patient must have a referral from a primary care provider inside the IHS system to access an outside provider through the CHS system. This provision is very similar to the gatekeeping functions of most managed care organizations. However, CHS has additional requirements: Each CHS program has a designated geographic area and only people who live inside that geographic area can access CHS-funded services. Thus, most urban Indians are not eligible for CHS since they live away from their home reservations, which are often designated as the geographic boundaries for contract health service delivery areas. Furthermore, the rules governing CHS exclude certain types of medical care, such as infertility treatment and procedures that are considered experimental.

Each CHS program has a limited annual budget. If the budget is fully expended before the end of the fiscal year, then nobody in the CHS area can access specialty care until the beginning of the next fiscal year. To prevent this from happening, the IHS creates categories of services that are prioritized.

Depending upon the amount of funding in the CHS budget, IHS beneficiaries may be able to access only Priority I services, such as emergency medical services. However, if more funding is available, people may be able to access lower priority services, such as non-emergency orthopedic surgery. Often, AI/AN do not have access to medical treatment under the CHS program that is otherwise commonly covered by private health insurance. For example, women who have mastectomies for breast cancer are not able to have reconstructive surgery in many parts of the IHS. And in times of budget shortfalls, routine screening mammograms may be delayed up to two years. Access to specialty care is highly dependent on Congressional funding for the CHS, which varies annually.[3]

Congress and the courts have stipulated that CHS is a "payer-of-last resort." This means that a person who has an alternate resource, such as private insurance or Medicare, must use these before CHS. Thus, CHS conserves it's funding by paying the deductible or co-payment on insurance rather than the full bill. Another example is that a veteran must go to a Veteran's Administration hospital or clinic, rather than using CHS. Going one step further, the IHS regulations require that a person who may be eligible for Medicaid must apply and be denied before they can use CHS.

To further conserve the CHS budget, many IHS and tribally operated programs have developed rather distinctive referral practices. For example, the IHS clinic may provide most prenatal care, waiting until the third trimester to refer the pregnant woman to a private sector physician who will deliver the baby at a reduced charge. The CHS program may limit the number of visits to a specialist and have the follow-up care provided by practitioners in the IHS or tribal clinic. Working with the private sector in this way requires finding medical specialists who understand the Indian health system, send their clinical summaries in a timely manner, and work cooperatively with Indian health physicians. Often these individuals are physicians who previously left the Commissioned Corps or the IHS for private practice or specialty training and still want to maintain their ties to the AI/AN community. However, this approach often causes fragmented care and situations where there may be inadequate follow-up. Because the CHS budget is so limited, a person with alternate resources usually has much greater access to specialty medical care than a person who is served solely by the Indian health system.

PHARMACY

There has been much discussion in the United States about the high cost of medicine and the lack of coverage for pharmaceuticals by Medicare and some types of private insurance. In fact, one of the greatest attractions of managed care for consumers is the inclusion of pharmacy benefits.

The Indian health system has extraordinary pharmacy services. Most IHS hospitals and clinics have pharmacies and offer medications for free. The cost

---

[3] It should also be noted that some tribes that are small or recently recognized have programs that are almost entirely CHS with no direct services. In these situations, CHS funding levels and rules also impact access to primary care services.

of pharmaceuticals is controlled by using formularies and federal purchasing mechanisms that result in volume discounts. Some Indian health pharmacies offer both over-the-counter medicines and prescription medicines to eligible AI/AN at no charge. In some places, CHS funding is used to assure after-hours access to pharmacy services by contracting with private-sector pharmacies.

IHS pharmacists also take a more active role in health care. They review patient medical records, actively participate in quality assurance, work closely with the medical team, and counsel patients about how to take their medications. Some Indian health pharmacies automatically re-fill prescriptions for medications for chronic conditions and mail them to the patients. The Mashantucket Pequot Tribe of Connecticut has even started a profit-making managed care pharmacy corporation (Dixon 1998b).

Although access to pharmacy services is excellent on most reservations, it is much more limited for urban Indians. Furthermore, because the IHS system uses a formulary, some patients who are under the care of medical specialists outside the IHS may not be able to have their prescriptions filled at IHS or tribally-operated pharmacies because newer or more expensive medications may not be available there. New medications that have proven more effective are now available for some of the illnesses that are commonly treated in IHS outpatient clinics, including depression, diabetes, high cholesterol, and heart disease. However, these prescription drugs are costly and there are often no generic substitutes, and the IHS budget has not kept pace with the demand for these pharmaceuticals. So the operating units with the lowest levels of per capita funding cannot afford to include these modern drugs in their formularies. As a result, patients in these areas have access to free, but substandard care.

LONG-TERM CARE

Accessibility of nursing home care is not only affected by the same factors as other types of health care—geographic location, low population density, and diseconomies of scale—but also by legal, financing, and licensing issues.

The IHS has never taken responsibility for long-term care, so there are no IHS nursing homes and no provisions for tribal contracting of long-term care services in the Indian health system. The IHS was originally built to handle acute illness in a much younger population. With the growing elder population and increasing prevalence of chronic health conditions, the need for long-term care has increased dramatically. However, there are only about a dozen tribally operated nursing homes in the country (See Chapter 6) and they rely predominantly on funding from Medicaid and tribal subsidies. Many tribes would like to have nursing homes, but they are blocked by state certificate-of-need requirements, Medicaid licensing requirements, and lack of commercial financing.

AI/AN who need nursing home care must rely on Medicaid and often they can only be served by facilities that are a significant distance from their families, friends, and communities. At a Regional Forum on Indian Health Care in Bismarck, North Dakota, in 1995, American Indian participants talked about these issues of access to nursing home care:

> Our tribal members do not have the financial resources to drive all the way to Aberdeen, South Dakota, spend a couple of nights in a hotel, and go back. They might be able to do that once a month, if they are lucky. They might be able to do that once every 2 to 3 months. But that is all they can do. If we have a nursing home on the reservation, it is a short trip right up to the nursing home and they can be with their loved ones. (National Indian Health Board 1996, p. 11)

Social isolation is not the only problem. The social environment of non-Indian nursing homes does not accommodate AI/AN cultural needs, as explained by another American Indian at the Bismarck forum:

> When you are 85 years old and you are laying in a nursing home—let's say you have spent your entire life at Cheyenne River. Now, all of a sudden, you are 180 miles away from home in Aberdeen, South Dakota. You are surrounded by people you don't know, non-Indian nurses who don't speak your language, who have no comprehension of your culture. They basically don't care about your culture. (National Indian Health Board 1996, p. 11)

Others talked about the need for their elders to speak their own language, and to eat their traditional foods while in long-term care facilities.

The desire for tribally operated nursing homes is very high. But, the economic realities make home- and community-based care a more feasible approach to long-term care. However, many of the types of services that are typically part of the continuum of long-term care are generally not available in AI/AN communities.

DENTAL CARE

IHS beneficiaries can receive dental care at most Indian health system hospitals and clinics. The IHS dental program evolved from an emergency care program staffed by itinerant dentists to an interdisciplinary community-oriented program that works closely with environmental health programs to assure that water is fluoridated. Nevertheless, dental disease is more prevalent among AI/AN than the U.S. population as a whole (Indian Health Service n.d.)

Limited funding means long waits for dental appointments at most Indian health facilities. Using the American Dental Association coding list, the IHS reports that 2.4 million dental services were provided in fiscal year 1996 (Indian Health Service 1997). While a survey of tribal health directors in 1997 found that nearly a quarter of the tribally-operated programs had expanded their dental programs to include such services as oral surgery, pediatric dentistry, and orthodontics, the results suggest that the majority of tribes do not have access to these dental specialties (Dixon et al 1998).

In places where funding is most limited, IHS dentists are pulling teeth rather than trying to save and restore them. New demands for dental care are resulting from ever increasing levels of diabetes. As the dentist-to-population ratio declines, it is increasingly difficult to recruit dentists to AI/AN communities.

MENTAL HEALTH AND SUBSTANCE ABUSE SERVICES

The need for mental health and substance abuse services is high in AI/AN communities. Compared to the U.S. All Races population, in 1993 the AI/AN age adjusted mortality rate was 579 percent greater for alcoholism, 70 percent greater for suicide, and 41 percent greater for homicide (Indian Health Service 1997). Furthermore, injury and poisoning are among the top five causes of hospitalization for AI/AN. Illegal drug use is a growing problem for AI/AN communities. The age-adjusted drug-related death rate increased from 3.4 deaths per 100,000 in 1979–1981 to 5.3 in 1992–94. When adjusted for miscoding on death certificates, the rate is 6.0, which is 18 percent greater than the U.S. All Races rate (Indian Health Service 1997).

The acute care medical system feels the impact of alcoholism and mental illness—nearly 5 percent of hospital discharges are for mental disorders. When comparing the number of discharges for persons 15 years old and older, the IHS and tribal hospitals have 60 percent more discharges with a first-listed diagnosis of alcoholism than other U.S. general short-stay hospitals (Indian Health Service 1997). The rate of hospital discharges for alcoholic psychosis at Indian health hospitals is more than twice that of other hospitals (Indian Health Service 1997). This probably means that AI/AN, with alcoholic psychosis have greater access to care than non-Indian people with a similar diagnosis who have become the homeless street people in many U.S. cities.

For years, the tribes and IHS have identified alcohol and substance abuse as the most significant health problem affecting AI/AN communities (Indian Health Service n.d.). Nearly all tribes have some alcohol and mental health services, and most are tribally managed. The Indian Alcohol and Substance Abuse Prevention and Treatment Act of 1986 authorized IHS to develop one regional youth treatment center in each IHS Area.

Nevertheless, the accessibility of mental health and substance abuse treatment continues to be a problem. One study found that the greatest unmet behavioral health needs for AI/AN were adult residential alcohol treatment, outpatient substance abuse counseling, inpatient psychiatric care, and outpatient mental health counseling (Provan and Carle 2000).

While people with chronic mental illnesses may qualify for Medicaid, the move to managed care makes it difficult for tribally-operated programs to receive Medicaid reimbursement for services provided. Many of those who qualify for Medicaid have dual diagnoses that include alcoholism. The unique staffing patterns of many tribally operated alcohol treatment programs may not meet the credentialing standards of managed care plans. Furthermore, behavioral managed care organizations frequently do not cover services such as intensive case management, family support and education, culturally sensitive therapies, supported employment, and other rehabilitation services (Provan and Carle 2000). Managed care organizations have reduced their costs by shifting to "brief therapy" and terminating benefits for non-compliant individuals. Overall, these policies have further reduced options for AI/AN Medicaid beneficiaries with behavioral health needs (Provan and Carle 2000).

HIV/AIDS PREVENTION AND TREATMENT

The prevalence of Human Immunodeficiency Virus (HIV) infection and Acquired Immunodeficiency Syndrome (AIDS) is difficult to assess for American Indians and Alaska Natives because people are often misclassified in databases. Many individuals with HIV/AIDS are diagnosed in urban areas and seek treatment outside the Indian health system; the IHS does not have a comprehensive database to track these cases. However, existing figures suggest that the annual AIDS case rate for AI/AN in 1996 was 10.7 per 100,000 and rising, with a 45 percent increase in AIDS-associated opportunistic illnesses from 1990 to 1995 (Rowell and Bouey 1997). A database compiled by the National Native American AIDS Case Management Network suggests that fewer than 15 percent of clients have private medical insurance, while a majority have alcohol abuse problems, 20 percent have mental illnesses, almost half have had drug abuse problems, and over 25 percent have been homeless (Rowell and Bouey 1997). It appears that the disease pattern for HIV/AIDS among AI/AN is different than the rest of the U.S. population with a higher rate of sexual transmission, a lower rate of needle transmission, and a higher rate of infection among women.

Advances in the treatment of HIV/AIDS have been extremely successful, but the cost of drugs is between $10,000 and $16,000 per person per year. A single HIV/AIDS case can have a huge impact on the budget of an Indian health facility. The Ryan White Care Act is designed to provide funding to states for treatment of HIV/AIDS, but few tribes or urban Indian health programs have been able to access this funding. While the needs for alcohol and drug treatment are great among this population, few Indian health treatment programs are prepared to accept people living with HIV/AIDS.

The Phoenix Indian Medical Center has been designated by the IHS as an HIV Center of Excellence and referral center (Wood et al 1997). The Centers for Disease Control and Prevention (CDC) has funded National Regional

Minority Organizations, such as the Intertribal Council of Arizona, to provide HIV/AIDS prevention and community education programs (Wood et al 1997). A culturally sensitive model for case management has been developed by the National Native American AIDS Prevention Center, located in Oakland, California, and replicated in several tribal and urban Indian settings. However, case management services are available for AI/AN who are HIV-infected in only about a third of the states with tribes.[4]

Access to medical care, drug therapy and substance abuse treatment are all problems for AI/AN who are HIV-infected. Case management is essential to help connect AI/AN to the services and funding they need that are outside the Indian health system. However, funding for case management programs is so limited that many AI/AN who are living with AIDS are not able to access the same types of services that are available for those living in cities with high rates of HIV/AIDS.

OTHER SERVICES

IHS and tribal programs have expanded their types of services as they re-prioritize needs depending on the level of funding by Congress and the availability of tribal subsidies. With more funding available for diabetes programs (See Chapter 8), there has been more emphasis on hiring nutritionists, diabetes educators, podiatrists, and ophthalmologists. A 1997 survey of tribal health directors found that Eye, Ear, Nose, and Throat (EENT) services, such as optometry and audiology, were added or expanded most frequently by tribes, with 30 percent of tribes reporting these types of improvements in their programs (Dixon et al 1998). Women's health care, including mammography and colposcopy, was expanded by 28 percent of the tribally operated programs and 19 percent of IHS-direct-service programs in the study (Dixon et al 1998). While these types of specialized services are reaching some tribes, not all tribes have access to these important screening and treatment procedures.

TRANSPORTATION

In most parts of America, transportation is considered an access issue when health care facilities are more than a 30-minute drive from a person's residence. AI/AN who live on reservations, in rural areas and in Alaska Native villages are frequently more than 30 minutes from most types of health care. Public transportation is generally limited or non-existent in these communities. People living in poverty may have an old vehicle that is in disrepair and cannot provide reliable transportation for long distances. Alaska Native people have even greater transportation issues since most Alaska villages are not on a highway system. Accessing all but the most basic health care may require an airplane ticket that costs several hundred dollars. Even when the CHS program decides to pay for specialty medical care, transportation can be a barrier to accessing

---

4 In 1997, HIV/AIDS case management programs were provided by at least one tribe and/or urban Indian clinics in each of the following states: California, Oklahoma, Texas, Alaska, Washington, Arizona, Kansas, Minnesota, Wisconsin, New York and North Carolina (Rowell and Bouey 1997).

care. Often, there are peculiar provisions, such as paying for transportation only one way.

The IHS contracts with national "centers of excellence" to provide some types of medical specialty care, but these are usually located far from the patient's community. Many American Indians and Alaska Natives are reluctant to travel alone to another state where they do not know anybody, yet families can rarely afford the costs of an airline ticket and hotel to send another family member as an escort to provide companionship and emotional support.

TRADITIONAL HEALING

Some I/T/U programs have embraced traditional healing more than others. Official policies of the Indian Health Service endorse the integration of traditional medicine and Western medicine; this is most often seen in alcohol and substance abuse treatment programs. Most Indian hospitals, as well as some private hospitals that contract with the IHS, allow their smoke detectors to be disconnected so that smudging can occur.

Cultural practices relating to traditional medicine vary from tribe to tribe. For some tribes, it would not be appropriate to conduct ceremonies and healing practices in the setting of a clinic or hospital. For other tribes, the legacy of government policies and missionary activity virtually eliminated the knowledge of traditional medical practices and the training of tribal healers. Occasionally, these tribes have adopted the healing traditions of other tribes (Dixon 1998b).

A study among the Navajo found that 62 percent of Navajo patients at an IHS facility had used traditional healers and 39 percent use them on a regular basis (Kim and Kwok 1998). In intensive interviews with AI/AN Medicaid recipients, 75 percent of those interviewed reported that they used traditional medicine, or Indian medicine, such as medicine men, traditional healers, herbs, and other types of healing that Indians used before there was Western medicine (Dixon, Lasky et al 1997). However, only 35 percent of those interviewed thought it was important to have traditional healing available in their health care clinic. Urban Indians were more interested in their clinics offering traditional healing than were AI/AN living in rural areas. This was explained by one rural American Indian who noted that medicine men work separately in his tribe and he would not expect to find them in a Western health care setting (Dixon, Lasky et al 1997). However, urban Indians are separated from their traditional healers and urban Indian clinics can often help to provide access to these types of services.

The study on the use of Navajo healers also found that the cost of ceremonies varied from $1 to $3,000 with an average cost per visit of $388 (Kim and Kwok 1998). In addition to paying for the services of a healer, a Navajo must also pay the costs for food for those involved in the ceremony. In 1998, the Veterans Administration (VA) adopted a policy to pay traditional Navajo medicine men $50 for a diagnosis from a hand trembler, crystal gazer, or stargazer and up to $750 for any of nine ceremonies that aim to restore harmony in a returning warrior. It is estimated that 6,000 to 10,000 Navajo veterans are unwell and in need of traditional medicine services (Donovan 1998).

To embrace traditional healing means that I/T/U clinics need to develop policies and procedures for credentialing traditional healers, granting them privileges, and paying them. They also have to consider issues of liability, charting and third-party billing. Although mainstream American health care plans are increasingly including alternative medicine in their benefit packages, some tribes find it easier to keep their traditional practices separate from their Western health care operations. The major obstacle, however, is that Contract Health Services funding is so limited that it is generally not available to pay for traditional healers.

ALTERNATE RESOURCES AND CONSUMER STRATEGIES TO MAXIMIZE ACCESS TO CARE

AI/AN who have alternate resources have the best access to both primary care and specialty care. Because they are eligible for the IHS at no charge, AI/AN people rarely purchase health insurance. However, they may have access to alternate resources as a result of employer-purchased health care, Medicaid, Medicare or Child Health Insurance Programs (CHIP). AI/AN are less likely to have Medicare Part B or CHIP if they have to pay a premium. If they meet the eligibility requirements for Medicaid, they may be able to obtain Medicare Part B without paying the premium as a Qualified Medicare Beneficiary (QMB) or a Selected Low Income Medicare Beneficiary (SLIMB), although these programs have not been well advertised in Indian country.

PATTERNS OF ACCESSING HEALTH CARE

AI/AN consumers with alternate resources who live in areas where both IHS-funded and private sector facilities are available have established patterns of accessing care that usually include both systems. These patterns were identified in a survey of 409 tribal employees in two different tribes that had both private health care benefits and access to the Indian health system (Dixon, Lasky et al 1997). Over 80 percent of the tribal employees went to the Indian health facilities for minor illnesses. Nearly 60 percent used private sector health care for surgery or treatment of a serious problem. And nearly 50 percent used the private sector for problems that could be considering embarrassing and for which they wanted greater confidentiality.

These patterns have been shaped by the CHS rules, co-payments on alternate resources, and consumer perceptions of the Indian health system. Because CHS rules force IHS recipients to use their alternate resources prior to CHS payment for private sector care, alternate resources are most often used to pay for medical specialty care. If the CHS program authorizes the care, then the AI/AN consumer will not incur any co-pays or deductibles. However, if the

CHS does not authorize the care, then the consumer must pay the deductible or co-pay and this often serves as a deterrent to using private sector medical care. Consumers are more willing to incur the expenses of co-pays and deductibles when they perceive a problem with the Indian health system, such as wanting a second opinion, not wanting to wait to see a doctor, or worrying about confidentiality for an embarrassing problem. For example, about 47 percent of the sample of tribal employees said they would go to the private sector for mental health or substance abuse treatment, and HIV or STD testing.

Another group of AI/AN patients with alternate resources that have no co-pays or deductibles to influence their decision-making are Medicaid recipients. Intensive interviews with 20 AI/AN Medicaid recipients showed a similar pattern of accessing care (Dixon, Lasky et al 1997). About 20 percent said that they always use the Indian health system and 15 percent said that they always use the private sector or county facilities and services. The other 65 percent used a mix of both types of services. For 60 percent in this sample, this mix consisted of using IHS for minor problems and using the private sector or county system for major problems, usually along the referral patterns established by the IHS. Another 10 percent said that they used the private sector to get a second opinion when they were not happy with IHS services. About 5 percent said that they use a private sector doctor, but go to the Indian health system for other services, presumably pharmacy, dental, and optical.

This mixing of Indian health and private services not only reflects the patterns established by the IHS, but it also indicates pragmatic consumer behavior. AI/AN consumers with alternate resources seek to maximize their choices and minimize their costs. Furthermore, for the majority of AI/AN in both samples with alternate resources that give them more choices, the Indian health system remains their primary care provider.

FACTORS AFFECTING AI/AN CONSUMER CHOICE OF HEALTH CARE PROVIDERS

The loyalty to the IHS as a primary care provider is somewhat difficult to explain. In a survey of tribal employees (Dixon, Lasky et al 1997), only 18 percent of the respondents ranked the IHS-funded health care services as excellent, while 49 percent ranked private sector health services as excellent. Those who prefer private sector health care were more likely to have had a bad experience with IHS (24 percent as compared to 5 percent among those who prefer IHS services). The primary attraction to IHS is that it is affordable (47 percent of sample), and accessible and convenient (20 percent of sample). Depending upon local circumstances, what attracted AI/AN consumers to private sector health care was less waiting time, quality of care, availability of medical specialists, and confidentiality.

CULTURAL VALUES THAT INFLUENCE CONSUMER BEHAVIOR

The items typically identified as evidence of culturally competent care were not a factor in selection of health care providers among the tribal employees who were surveyed (Dixon, Lasky et al 1997). That tribal language was spoken and the availability of traditional Indian healers were minor considerations, only somewhat important to most of the survey respondents. For the tribal employees, these ranked last in a list of 19 factors in selecting a health care provider.[5] While the respondents do not generally choose a health care provider on the basis of the availability of traditional healers or tribal language, they do want to be treated by providers who understand and accept their culture. A doctor's experience with Indians was considered somewhat important or very important among 52 percent of the tribal employees surveyed and 85 percent of the Medicaid consumers interviewed.

The survey of tribal employees (Dixon, Lasky, et al 1997) included an open-ended question: "What makes you want to use IHS-funded facilities?" A small, but significant, portion of the sample (16 percent) cited government commitment and trust responsibility, family history of use, habit, and familiarity. In the interviews with Medicaid consumers, most people talked about wanting to use IHS-funded facilities for social and cultural reasons. These included knowing the staff, seeing friends and socializing, feeling more comfortable, and liking the more relaxed atmosphere. Some said that they went to the IHS-funded facilities because their family did and it was a "habit." About 25 percent of the Medicaid recipients interviewed spoke about prejudice against Indians being a factor in their desire to find health care providers and organizations that would treat them with respect.

Some important cultural factors relating to choice of health care providers deserve further exploration. While the study, *Factors Affecting Consumer Choice of Health Care Providers* (Dixon, Lasky et al 1997), looked at consumer behavior from an individual perspective, further research is needed on cultural factors that are related to tribal membership and the sense of responsibility for others in the family, clan, and tribe. Interviews with tribal leaders (Dixon, Bush, Iron 1997) indicate a widespread belief among American Indians that it is important for Indian people to have a separate health care delivery system from other people for reasons that include tribal responsibility for its members, tribal sovereignty, preserving and maintaining the federal trust responsibility, employment opportunities, community development, empowerment, and tribal identity. These cultural values may influence consumer behavior.

ECONOMIC CONSEQUENCES OF CONSUMER CHOICES

Consumer choices of health care providers can help perpetuate the Indian health system for others in the community who do not have alternate resources. When AI/AN consumers with alternate resources choose to use IHS

---

[5] This is not to say that traditional healing is not important. In the interviews with AI/AN Medicaid recipients, 75 percent of the people reported that they used traditional medicine.

or tribally operated clinics and hospitals, this increases third-party income and therefore helps generate resources to meet the needs of all tribal members.

However, interviews with American Indian Medicaid recipients indicated that they did not understand the economics of this situation. Most thought that the Indian health care system was fully funded by the federal government. Among AI/AN Medicaid recipients in rural areas interviewed, only half thought that Medicaid would pay for services provided in IHS-funded facilities and 70 percent thought it was wrong for IHS-funded programs to bill Medicaid (Dixon, Lasky, et al 1997). They perceived this as IHS being paid double:

> Typically, rural people said, "I don't think it is right, because Indians deserve to be treated for free," and "we shouldn't have to show our [Medicaid] card— the Indian card should be enough," and "they are getting paid double." (Dixon, Lasky, et al 1997, p. 112)

Thus, people with alternate resources who choose to use IHS-funded facilities often do not provide the clinic with information that would enable the clinic to bill the third party. This is less of a problem for urban Indian clinics because they have sliding-scale fee structures that motivate people to report their alternate resources.

Despite Congressional intent to enhance the IHS budget through Medicaid and Medicare collections, there is still a large amount of lost revenue. Some Indian health clinics have worked with their states to obtain lists that would enable them to check for Medicaid status regardless of the patient's reporting. However, IHS-funded clinics are generally unable to compel their patients to reveal their Medicare and private insurance status.[6]

Because the CHS rules require the use of alternate resources, there is a greater success rate in identifying those resources for people who are referred outside the IHS system to receive services from the private sector. This helps to preserve the CHS funding for those who do not have alternate resources, thus increasing access to specialty care for the community as a whole.

THE IMPACT OF MANAGED CARE ON ACCESS TO CARE

Managed care has affected tribes in a variety of ways (Dixon 1998b): Tribes can be the purchasers of managed care plans for their tribal members or tribal employees; tribes can own managed care plans (although the only evidence of this to date is the Pequot Pharmaceutical Network (PRxN) owned by the Mashantucket Pequot Nation of Connecticut.); tribes, as well as urban Indian clinics and IHS facilities, can become providers under managed care plans. Tribes also serve in an advocacy role for their tribal members who are enrolled

---

[6] Even when patients report their alternate resources, the IHS cannot always bill private insurance. While an AI/AN may have employer-purchased health insurance, if their employer is a tribe that is self-insured, the IHS is prohibited from billing the tribe.

in managed care plans.

Federal anti-deficiency laws generally prohibit the IHS from entering managed care contracts in which the federal government assumes a risk that the cost of providing care will exceed the Congressional appropriations. So, for the most part, the IHS is unable to become a provider in a managed care organization with capitated payment systems that involve risk. While tribes and urban Indian clinics could accept capitated payment, few managed care organizations expect these types of providers to assume risk because their patient numbers are simply too small. So, most Indian health providers that are receiving any compensation from managed care organizations are being paid on a fee-for-service basis. Some may also be receiving non-risk capitated payments for primary care case management.

Private sector managed care organizations generally have not penetrated the remote rural areas where most tribes are located for the same economic reasons that private sector medical care is generally not available. Thus, the greatest impact of managed care on Indian health consumers and providers may be expected to come from government sources, such as Medicaid and Medicare, but Medicare managed care options are generally not available in rural areas. Furthermore, the main impetus for Medicare recipients to join managed care plans is the addition of pharmacy benefits. Since American Indians can receive their medicines free from the IHS, there is little incentive for them to enroll in Medicare managed care plans that would limit their choice of providers, unless they are living in urban areas where access to IHS-funded pharmacies is limited.

The major impact of managed care on Indian health consumers and providers is from Medicaid programs. The discussion that follows explains some of the dynamics of Medicaid managed care that ultimately affect access to care for American Indians and Alaska Natives.

MEDICAID MANAGED CARE MODELS

Medicaid is a federal-state program intended to serve the poor. Each state decides the types of services that will be covered and sets eligibility requirements for programs within federal guidelines. Thus, each state has a different Medicaid program. Initially, the federal government required that Medicaid recipients be given the freedom to choose their health care providers, and Medicaid functioned like traditional indemnity insurance with states paying private sector providers a fee for service. However, the Social Security Act that authorizes Medicaid has provisions that allow states to apply for waivers.

As private employers found that they could control health care costs through managed care plans, state governments decided that they could control Medicaid costs through managed care as well. Because managed care organizations restrict access to providers, the states that wanted to convert their Medicaid programs to managed care had to apply to the federal Health Care

Financing Administration (HCFA) for waivers. Two types of waivers have been used: the Section 1115 waiver provides for statewide demonstration projects, while the Section 1915(b) waiver removes the "Freedom of Choice" provisions, allowing state Medicaid programs to restrict access to the panel of providers in a given managed care plan and to implement the primary care physician (PCP) and gatekeeping features of managed care.

The study, *Indian Health in Nine State Medicaid Managed Care Programs* (Dixon 1998a), identified three models used by the states as they developed ways for the Indian health care system to interface with Medicaid managed care in the mid 1990s. {States included in the study were Arizona, California, Michigan, Minnesota, New Mexico, New York, Oklahoma, Oregon and Washington.) Model 1 involved keeping a fee-for-service option for American Indians; there were two variations on this model. The first variation made managed care voluntary for American Indians and gave them a choice of a traditional fee-for-service Medicaid programs. Both "opt in" and "opt out" approaches have been used. "Opt in" means that American Indians are put into a fee-for-service category unless they choose to enroll in a Medicaid managed care plan. "Opt out" means that all American Indian Medicaid recipients are enrolled in managed care plans unless they specifically request to be placed in a fee-for-service category. Generally, those states that allow American Indians to choose a fee-for-service option do not pay for off-plan services for those who choose to enroll in managed care plans. The second variation on this model creates a special "plan" for American Indians that is a fee-for-service program in which Indian health providers serve as primary care physicians (PCPs) and gatekeepers to specialty care.

Model 2 required mandatory enrollment in managed care plans. Variations of this model involved methods of paying for off-plan services delivered by Indian health providers. Virtually all off-plan services are paid on a fee-for-service basis using the IHS rates. Some states require the Indian health providers to bill each individual plan, while in other states the Indian health providers bill the state directly.

Model 3 was a combination of Model 1 and Model 2, usually involving mandatory enrollment in managed care plans for American Indian Medicaid recipients residing in the more densely populated geographic areas of the state and a fee-for-service approach for those living in rural areas.

IHS AND TRIBES AS PROVIDERS IN MANAGED CARE PLANS

In any of the above models, the IHS and tribes usually are reimbursed for the services that they provide to AI/AN Medicaid recipients. The IHS and tribes may be paid in three different ways: (1) as a provider in managed care plans; (2) by billing for off-plan services provided to AI/AN who are enrolled in a plan; and/or (3) as providers in a fee-for-service system that has been carved out for AI/AN.

Getting paid as a provider in a managed care plan is the most difficult of the three approaches. While some states have mandated that their Medicaid managed care plans contract with Indian health system facilities, tribal health directors have reported (Dixon 1998a) a number of administrative problems that make it difficult for tribes to become providers under managed care plans:

1. Because the Federal Tort Claims Act (FTCA) is extended to tribal contractors, many tribes do not purchase liability insurance. A managed care plan may not recognize the FTCA as meeting their insurance requirements for providers.

2. Many tribes are able to hire health care professionals who are licensed in another state, particularly Commissioned Corps and federal employees who are on Intergovernmental Personal Act (IPA) agreements. Managed care plans usually require providers to be licensed in the state in which they are practicing.

3. Most tribes only serve IHS beneficiaries. Managed care plans have non-discrimination clauses that would require tribes to serve non-Indians.

4. There has been a long tradition of IHS receiving accreditation through the Joint Commission for Accreditation of Health Care Organizations (JCAHO) and this is how most tribally operated clinics and hospitals are accredited. However, most managed care plans use the National Council on Quality Assurance (NCQA) for accreditation.

5. Some Indian health facilities may not meet codes, such as the standard set by the Americans with Disabilities Act (ADA) with which compliance is required by managed care plans.

6. In smaller Indian health clinics, medical staff do not have hospital privileges and are not on 24-hour call, both of which are usually required by managed care plans.

These obstacles often cause lengthy delays in reaching agreements, during which time the Indian health system may not be compensated for the services they continue to provide to AI/AN managed care Medicaid beneficiaries. Tribes that do manage to overcome these obstacles and become providers in managed care plans find the costs of meeting these and other administrative requirements burdensome. Furthermore, they must interface with plan administrators and clerks who do not understand the unique aspects of the Indian health system and the needs of AI/AN consumers. Also, tribally operated programs that are providers in managed care plans reported that they were not paid in a timely way.

For tribal health programs that will be paid at the IHS rate under the IHS/HCFA Memorandum of Agreement (See chapter 4) regardless of the system in which they are operating, becoming a provider in a managed care plan increases the administrative costs of doing business without increasing income. In the private sector, this is seen as a loss of profits. In the Indian health system, the increased administrative costs mean fewer resources to meet the needs of a growing population. This translates into reduced access to care for the tribe as a whole.

URBAN INDIAN CLINICS AS PROVIDERS IN MANAGED CARE PLANS

Urban Indian clinics face many of the same obstacles in their efforts to become providers in managed care plans. There are 34 urban Indian clinics in the nation and about 20 of them bill Medicaid for the services they provide (Dixon 1998a).

Urban Indian clinics are not covered under the IHS/HCFA MOA. Therefore, they are not entitled to receive the IHS Medicaid reimbursement rates. As with other community health centers, the urban Indian clinics have relied on reimbursement rates that were provided to Federally Qualified Health Centers (FQHCs) using their audited cost reports. FQHC rates tend to be higher than the usual Medicaid rates, because they are based on the premise that FQHCs cannot shift costs to other third-party payers since they have very few patients with private health insurance. However, the Balanced Budget Act of 1997 is phasing out the FQHC rates, resulting in greater costs and less Medicaid income for urban Indian clinics. This threatens the very survival of some urban Indian clinics as medical providers (Dixon 1998b).

Some states do not value the unique cultural role of community health centers and see only the cost savings of rolling all Medicaid recipients into less expensive managed care plans. This often means AI/AN must travel across town to an assigned provider who lacks cultural sensitivity. While the financial barriers to care may be diminished, cultural issues relating to access may become more significant.

CONSUMER CHOICE OF PRIMARY CARE PHYSICIANS

Primary care physicians (PCPs) in a managed care system are designed to increase access to care by creating a "medical home-base" for patients. This cornerstone of managed care is intended to lower costs as the PCP acts as a "gatekeeper" to decrease the inappropriate use of emergency room care and specialty medical care. However, for the AI/AN consumer, the PCP becomes the medical equivalent of the "home away from home."

The savvy AI/AN consumer will maximize his or her options by selecting a PCP who is not part of the IHS or tribal health care delivery system, allowing the AI/AN consumer a choice of seeing either their IHS or tribal provider at no cost, or seeing their private sector primary care provider who is paid by Medicaid. According to established patterns, 60 percent of these consumers will continue to see their IHS or tribal provider for most of their basic health care needs. In fact, a study of AI/AN Medicaid recipients indicated that 40 percent of those who had been assigned a PCP outside the IHS system did not even know the name of their PCP (Dixon, Lasky et al 1997). However, capitation payments continue to go to the private sector PCP. The IHS and tribal providers will not get paid for the services they provide to Medicaid beneficiaries, unless the state pays the Indian health system for off-plan services.

Under the IHS/HCFA MOA, states would get 100 percent federal funding for any services that were delivered off-plan by IHS or tribal providers. Yet, 5 of the 9 states studied did not pay IHS or tribal providers for off-plan services (Dixon 1998a). This is less of a problem for urban Indian clinics because they normally charge patients for their services. So, AI/AN who go to urban Indian clinics have a choice of paying for their service or changing their PCP to the urban Indian clinic. This is a powerful incentive for consumers to select the Indian health provider. However, IHS and tribal clinics do not charge for their services, so there is no incentive to change PCPs.

Even when AI/AN consumers are willing to change their PCP to an I/T/U provider, the I/T/U may be a provider under a different plan from the one in which the consumer is enrolled. State Medicaid programs often have lock-in policies that do not allow the consumer to change plans for 6 or 12 months.

Thus, the combination of lock-in rules and refusal to pay for off-plan services can reduce Medicaid income for Indian health providers. While this is not an access problem for AI/AN consumers who are on Medicaid, it is a problem for the health care delivery system that is already under-funded. Medicaid funding is needed to provide access to care for the tribal members who are not on Medicaid. Many of those who are on Medicaid today may not be on Medicaid tomorrow, so it will be their problem as well.

Furthermore, the assignment of a PCP does not necessarily guarantee access to care in a timely way. Among a sample of AI/AN Medicaid recipients who were enrolled in managed care plans, only 14 percent could get same day appointments with their PCP, nearly a third had to wait 1–2 weeks for an appointment, and over 20 percent said they had to wait at least 3 months to see their PCP (Dixon, Lasky, et al 1997).

REFERRAL PATTERNS

One of the great benefits of Medicaid for AI/AN consumers is increased access to medical specialty care, including physicians, diagnostic tests requiring sophisticated technology, outpatient procedures, hospitalization, surgery, physical therapy, and just about anything else that is not part of a routine visit to a PCP. One of the issues for the U.S. population as a whole is that of managed care plans denying services; ironically, this complaint has not surfaced in regard to Indian health.[7] Rather the problem seems to be the complicated referral patterns.

Most managed care plans create a gatekeeping function for the PCP. This means that the patient must see the PCP first to get a referral to a specialist. Sometimes the PCP has to obtain prior authorization from a utilization review office within the plan. Then the patient is limited to the panel of specialists and hospitals that are providers under the plan.

If the patient is seeking care at an I/T/U facility that is not their PCP, he/she may have to go to their private sector PCP to get a referral to a specialist. When the state Medicaid managed care program rules allow AI/AN to go off-plan to I/T/U providers, they may also give those providers the authority to determine the medical necessity of the referral. However, getting authorization from a utilization review office is rarely quick or easy—it can take up to two weeks to notify the doctor that the referral has been approved. When AI/AN patients are homeless or living without a telephone, it is especially difficult to notify them and arrange the follow-up appointment.

Access to specialty care would be so much easier for AI/AN patients (as well as other people enrolled in managed care plans) if they could have a referral, authorization, and appointment in hand when they leave their physician's office. This is usually done through the CHS program. However, Medicaid managed care often makes it much more bureaucratic and time-consuming.

While the I/T/U would prefer to be in a fee-for-service carve out, some states keep their fees so low that it is difficult to find specialty medical providers who are willing to accept Medicaid patients. Access to specialists is sometimes used as an incentive to get AI/AN to enroll in managed care plans even though they may have a choice to opt-out. The managed care plan is required to provide a network of specialists and those specialists are required to see all referrals through the plan. However, if the payments to the specialists in the network are too low, the specialists may subvert the process by limiting the number of appointments they take each month from Medicaid patients and those patients may have to wait a long time for an appointment.

SUMMARY

American Indians and Alaska Natives have many of the same problems accessing health care as other people living in remote rural areas, including poverty, unemployment, low education, population density too low to support private sector health services, and lack of public transportation. The Indian Health Service was intended to improve access to care for AI/AN by providing services in rural communities at no cost to tribal members. The IHS developed

---

[7] Dixon (1998a) offers the following possible explanations for this difference in perceptions: (1) the Indian health system has always rationed care through CHS and people are used to the idea of services being denied; (2) Indian health providers are less likely to make referrals for sophisticated tests and procedures because they are not offered in most I/T/U facilities; (3) Medicaid covers more services than IHS so it is seen as an expansion of services; (4) if the managed care plan denies a service, then CHS pays for it; (5) there is less denial of services because the costs are reimbursed through the 100 percent FMAP.

creative ways to use mid-level practitioners, paraprofessionals, and local people as health workers to overcome the diseconomies of scale in rural areas and the difficulty in recruiting sufficient numbers of health professionals. Overall, the Indian health system has excelled in primary care, prevention, and community outreach.

Funding deficiencies have resulted in restricted access to medical specialty care. Furthermore, the IHS does not fund long-term care. Access to some types of primary care, such as screening that requires expensive diagnostic equipment and trained technicians, is limited. While Indian health care includes pharmacy, dental care, eye care, mental health, and substance abuses services, the level of these services and waiting times for appointments are dependent on funding from Congress. There is insufficient funding to meet even the most basic primary care needs of a growing AI/AN population.

Patients are more likely to access the full range of health services if they have alternate resources, such as Medicaid, Medicare, or private health insurance. However, AI/AN participation in Medicaid, Medicare, and private health insurance is disproportionately low. Patients with alternate resources provide an opportunity for the Indian health system to bill third parties, increase their resources and improve access to care for all tribal members.

While a majority of tribal members who have alternate resources continue to use IHS-funded facilities for their primary care, managed care has made it more difficult for Indian health facilities to bill Medicaid. Managed care also has reduced access to care for AI/AN Medicaid patients by creating more complicated referral patterns and setting fees for private sector medical specialists too low. The administrative burdens of managed care have consumed a portion of the Medicaid income received by Indian health facilities and thereby reduced the amount available to improve access to care for all tribal members.

More efforts are needed to understand the complicated issues of access to care. Reducing the barriers to care is a prerequisite for improving health services for American Indians and Alaska Natives.

ACKNOWLEDGEMENTS

This chapter draws extensively on my work as a Policy Analyst at the National Indian Health Board and studies conducted with funding from the Henry J. Kaiser Family Foundation, the Indian Health Service, the National Indian Council on Aging, and the National Heart, Lung and Blood Institute.

REFERENCES

Dixon M. *Indian Health in Nine State Medicaid Managed Care Programs.* Denver, CO: National Indian Health Board; 1998a.

Dixon M. *Managed Care in American Indian and Alaska Native Communities.*

Washington, D.C.: American Public Health Association; 1998b.

Dixon M, Bush JK, Iron PE. Factors Affecting Tribal Choice of Health Care Organizations. In: *A Forum on the Implications of Changes in the Health Care Environment for Native American Health Care*. Washington, DC: the Henry J. Kaiser Family Foundation; 1997.

Dixon M, Lasky PS, Iron PE, Marquez C. Factors Affecting Native American Consumer Choice of Health Care Provider Organizations. In: *A Forum on the Implication of Changes in the Health Care Environment for Native American Health*. Washington, DC: The Henry J. Kaiser Family Foundation; 1997.

Dixon M, Shelton BL, Roubideaux Y, Mather DT, Smith C. *Tribal Perspectives on Indian Self-Determination and Self-Governance in Health Care Management*, Vol 4. Denver, CO: National Indian Health Board; 1998.

Donovan B. Traditional Navajo care gets VA nod. *The Arizona Republic*. April 8, 1998.

Flores G, Bauchner H, Feinstein AR, Nguyen UDT. The Impact of Ethnicity, Family Income and Parental Education on Children's Health and Use of Health Services. *American Journal of Public Health*. July 1999, 89:7: 1066-1071.

Fielding J E. Public Health in the Twentieth Century: Advances and Challenges in *Annual Review of Public Health, Volume 20, 1999*, Fielding JE, Lave LB, Starfield B, eds, *Annual Review of Public Health, Volume 20, 1999*. Palo Alto, CA: Annual Reviews; 1999.

Giroux J, Takehara J, Asetoyer C, Welty T. HIV/AIDS Universal Precaution Practices in Sun Dance Ceremonies. *The IHS Primary Care Provider*. 1997, 22:4.

Green LW. Health Education's Contributions to Public Health in the Twentieth Century: A Glimpse Through Health Promotion's Rear-View Mirror in *Annual Review of Public Health, Volume 20, 1999*, Jonathan E. Fielding, Lester B. Lave, and Barbara Starfield (eds). Palo Alto, CA: Annual Reviews; 1999.

Indian Health Service, U.S. Department of Health and Human Services. *Trends in Indian Health*. Rockville, MD: Indian Health Service, DHHS; 1997.

Indian Health Service, U.S. Department of Health and Human Services. *Comprehensive Health Care Program for American Indians & Alaska Natives*. Washington, DC: Indian Health Service, DHHS; no date.

Kauffman JA, Johnson E, Jacobs J. Overview: Current and Evolving Realities of Health Care to Reservation and Urban American Indians. In: *A Forum on the*

Implications of Changes in the Health Care Environment for Native American Health Care. Washington, DC: The Henry J. Kaiser Family Foundation; 1997.

Kim C and Kwok YS. Navajo Use of Native Healers. *Archives of Internal Medicine.* November 9, 1998, 158:2245–2249.

Mueller KJ, Ortega ST, Parker K, Patil K, Askenazi A. Health Status and Access to Care Among Rural Minorities. *Journal of Health Care for the Poor and Underserved.* May 1999,10:2.

National Indian Health Board. *Regional Forum on Indian Health Care: Aberdeen Area,* Bismarck, North Dakota, July 19-21, 1995, Denver, CO: National Indian Health Board. 1996.

Provan KG, Carle N. *A Guide to Behavioral Health Managed Care for Native Americans.* Tucson, AZ: Center for Native American Health, University of Arizona; 2000.

Rosenbaum S. Medicaid and Indian Populations: Issues and Challenges. In: *A Forum on the Implications of Changes in the Health Care Environment for Native American Health Care.* Washington, DC: The Henry J. Kaiser Family Foundation; 1997.

Roubideaux Y. *Native American Health and Welfare Policy in an Age of New Federalism.* Tucson, AZ: Udall Center for Studies in Public Policy, University of Arizona; 1998.

Rowell RM, Bouey PD. Update on HIV/AIDS Among American Indians and Alaska Natives. *The IHS Primary Care Provider.* 1997, 22:4.

Scutchfield FD, Williams SJ. The American Health Care System: Structure and Function. In: Wallace RB, ed, *Public Health and Preventive Medicine.* Stamford, CT: Appleton & Lang. 1998.

Wood G, Albert A, Claus C, Rousey B, James C, Davis D. HIV Center of Excellence. *The IHS Primary Care Provider.* 1997; 22:4. 1997.

Yen IH, Syme SL. The Social Environment and Health: A Discussion of the Epidemiologic Literature. In: Fielding JE, Lave LB, Starfield B, eds, *Annual Review of Public Health, Volume 20, 1999.* Palo Alto, CA: Annual Reviews. 1999.

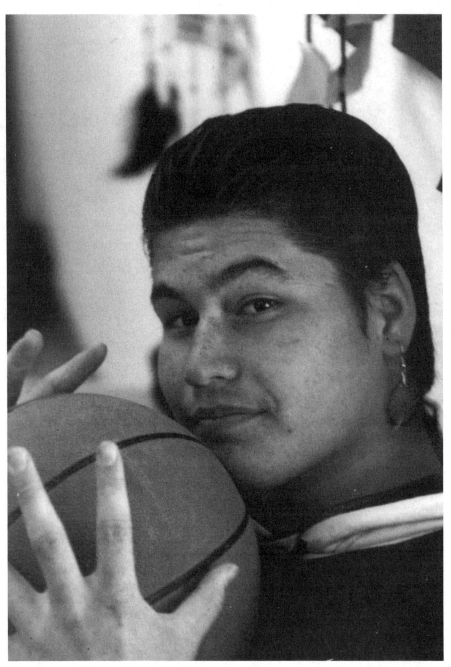

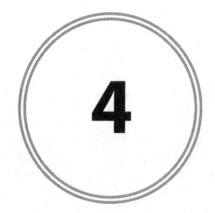

Organizational and Economic Changes In
Indian Health Care Systems

Mim Dixon, David T. Mather, Brett L. Shelton
and Yvette Roubideaux

A s we move into the 21st century, both the Indian health system and the mainstream American health care system are in flux. Indian health care in the United States is evolving into a more complex and sophisticated health care delivery system. After 25 years of steadily increasing numbers of tribes that operate health programs, the federal government has become more of a funding agency and less of a direct provider of health services. Federal funding streams now include not only appropriations to the Indian Health Service (IHS), but also funding through Medicaid, Medicare and block grants from various federal agencies.

Like Indian law, the economic and organizational aspects of Indian health care involve a multitude of special provisions that apply only to American Indians and Alaska Natives (AI/AN). This chapter attempts to explain some of the distinctive characteristics of the Indian health care system that are layered on top of the already complex economic and organizational structures of the mainstream American health care system. The factors that have influenced tribal decisions regarding the management of health care systems include unique historic circumstances in various regions of the country, the development of federal regulations, the provision of technical assistance to tribes, the opportunity to capture administrative costs through tribal shares, and funding for contract support costs.

Tribes that operate their own health care systems generally view contracting and compacting as creating improvements in health care for tribal members. However, this trend has also led to changes in the IHS, including a redesign of the agency and downsizing of administrative functions as a result of the withdrawal of administrative resources from headquarters and Area offices. The evolution of the Indian health care system in the past quarter century must be viewed in the context of the financial constraints imposed by Congress. Because the IHS is not considered an entitlement program and Congress has chosen not to fully fund the health care needs of Indian people, there is a greater reliance on Medicaid, Medicare, and other third-party resources. It is difficult to assess the level of funding needed for Indian health because there is no defined benefit package; the IHS uses a public health model unlike other health care delivery systems in our country, and the method of financing facility construction is different from mainstream health care. The most recent attempt to assess the financial requirements of providing an adequate level of health care to American Indians and Alaska Natives (AI/AN) is the Level of Need Funded (LNF) Study. This could be a useful tool for Congress to exercise its federal trust responsibility and reduce the disparities in health status in the AI/AN population.

CONTRACTING AND COMPACTING

Before the Indian Self-Determination and Education Assistance Act of 1975 (P.L. 93-638) was passed into law, the federal government operated nearly all of the health programs and facilities that served American Indian and Alaska Native people. By 1996, IHS was operating only 37 of the 49 hospitals and 113 of the 492 ambulatory facilities in the Indian health system. At the turn of the century, all tribes were operating at least some of their own health care programs, such as Community Health Representatives (CHR) and Community Health Nursing (CHN) programs, and more than 70 percent were operating outpatient medical clinics (Dixon et al, 1998). A 1997 survey of tribal leaders projected that within 5 years only 6 percent of tribes would have their outpatient medical services provided directly by the federal government (Dixon et al 1998).

P.L. 93-638 provides two mechanisms that enable tribes to operate their own health care systems (See chapter 1). Title I allows tribes to contract with the federal government to manage any part of their health care program that would otherwise be provided by the IHS. Title III allows tribes to develop more comprehensive compacts with annual funding agreements (AFAs); compacts are more flexible than contracts and allow tribes to reallocate funds and redesign programs without federal approval.

GROWTH OF CONTRACTING AND COMPACTING

Initially, the federal government tried to maintain the status quo and subsequently created many obstacles for tribal contracting. Most tribes were reluctant to contract their programs in the 1970s. Factors that influenced the growth of contracting and compacting included historical circumstances, development of regulations, provision of technical assistance, and funding of administrative costs. As these challenges were surmounted, the trend over time was for more and more tribes to operate their own health care programs.

HISTORICAL CIRCUMSTANCES THAT CREATE REGIONAL VARIATIONS

The unique history of tribes has affected the patterns of contracting and compacting in various Areas. In California, the federally recognized tribes did not receive health care funding from the IHS until the California Rural Indian Health Program was started as a demonstration project in 1969. In 1977, two years after passage of the Indian Self-Determination Act, the IHS established the California Area Office. From the very beginning, the California tribes received their health care through tribal contracting. And also from the beginning, the California Indian health system was funded at a lower level than the rest of the nation. While the 100 tribes in California comprise a significant portion of the tribes that contract for their health services in the U.S., the paucity of their funding at least partially explains why they are among the least satisfied with their health services (Dixon et al, 1998).

In places where the IHS did not invest in the bricks and mortar to build hospitals and clinics, tribes were not given the choice to receive IHS direct services. Instead, the IHS managed Contract Health Services (CHS) programs to purchase health care services from private medical care providers for those tribes. Under P.L. 93-638, the tribes then contracted with the IHS to manage the CHS programs. From the beginning of tribal self-determination, there was a disproportionately high percentage of contracting among tribes that were relatively recently recognized by the federal government, including those east of the Mississippi River, in the Great Lakes region, and in the Pacific Northwest.

Alaska also skews the numbers when looking at contracting and compacting. Every village named in the Alaska Native Claims Settlement Act is considered to be a tribe by the IHS. Thus, 237 of the 558 federally recognized tribes are in Alaska, about 40 percent of the total. Most of the tribes in Alaska receive their health care through regional non-profit Native corporations that began contracting with the IHS in 1969, before the Indian Self-Determination Act was passed. When the IHS self-governance demonstration project started, the number of compacts was limited to 17 tribes. Rather than compete for a limited number of slots, the regional Native health corporations and some independent village health providers cooperated in the development of a proposal for a combined compact. With encouragement from the IHS Alaska Area office, the tribal organizations in Alaska have been on the cutting edge of tribally operated health care. Not only are all the nonprofit Native corporations operating their own outpatient medical services and hospitals, but a statewide consortium of tribal organizations manages the Alaska Area Office and the Alaska Native Medical Center, a statewide tertiary care facility in Anchorage.

In other areas of the country, tribes have moved toward contracting and compacting in a more cautious manner. A 1984 assessment of the impact of the Indian Self-Determination Act implementation found:

> Reasons given by tribes for not wanting to contract include the administrative burdens that must be assumed in contracting and the fact that indirect costs are not adequately covered. Tribes who were generally satisfied with the IHS delivery of services also expressed that they are less interested in contracting these services. (National Indian Health Board et al 1984)

Despite these concerns, the number of tribes that consider contracting and compacting is increasing over time. As they weigh their options, tribes consider the regulations allowing programs to be redesigned to better meet local needs and to provide generally higher levels of funding at the local operating level due to the availability of tribal shares and contract support costs.

DEVELOPMENT OF REGULATIONS

The federal government was slow to promulgate regulations to implement the tribal contracting provisions of Title I after the passage of P.L. 93-638 in 1975, and over time tribal leaders became dissatisfied with this burdensome process. In 1988, Congress passed amendments that not only created the Title III Self Governance Demonstration Project (compacting), but also created changes in the contracting process. The 1988 amendments provided that tribes could recover both direct and indirect costs of contracting, so that services would not be diminished as they were transferred from federal to tribal management.

However, it was not until 1994 when Congress passed the Indian Self-Determination Contract Reform Act (P.L. 103-413) that contracting became a more desirable option for many tribes. For the first time, Congress imposed a "negotiated rulemaking" process on the Secretaries of the Department of the Interior (DOI) and the Department of Health and Human Services (DHHS). Representatives of 48 tribes participated in the development of government regulations that were published in the *Federal Register* on June 24, 1996. A number of advantages that had previously been extended to compacting tribes were now also available under contracts, including policies about administrative resources. That same year, technical amendments were added to the Indian

Self-Determination Act through P.L. 104-109, which allowed tribes to incorporate any provision of Title I into Title III. So, by 1996 tribes had a more accommodating legal framework in which to enter into contracts or compacts with the federal government.

TECHNICAL ASSISTANCE FOR TRIBES

When tribal contracting began, the IHS Area Offices provided technical assistance to tribes. It is possible that some of the Area Offices had a conflict of interest in this effort, since increased tribal contracting and compacting was likely to result in a reduction in the number of jobs in the Area Office. However, a survey of tribal leaders and tribal health directors by the National Indian Health Board (NIHB) in 1997 found that tribes in 10 of the 12 IHS Areas believed their Area Office was either encouraging or neutral toward contracting and compacting (Dixon et al, 1998).

The Tribal Self-Governance Demonstration Project Act of 1991 directed the IHS to begin planning activities with the 17 tribes that had compacts with DOI. In 1992, Congress added $2 million to support the administrative costs for self-governance planning, negotiations, implementation, and technical assistance. Technical assistance for compacting took a very different course than the technical assistance provided for contracting. In the spirit of tribal self governance, a tribally-operated technical assistance program was established. The Lummi Nation in Washington has been the location of the Self-Governance Communication and Education initiative. In addition, the Tribal Self-Governance Advisory Committee (TSGAC), which represents all of the compacting tribes, meets quarterly. Their agenda is set by the tribes and usually includes briefings and talks by high-level officials from the IHS and DOI.

ADMINISTRATIVE COSTS

The Indian Health Service budget includes funding for both the direct delivery of health services at the Service Unit level and administrative support for those services at the Area and Headquarters levels. As tribes assumed management for their health care systems via contracting and compacting, some felt that they did not need the oversight and administrative support that was built into the IHS budget at the Area and Headquarters levels, and could incorporate those same functions into their tribal operations. Thus, they believed that they should be able to take a portion of the funding for those Area and headquarters positions and services and add it to their tribal budgets. A tribe's portion of these Area and headquarters administrative costs is commonly called their "tribal share."

Tribes that were receiving services directly from the IHS were concerned that compacting tribes would take more than their fair share of the Service Unit, Area and/or Headquarters budgets, leaving the Agency with inadequate resources to support the directly operated programs. This concern generated the need to determine what proportion (or tribal share) of the Area office's and

Headquarter's resources could be allocated to the individual tribal health program under a compact or contract. The task was more than a financial accounting; it was also a philosophical dilemma. Some activities of the IHS Headquarters and Area offices administrative staff could be apportioned to the tribes, but others were inherent to the federal function (such as submitting a budget for the agency to Congress) and/or could not be undertaken in a piecemeal way (such as compiling statistics on the entire Indian health system).

Initially, the tribes and the federal government had very different ideas about which functions could be eliminated at Headquarters and the Area offices and which must continue to be provided by the IHS directly (referred to as "residual" functions and services). Tribes driven to maximize control and resources at the local level argued for a dramatic reduction in the size and costs of the IHS Headquarters and Area infrastructure. This tribal challenge to the mission of the IHS Area and Headquarters offices stimulated a major reassessment and redesign of these functions within the IHS.

CONTRACT SUPPORT COSTS

As tribes assumed federal contracts, they encountered a number of additional costs that were not part of the federal program budget (Sizemore 1997). For example, the federal government is self-insured for Workers Compensation and does not need to purchase insurance, but contracting tribes are required by law to provide this protection. Also, tribal contractors are required to meet standards from which the federal government exempts itself, such as accessibility of facilities under the Americans with Disabilities Act. These additional costs associated with contracting and compacting are called "contract support costs." If the tribes are not reimbursed by the federal government for these contract support costs, resources must be diverted from health care programs, and services are then diminished.

In 1988, Congress directed the federal government to provide contract support costs and established an Indian Self-Determination (ISD) Fund to help tribes defray the start-up costs of contracting. However, the demand for contract support costs far exceeded the availability of ISD funds, and the IHS chose to distribute the funds on a first-come-first-served basis. As a result, a long waiting list developed with many tribes unable to begin the contracting process unless they used tribal funds to cover these costs. In 1997, the ISD fund had $7.5 million, but an additional $36 million had been requested by tribes (Sizemore 1997). As more tribes wanted to enter into contracts and compacts, the list grew longer.

A survey of tribal health directors in 1997 found that most tribes were not receiving full funding for contract support costs (Dixon et al 1998). One tribal health director from the Aberdeen Area explained his tribe's reluctance to contract their programs this way:

If we were to contract, it would take 3–5 years to get contract support dollars and as previously mentioned the Tribe does not have operating capital to wait that long. (Dixon et al, 1998, p. 136).

Some tribes in the survey estimated that the government owed them over $3 million in unpaid contract support costs. As frustration with the lack of federal funding for contract support costs mounted, some tribes sued the federal government to enforce the provision for contract support costs in self-determination contracts and self-governance compacts.[1]

The real problem was that Congress refused to provide adequate appropriations for the ISD fund. In 1998, Congress actually applied a moratorium on new federal contracts and compacts until a solution could be found to the contract support costs problem. In fiscal years 1998 and 1999, Congress provided a $60 million increase in contract support appropriations in the IHS budget to bring funding for contract support costs to a level that would cover approximately 90 percent of the negotiated requirement. The moratorium on new contracts was lifted in the fiscal year 2000 Appropriation Act.[2] While this additional appropriation for tribal contract support costs enables tribes to continue contracting and compacting for IHS programs, it does not solve the more serious problem of inadequate funding for the direct costs of health care services in the Indian health system.

TRENDS IN COMPACTING AND CONTRACTING

Prior to implementation of the Indian Self-Determination Act in 1976, there was some tribal contracting in California, Alaska and other places. But tribal contracting increased threefold (from $32.6 million to $130.7 million) in the next five years, and there was a 50 percent rate of growth in contracting during the subsequent five years. From 1986 until 1991, the dollar amount of tribal contracting doubled again, from $199 million to $410 million. During that same period, compacting was introduced; by 1996, tribes were managing $371 million in contracts and $345 million in compacts. In the 20 years after passage of P.L. 93-638, tribally operated programs grew to $716 million, nearly one-third of the IHS budget. Figure 4.1 shows this astounding growth in tribal operations in 5-year increments.

---

[1] These cases include: *Ramah Navajo School Board v. Babbitt*, 87F.3d 1338 (D.C. Cir. 1996); *Ramah Navajo Chapter v. Lujan*, 112 F.3d1445 (10th Cir. 1997); *Shoshone-Bannock Tribes v. Shalala*, 988 F. Supp. 1306 (D.Or.1997) (Shoshone-Bannock I) and *Shoshone-Bannock Tribes v. Shalala*, 999 F. Supp.1395 (D.Or.1998) (on reconsideration) (Shoshone-Bannock II); Appeal of Alamo Navajo school Board, Inc. and Miccosukee Corp., IBCA 3463 (Dec. 4, 1997); *Babbitt v. Miccosukee Corp.*, Federal Circuit No. 98-1457; and *California Rural Indian Health Board v. Shalala*, No. C-96-3526 (N.D. Cal.).

[2] Actually two moratoriums were imposed on tribal contracting in the FY 98 and FY99 Appropriation Acts. One was a national moratorium on new contracting for a one-year period in FY 98 and extended for another year in FY99; however, this was not included in the FY2000 Appropriation Act. The other moratorium was applicable to Alaska Native villages that were currently members of consortia and prohibited these villages from contracting for the consortia services directly from the IHS. This moratorium was imposed for 3 years, through FY2001.

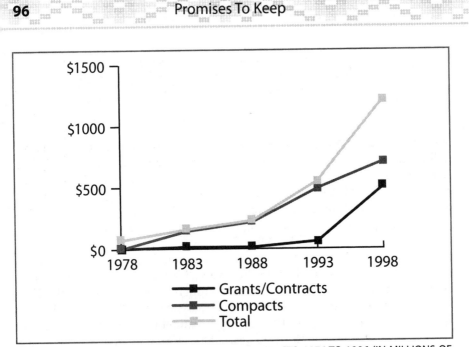

FIGURE 4.1 GROWTH IN IHS CONTRACTS AND COMPACTS, 1976 TO 1996 (IN MILLIONS OF DOLLARS)
SOURCE: IHS 1997 TRENDS, TABLE 5.1

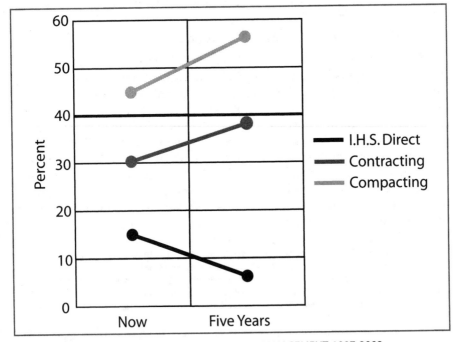

FIGURE 4.2 PROJECTED TRENDS IN HEALTH CARE MANAGEMENT, 1997-2002
SOURCE: DIXON ET AL, 1998, FIGURE 9.3.

The NIHB survey of tribal leaders and tribal health directors in 1997 indicated that the trend toward more contracting and compacting would continue as half the tribes in the study expected to change their health care delivery systems within 5 years as indicated in Figure 4.2 (Dixon et al, 1998).

It should be noted that while only 6 percent of tribal leaders predicted that they would remain IHS direct-service tribes under the definitions of the study, this does not mean that the contracting and compacting tribes will provide a full complement of IHS health services to their members. Tribal operation of entire Area Offices, large IHS hospitals, and complex medical centers that serve many tribes requires political agreement among the tribes involved and political support for an inter-tribal entity to operate the facility. This has been possible only in the Alaska Area, where a multi-tribal consortium operates the Alaska Native Medical Center and contractable portions of the Area office. In most Areas, the IHS still directly operates these larger facilities and is expected to do so for some time. As a result, the IHS is expected to retain substantially more than 6 percent of the IHS budget in the foreseeable future.

SUCCESS OF TRIBALLY-OPERATED HEALTH SERVICES

Many of those who worked for the IHS doubted that tribes could successfully manage their own health programs and believed that a diminished role for the federal government would undermine the progress made by the IHS in eradicating infectious diseases like tuberculosis, improving maternal and child health, and increasing AI/AN life expectancy (Jorgenson 1996, Kunitz 1996, Rhoades 1997a, 1997b). However, after the passage of P.L. 93-638, there was continued improvement in all of these areas, despite reduced per capita spending by Congress on Indian health (Dixon et al, 1998).

In 1997, the National Indian Health Board (NIHB), a national health policy organization representing all federally recognized tribes, conducted a survey of 210 tribal leaders and tribal health directors (Dixon et al 1998). The purpose of this survey was to gather tribal leaders' perspectives on the health systems serving their tribes and to compare results among tribes with different types of health care delivery systems. While the results of this survey only represent the perspectives of those tribes that responded, and may therefore be subject to selection/respondent bias, this survey is the only study of its kind.

To analyze the results of the survey, the tribes were divided into three groups: every tribe that had a negotiated Title III self-governance compact with the IHS, regardless of the types of services included in that compact, was considered a "compacting tribe"; tribes that did not have a Title III compact with the IHS and that managed at least one outpatient medical clinic through a Title I contract were considered "contracting tribes"; and tribes that did not have a Title III compact with the IHS and did not manage their outpatient medical clinic were considered "IHS direct-service tribes."

Overall, the survey found that tribally-operated health systems were faring better than the federally-operated systems in a number of dimensions. Results of the survey indicated that compacting and contracting tribes more commonly added new programs (Figure 4.3) and new facilities (Figure 4.4) compared with IHS direct service tribes.

Furthermore, a greater percentage of compacting and contracting tribes added prevention programs and community based health programs than the systems operated by the IHS.

According to the NIHB survey, tribal leaders and tribal health directors more commonly perceived that the overall quality of their health care had improved if they were operating their own health care systems as compared to those who received IHS direct services. Also, a greater proportion of tribal leaders of compacting and contracting tribes perceived improvements in waiting time, types of services, and number of people served, than tribal leaders from tribes with direct IHS services (Figure 4.5)(see chapter 11).

The addition of new services and facilities by tribally-operated programs was made possible by changes in management that either generated more income or reduced costs, or both. The study found the most prevalent management improvement to be negotiation of purchasing agreements that reduced the cost of supplies. About 20 percent of contracting tribes reported that they had acquired new computer systems and/or financial management

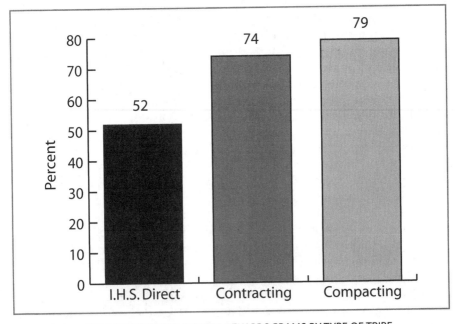

FIGURE 4.3 PERCENT OF TRIBES ADDING NEW PROGRAMS BY TYPE OF TRIBE
SOURCE: DIXON ET AL, 1998, FIGURE 5.1.

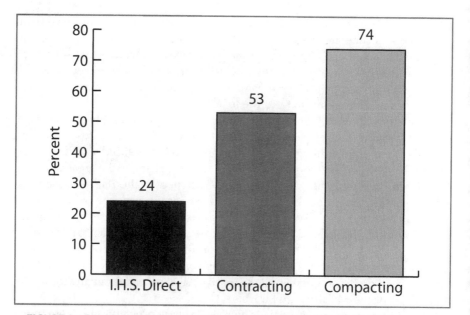

FIGURE 4.4 PERCENT OF TRIBES ADDING NEW FACILITIES BY TYPE OF TRIBE
SOURCE: DIXON ET AL, 1998, FIGURE 5.7.

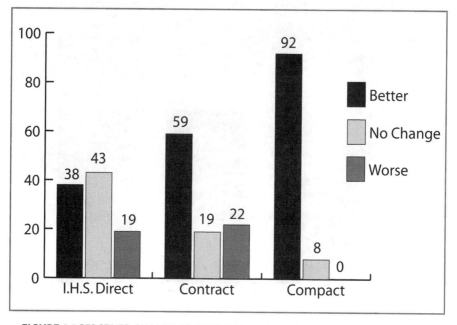

FIGURE 4.5 PERCEIVED QUALITY OF CARE BY TYPE OF HEALTH CARE DELIVERY SYSTEM
SOURCE: TRIBAL LEADERS SURVEY (EXCLUDING ALASKA), FROM DIXON ET AL, 1998, FIGURE 7.5.

systems, and 16 percent created new billing office positions that improved their capabilities to generate third-party income. Tribes also initiated quality assurance programs and chose to eliminate some services or facilities that were perceived as low priority or under-used. As tribes moved into compacting, about 10 percent reported that they reorganized to create fewer supervisory positions and shifted more responsibility to the local level.

The study showed that in tribally-operated programs a higher percentage of the operating budget came from non-IHS sources (Figure 4.6). Mather (1998) found that although tribes increased their Medicaid and Medicare income by 400 percent from fiscal year 93 to fiscal year 97, the greatest dollar increase in Medicaid and Medicare income accrued to the IHS because they were operating the hospitals that generated the most revenue.

In addition, the survey found that tribes operating their own programs more commonly subsidized Indian health care with income from tribal profit-making ventures. While the Alaska non-profit regional Native corporations generally do not receive tribal subsidies, approximately 40 percent of the tribally-operated programs outside Alaska receive tribal subsidies ranging from 2 to 45 percent of their health care budgets.

Tribes that were operating their own health care programs also were more likely to subsidize the construction of new health facilities. The survey found that tribes contributed non-IHS funding to 29 percent of the new facilities

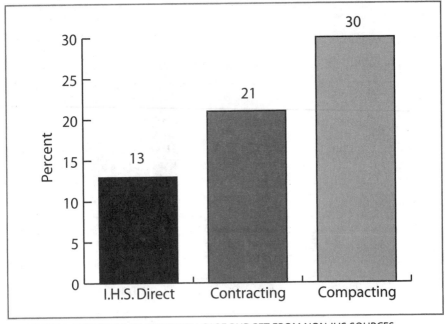

FIGURE 4.6 PERCENTAGE OF HEALTH CARE BUDGET FROM NON-IHS SOURCES
Source: Dixon et al 1998, Figure 6.1.

built for IHS direct service tribes, 62 percent of new facilities for contracting tribes, and 75 percent of new facilities for compacting tribes.

IMPACT OF TRIBAL OPERATIONS ON THE INDIAN HEALTH SERVICE

The growth in contracting and compacting resulted in the reduction in IHS administrative resources as these resources were transferred to tribes involved as "tribal shares." This involved tribal consultation at the Area and national levels to reassess the future role of the IHS, as the Clinton Administration was downsizing the federal government. Faced with all these challenges, the IHS began to re-think its mission for the first time since the agency was created by the Transfer Act of 1954.

INDIAN HEALTH DESIGN TEAM

An Indian Health Design Team (IHDT) was created in 1995 to consider how to redesign the IHS in the context of tribal self-determination, self governance, and federal downsizing. With broad-based participation including tribes, urban Indian representatives, and federal employees, the IHDT worked for 2 years and developed 50 recommendations for changes in the IHS.

The results of the IHDT were not as sweeping as some may have envisioned. When the final report was written, the recommended organizational structure still included Headquarters, 12 Areas, and 150 Service Units.[3] However, it provided a new vision of the Indian health system that included more power sharing between the federal government, tribes, and urban Indian programs. A new term was coined: I/T/U. The I/T/U represents the three parts of the Indian health system: the IHS (I), tribally-operated programs (T), and urban Indian clinics (U). Under the leadership of Michael Trujillo, MD, MPH, Director of the Indian Health Service, the implementation of the I/T/U concept has meant that all three parties are at the table for decision-making, rather than decisions being handed down to the tribes and urban Indian clinics by the IHS.

Through the IHDT process, the IHS changed its mission from one of direction and control to one of support. The Area Offices and Headquarters Offices were envisioned as suppliers to the I/T/U. This ushered in a very different corporate culture, as the role of service supplier replaced the old role of "controlling and giving permission" (Indian Health Design Team 1997). The IHDT tried to replace the federal style of paternalism with a commitment to empower tribes and tribal organizations.

Tribes worked with the IHDT to achieve a consensus on the core functions of IHS Headquarters:

> Because most of the resources for Indian health come from the federal government, it is vital that IHS Headquarters advo-

---

[3]In 1996, 66 of the Service Units were operated by the IHS and 84 were operated by tribes or tribal organizations (IHS 1997).

cate for Indian health, advance our community based
approach, support a nation-wide Indian health network, document our health needs, and furnish a strong voice for tribes
and Indian people. (Indian Health Design Team 1997, p. 9)

It was anticipated that routine oversight functions would be delegated to field
offices. Headquarters was seen as providing advocacy, on behalf of all tribes,
within the Administration and Congress to obtain the resources necessary to
meet the health needs of Indian people.

Many of the IHDT recommendations were patterned on the business
model of the private sector, rather than on a governmental bureaucracy model.
A Business Plan Workgroup was created and charged with developing new
ways to increase revenues through third-party collections; control cost increases and maintain financial solvency; manage transfers of IHS components and
resources to tribes; and other "useful business-like approaches to internal management and operations" (Indian Health Design Team 1997). In some ways,
the IHS was trying to catch up to the tribally-operated programs that had
already been using the private sector as a benchmark for management and services.

As business and government went through a process of downsizing and
streamlining organizations in the 1990s, so too did the IHS. The IHDT recommendations called for consolidating administrative offices into three
Headquarters: Office of the Director, Office of Public Health, and Office of
Management Support. The number of divisions and branches was to be
reduced from 132 to less than 50; these changes were intended to result in
fewer people in management positions. IHS Headquarters was expected to
retain only a small portion of its existing budget, with the rest of the budget
and many positions being transferred to Area Offices and tribal programs.

IMPACT OF WITHDRAWING ADMINISTRATIVE RESOURCES

By 1997, compacting tribes had elected to move an estimated $48.3 mil-
lion in administrative resources from Headquarters and Area Offices into their
annual funding agreements (Mather 1998). These Headquarters and Area
"tribal shares" represented about 12 percent of the funding that went to tribes
under self-governance compacts. The impact of withdrawing these resources
has varied from Area to Area. In general, the Areas with the greatest tribal participation in self governance showed the largest reductions. The Alaska and
Portland Areas, which have the highest proportion of compacting, experienced
the greatest decline in Area Office funding and staffing.[4] Four Areas had no
tribes with self-governance compacts (Aberdeen Area, Albuquerque Area,
Navajo Area, and Tucson Area); but two of these Areas showed significant
downsizing (Albuquerque Area and Tucson Area).

---

[4] Mather (1998) found a 33.7 percent reduction in Alaska Area Office funding and a 25.2 percent reduction in Portland Area funding from FY93 to FY97.

Mather (1998) found that this withdrawal of tribal shares had very little impact on Headquarters or Area Office funding through fiscal year 1997. When adjustments were made for inflation and population growth, the per capita funding for Headquarters and Area operations declined 13 percent from about $111 to about $97 from fiscal year 1993 to fiscal year 1997. This is actually less than the 18 percent decline in per capita inflation-adjusted appropriations for the IHS as a whole. However, it should be noted that this study was completed before the planned implementation of the IHDT recommendations to downsize Headquarters by 80 percent. In the federal system, it takes 2 to 3 years to realize an economic benefit from staff reductions, because those reductions create substantial initial costs, such as separation pay, leave payments, and moving costs.

IMPACT ON IHS DIRECT SERVICE TRIBES

The NIHB study, *Tribal Perspectives on Indian Self-Determination and Self-Governance in Health Care Management* (Dixon et al, 1998), sought to answer the question, "Does compacting hurt other tribes?" The study offered this conclusion:

> While many tribes in this study said that they were hurting from lack of adequate federal funding, few reported that they were hurting as a result of other tribes compacting. Overall, most of the tribes that were not compacting reported improvements in services, management and quality of care.

> One of the negative impacts cited (which could be related to withdrawal of tribal shares, or reductions as a result of the implementation of IHDT recommendations, or inadequate federal funding) included the shift of responsibilities from IHS Headquarters to Area Offices and from Area Offices to Service Units; but, this was also perceived in a positive way as resulting in more local control. Another negative impact cited was the reduction in Area Office discretionary funds to cover shortfalls at the end of the fiscal year. (Dixon et al 1998, p. 166)

As noted in the report, more responsibilities shifted to the local level, but the resources were not provided to pay additional operational costs at the local level, such as charges for the federal telephone system, unemployment insurance, workers compensation insurance, and other costs.

Many IHS direct service tribes feared that their resources would be taken away to support tribally operated programs, but Dixon et al, (1998) found no evidence for this. While most IHS direct service tribes did not report that services were diminished during the study period, they did not fare as well as compacting tribes. Some of this difference may be attributed to the availability of contract support resources to tribally-operated programs and some is probably attributable to increased local involvement in the design and operation of health services. Another portion of this difference may relate to economic development and subsequent levels of tribal subsidies to health care programs, although this is difficult to quantify.

DISINTEGRATION OF HEALTH SERVICES

Another concern about contracting and compacting was that the Indian Health System would disintegrate. The former Director of the IHS, Everett R. Rhoades, MD, called it "balkinization" (Rhoades 1997a); this was a concern expressed more often by employees of the IHS than by tribes.

Increased tribal management of health care not only involves dismantling portions of the federal bureaucracy, but it also involves more local control and empowerment of tribes. This is sometimes frustrating for state officials and other federal agencies that are not accustomed to tribal consultation. They find it easier to talk to one person in a federal bureaucracy whom they presume can represent the interests of all tribes concerned with an issue, rather than consulting with each tribe. Tribes, however, want a government-to-government relationship that respects each tribe's sovereignty.

Despite fears of disintegration, there was a high degree of consensus among tribes regarding the need for some integrated functions to continue. The IHDT addressed the need for an integrated system by recommending a strong role for IHS Headquarters to represent all tribes in advocating on behalf of the I/T/U. Also, tribes have repeatedly endorsed the need for an integrated health data system and continued public health surveillance on both the national and local levels. While the Baseline Measures Workgroup developed recommendations for tribal reporting of data (IHS 1996), there have been insufficient resources to develop standards and training to enable tribes to fully implement this idea. Roubideaux (1998a) found that while Indian health facilities collected quality assurance data, they analyzed and reported it in different ways.

Ironically, the glue that holds the system together is a lack of funding. Because tribes do not have sufficient resources to provide the full range of health services to their members, they continue to use the IHS referral system to access tertiary-care hospitals that are operated by the IHS and other federal agencies. While some have suggested that tribal operations would lead to diseconomies of scale (Kunitz 1996), tribes have reported more cost-efficient and income-producing operations than the federal government (Dixon et al, 1998). Some tribes are entering into multi-tribal agreements for purchasing and delivering services that create economies of scale.

Furthermore, many tribes recognize the value of cooperation and unity. Tribally controlled Area Health Boards are providing coordination, communication, training, and technical assistance to tribes.[5] These multi-tribal organi-

---

[5] Variation in funding for Area health boards means that some are more active and effective than others.

zations are filling the role that was previously filled by the IHS Area Offices. So, while there is a disintegration of the federally controlled system, there is growing integration within tribally controlled systems.

FINANCIAL CONSTRAINTS ON THE INDIAN HEALTH SYSTEM

The evolution of the Indian health system toward tribal management is a result of persistent unmet health care needs. The growth of contracting and compacting came at a time when the Indian health system was acutely under-funded. Many tribes regarded self-determination and self-governance as an opportunity to deliver better health services in a more cost-effective manner while exercising their sovereignty (Dixon et al, 1998). The opportunity to claim administrative resources from the Area Office and Headquarters also enabled tribes to obtain more resources at the local level for their health services. However, for other tribes, the lack of funding for the Indian health system serves as a powerful disincentive to contract because they do not have the resources to absorb ailing, under-funded programs.

CONGRESS DOES NOT REGARD INDIAN HEALTH AS AN ENTITLEMENT PROGRAM

Despite the long history of federal trust responsibility and federal laws that authorize the United States to provide health care to American Indian tribes, Indian health care is not considered an entitlement program by Congress. An entitlement means that the government defines eligibility for a program and the services that are covered, and pays for the cost of those services to the eligible population. If the services cost more than the budget for a year, then Congress does a supplemental appropriation to cover cost overruns. Medicaid and Medicare are both entitlement programs, and there is no possibility that they will "run out of money." However, Congress has been concerned about the high costs of Medicaid and Medicare, they control them by manipulating eligibility, covered services, or fees to providers for care.

In contrast, the Indian Health Service (IHS) is not an entitlement program. Congress sets the budget for the year and there is seldom a supplemental appropriation to cover cost overruns. When allotted funds are spent, the services cease to be provided. Because eligibility is generally fixed for Indian health care, the amount of the budget determines the level of the services. Historically, the Indian Health Service has been funded at a level far below the health care needs of the American Indian and Alaska Native (AI/AN) population.[6]

In the last quarter of the 20th century, the U.S. political process placed a priority on limiting the growth of the domestic portion of the federal budget,

---

[6] The DHHS (1986) reported that the per capita expenditure for IHS was 75 percent of national expenditure levels in 1975 and 69 percent in 1986. In the FY99 budget submission to the DHHS, IHS reported that its FY97 appropriations were less than 34 percent of the per capita expenditure for the civilian US population (Mather 1998). The Level of Need Funded Study (IHS 1999) found that the IHS has only 60 percent of what it would cost for a comparable federal employee benefit package.

including the non-defense portion of the federal government, in an effort to reduce the deficit without increasing taxes. To accomplish these objectives, Congress enacted Balanced Budget Acts that provide a disciplined approach to the creation of federal budgets. This budgetary process usually involves estimating the federal revenues for the year, deducting the fixed cost of government including entitlement programs, and forcing all other programs to stay within the remaining available funding. Thus, as entitlement programs grow, the non-entitlement programs must shrink to keep the total cost of government constant. To make this system work, both the Administration and Congress agree on general budgetary guidelines for a given fiscal year. They usually agree to a percentage increase over the previous year that can cover the cost of overall inflation (as opposed to medical). Agencies then are asked to prepare budgets using the baseline of the previous year and adding the specified increments. This approach is devastating for Indian health. Because the IHS has been historically under-funded, small annual increases can never bridge the gap between existing appropriations and the funding necessary to meet the needs. Furthermore, medical inflation has exceeded overall inflation for the past several decades. This has hurt the IHS in two ways: First, the government sets its annual increments in budgeting on the lower overall inflation rate, while the IHS is experiencing the higher medical inflation rate, therefore it falls further behind in real spending. Second, the huge entitlement programs like Medicaid swallow more of the budgetary pie as medical inflation increases, so there is less available to the non-entitlement programs like the IHS.

Population growth further compounds this problem. Because IHS is not an entitlement program, it does not automatically get more funds when it has to serve more people. The AI/AN population is growing through high birth rates, lower death rates, longer life expectancies, more tribes being recognized by the federal government, and higher tribal enrollment. In the next 50 years, the AI/AN population is expected to nearly double (Roubideaux 1998b). Yet, the agency must still prepare budgets according to the rules that are designed to limit the growth in the federal government and federal expenditures.

There is one way to get more resources than the federally designated increment allows. This involves a program and budget initiative by the President that would be endorsed by Congress. Typically, these types of initiatives occur to further the political agendas of elected officials, such as making good on campaign promises to put more teachers in classrooms, to put more policemen on the streets, to promulgate a war on drugs, or to find the cure for breast cancer. Because American Indians and Alaska Natives are one of the smallest minority groups in our country, they generally cannot command the political clout for a new spending initiative—the spending simply does not translate into enough votes in the next election to justify it on political grounds. National politicians rarely act on moral grounds when there are insufficient votes to create a political justification.

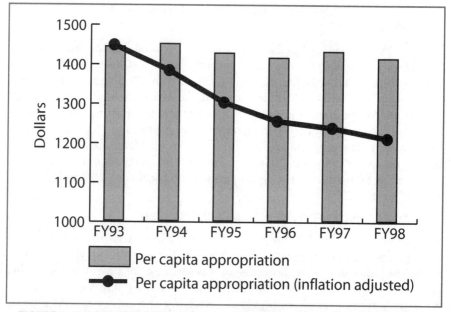

FIGURE 4.7 IHS PER CAPITA APPROPRIATIONS ADJUSTED FOR INFLATION 1993-1998
SOURCE: DIXON ET AL, 1998, FIGURE 4.3

The end result of the balanced budget approach without an entitlement is a downward spiral in which the IHS receives less real funding per capita each year and this necessarily results in increased rationing of health care services. If IHS had been an entitlement program, its funding likely would have grown at 4 times its rate of growth in the 1990s.[7]

DECLINE IN IHS PER CAPITA APPROPRIATIONS

For the five-year period from fiscal year 1994 to fiscal year 1998, Congressional appropriations for the Indian Health Service grew by 8 percent from $1,943,068 to $2,098,612, and medical inflation increased by 20.6 percent. At the same time, the IHS service population jumped from 1,299,415 to 1,466,354, an increase of 12.8 percent (Mather 1998).So, when Congressional appropriations are adjusted for inflation and considered on a per capita basis, the funding actually declined by 18 percent over the five-year period. IHS per capita appropriations adjusted for inflation fell from $1,382 in fiscal year 1994 to $1,183 in fiscal year 1998, as shown in Figure 4.7.

In the fiscal year 2001 budget, IHS received its largest increase ever: $213 million. This 9 percent increase will raise IHS's spending power by barely one percent, since the typical managed care plan is expected to increase its premiums by 8.5 percent for 2001.[8]

---

[7] Based on the Medicaid growth rate from 1992 to 1996, averaging 10 percent per year, which was 4 times the level of growth in the IHS budget over the same period (Mather 1998).

[8] In addition to the IHS budget that is in the DOI appropriation, the DHHS budget had new funding for AI/AN programs including $70 million for diabetes and $30 million for alcohol and drug abuse programs.

INCREASING RELIANCE ON MEDICAID, MEDICARE, AND OTHER THIRD-PARTY RESOURCES

Like the Veterans Administration and other federal health care programs, the IHS was prohibited from collecting reimbursement from Medicare and Medicaid, until the passage of the Indian Health Care Improvement Act (IHCIA) in 1976. The growth in Medicaid and Medicare funding for the IHS has paralleled the growth in tribal contracting and compacting. At the same time, the decline in adjusted per capita appropriations to the IHS has resulted in a greater reliance by the Indian health system on Medicaid, Medicare, and other third party resources. The amount of third party income to the IHS increased by 80 percent in the 5 year period from fiscal year 1993 to fiscal year 1997 (Mather 1998).

MEDICAID RATES FOR THE INDIAN HEALTH SYSTEM

Initially, the IHS did not have an accounting system that enabled the agency to establish billing rates. Rates were set for Medicaid services by inter-agency negotiation with little concern for actual costs of providing care. This generated an exceedingly low flat-rate per visit or hospital day, regardless of the number or types of services provided. Recently, the agency has been more aggressive in the collection of cost data to support a somewhat higher rate.

The rates, which are negotiated with the Health Care Financing Administration (HCFA), were commonly called the "HCFA rates" or the "IHS rates." Under the Indian Health Care Improvement Act (P.L. 93-437), there are rates for outpatient and inpatient care; the rate for Alaska is negotiated separately due to the higher costs of health care in the state. The IHCIA also stipulated that the federal government would provide 100 percent Federal Medical Assistance Percentage (FMAP) for covered services delivered to Medicaid recipients in IHS-owned facilities.

The changes to the Social Security Act in the IHCIA applied only to the IHS facilities and not to those owned by tribes. Initially, contracting tribes were operating programs in IHS facilities. However, the constraints on federal construction of Indian health facilities led tribes to seek other approaches to financing and constructing new clinics. The IHS worked with HCFA to find a way to assure that tribes would not be penalized as they took more responsibility for their health care.

In 1996, IHS and HCFA signed a Memorandum of Agreement (IHS/HCFA MOA) that changed the payment policies for tribally-owned facilities. The MOA extended the 100 percent FMAP to covered services provided to Medicaid beneficiaries through tribally owned facilities.[9] The MOA provided for three different reimbursement approaches that could be used with tribally-owned facilities: (1) the IHS rate; (2) the rate established by the tribe

---

[9] The word "through" in the MOA has been subject to various interpretations that may or may not include outreach services or off-site facilities.

as a Federally Qualified Health Center (FQHC)[10]; or (3) another Medicaid rate that is used by the state. The MOA also tackled the controversy of state licensing requirements for Medicaid. According to the MOA, tribally owned facilities must meet all state licensing requirements, but as sovereign tribal nations they do not have to be licensed by states.

Because states were not signatories to the IHS/HCFA MOA, some states were slow to implement it. Dixon (1998a) found that the MOA was interpreted differently by different states and regional HCFA offices with regard to the definition of an encounter, the number of encounters allowable per day, the application of the 100 percent FMAP, the state role to assure that standards are met, and the choice of reimbursement. Also, the IHS/HCFA MOA did not extend to urban Indian clinics facing the prospect of FQHC rates being phased out by 2003 under the Balanced Budget Act of 1997.[11]

MEDICAID, MEDICARE AND OTHER THIRD-PARTY RESOURCES AS A PERCENTAGE OF INDIAN HEALTH SYSTEM BUDGET

Medicaid income to tribes grew significantly after 1996. The 100 percent FMAP in the IHS/HCFA MOA created the incentives for states to be more flexible in dealing with tribes (Dixon 1998a). At the same time, many states expanded their eligibility for Medicaid services under more generous federal guidelines, waivers, and the Child Health Insurance Program that was initiated in the Balanced Budget Act of 1997. Also, after nearly two decades of stagnant rates, the Medicaid rates for IHS inpatient and outpatient services increased by over 50 percent in 1997.

Still, Medicaid spending for AI/AN lags behind Medicaid spending for other Americans. There are several reasons for this. First, approximately 70 percent of Medicaid spending is for nursing home care and nursing homes generally are not utilized as much by older AI/AN because of cultural and accessibility issues. Second, with welfare reform under the Personal Responsibility and Work Opportunity Reconciliation Act of 1996, Medicaid is no longer linked to public assistance (Schneider and Martinez 1997). Since their health care is already provided by the IHS free of charge, most AI/AN will not apply for Medicaid unless they are required to do so under Contract Health Services rules. And, third, as states have converted their Medicaid programs to managed care, there has been confusion by both AI/AN patients and I/T/U providers regarding accessing services and recovering reimbursement under Medicaid (Dixon 1998a, 1998b).

In fiscal year 1997, the IHS system received approximately $290 million in third party revenues. This represents about a 14 percent increase in IHS funding over the fiscal year 1997 appropriation level. It is assumed that some tribally operated health programs are receiving third party income that is not reg-

---

[10] FQHC rates were based upon Medicare cost reports that establish a full cost (or reasonable cost) reimbursement, rather than the discounted rates based upon the assumption that health providers can shift costs from public programs to private insurers.

[11] In 1999, bills were introduced in Congress to apply the 100 percent FMAP to urban Indian clinics.

istered in the IHS accounting system. Grants from other governmental agencies and private philanthropy, as well as contributions by tribes to both programs and the construction of new facilities, may be supplementing IHS funding in some tribally-operated programs.

The total extent of non-IHS resources is difficult to estimate for a variety of reasons. Tribally-operated programs are generally reluctant to report their sources of income for fear that Congress will cut their budgets by a corresponding amount. None of the national databases on health care resources adequately sample the reservation-based AI/AN population to create an independent source for this type of information. For example, a study that analyzed data from the major national data bases on health expenditures[12] estimated that only 35 percent of AI/AN were using the IHS[13] and that 28 percent had private insurance (Cox et al, 1999). This study might be able to describe the health resources of Americans who identify themselves as AI/AN, including urban Indians and those who are not enrolled in federally recognized tribes. However, even the authors of the study acknowledge that it does little to clarify the funding situation for the core users of the IHS services, who are members of federally-recognized tribes living in remote areas, such as reservations, pueblos and Alaska Native villages.

SHIFT TO MEDICAID FUNDING AS DE FACTO MEANS TESTING

During the 1990s a conservative faction in Congress tried to eliminate several aspects of tribal sovereignty. There was a misperception that American Indians were getting rich from casinos, which was true for only a very small portion of the tribes.[14] Reasoning that rich Indians did not need federally subsidized health care, some members of the U.S. Congress wanted to impose a means test. Under this plan, only less affluent Indians would receive federal subsidies for health care. Tribal leaders argued that health care was part of the federal treaty and trust responsibilities that exist regardless of tribal economic development. Also, tribes with profitable economies from gaming, natural resources, or other sources, are using their profits to subsidize health care and other community services.

Congress appears to be making a conscious decision to shift the funding for Indian health from direct appropriations for the IHS to the more indirect billing of Medicaid and Medicare. It could be argued that the declining per capita appropriations from Congress and the increased reliance on Medicaid funding is de facto means testing. Through this mechanism, the poorer tribes

---

[12] The Cox et al (1999) analysis used the following data bases: 1998 Current Population Study, the 1987 Survey of American Indians and Alaska Natives, the 1987 National Medical Expenditure Survey, the 1998 NMES Projection File and the HCFA 1998 National Health Expenditure Projection.

[13] The study cites IHS figures that 1.3 million of the estimated 2.4 million AI/AN use IHS services, which is 54 percent of the AI/AN population. This group is significantly under represented in sample in the databases, as only 35 percent of the samples reported using IHS services.

[14] Kalt (1998) reports that only one-third of tribes are engaged in any type of gaming and that most of those are not very profitable. He states that 8 of the most successful gaming tribes account for more than half of all Indian gaming revenues.

with more tribal members eligible for Medicaid are receiving more federal health care dollars. Of course, this is only true to the extent that the tribes manage their own Medicaid reimbursable services.

COMPARISON OF IHS FUNDING WITH OTHER HEALTH SYSTEM FUNDING

One of the most significant public health policy issues that affects American Indians and Alaska Natives is the level of funding for the Indian health system. Several approaches have been used by advocates to demonstrate that the current funding levels are insufficient. These approaches include comparing IHS funding with other health systems' funding; demonstrating that health outcomes demand increased funding levels to close the gap between AI/AN health and that of the U.S. population as a whole; assessing the quality of care in the Indian health system to show the need for greater funding to improve quality; and estimating the cost of meeting the needs identified by tribes.

While each of these approaches is persuasive and each document the dramatic under-funding of the IHS system, it is difficult to develop a method to accurately estimate the amount of funding from Congress that would meet the health needs of American Indians and Alaska Natives. For many years, the IHS used a complicated formula called the "Resource Allocation Methodology," or "RAM," to determine the budgetary needs of each Service Unit. As the IHS began implementing tribal consultation in the development of its budgets, the Area Budget Formula Teams used a variety of methods to estimate the needs of the tribes in their areas. Finally, Congress requested a consistent and standard way of measuring the level of need.[15] In 1998, the IHS established a Level of Need Funded (LNF) Workgroup that used the Federal Employees Health Benefits Program as the basis for their calculations. The study concluded that "the current IHS budget for personal health care services falls short of parity with other Americans by an estimated 46 percent" (I & M Technologies et al 1999). The LNF Workgroup (1999) estimated that it would take an additional $12 billion to bring the Indian health system to the same level of services as the health care provided to federal employees. They used a $2,980 per person cost to estimate a total cost of $7.4 billion annually for personal health benefits, with additional amounts needed for the public health services that comprise a large portion of the Indian health program. This figure does not take into account expenditures that would be necessary to bring

---

[15] While Congress requested the level of need study to measure the unmet needs, this is not the same methodology that is used to construct the Administration's budget request that is sent to Congress. The IHS must respond to Office of Management and Budget (OMB) budget formulation directives that are often called the "rules based budget." The OMB rules have been developed largely in response to Congressional budget limitations that are set forth in the Balanced Budget Act of 1997. In recent years, tribes have advocated for a "needs based budget" rather than a "rules based budget." However, Congress and the Administration continue to construct budgets by following the rules that add specified percentages to previous budgets.

infrastructure into parity, such as replacing deteriorating health care facilities and construction of new facilities when needed.

This way of highlighting the magnitude of under funding of the Indian health care system has also been used to compare the IHS per capita funding with that of other health care programs, such as Medicaid, Veterans Administration, military health care spending, or private sector managed care plans. While the results always show a significant difference in expenditures, methods of comparison are always problematic. For example, the Medicaid population has several subgroups with widely varying health needs, from healthy children who are relatively inexpensive to serve to those in nursing homes who are extremely expensive to serve. On the other hand, the military population and other types of federal employees are a relatively healthy group that would be expected to be less costly to serve than a tribal population with a higher than average rate of injuries and diabetes. Furthermore, the IHS is located primarily in manpower shortage areas that require unique approaches for training, recruiting, and retaining health professionals (such as service by the Commissioned Corps of the U.S. Public Health Service and scholarship programs) that make it difficult to compare with private sector health care delivered primarily in urban areas.

Also, it is difficult to compare the IHS per capita funding with funding for other health care delivery systems because the funding approaches are so different. Three fundamental differences between the IHS and all other health care systems are the absence of a defined benefit package, inclusion of public health services, and federal restrictions on facilities funding.

ABSENCE OF A DEFINED BENEFIT PACKAGE

Because the IHS is not an entitlement program and Congress has chosen not to fully fund it, there is a continual process of health care rationing. The amount of funding to each Service Unit in the IHS and needs assessments by tribes affect the types and amounts of services provided to the AI/AN people who live there. For some regions of the country, the Indian health system has tertiary-care hospitals that provide multi-specialty care, but other regions have such limited resources that they receive no inpatient care at all. One tribe may provide eyeglasses and orthodontia, while another tribe that does not offer these services may provide traditional healing. While most tribes have some type of pharmacy benefits, the formulary varies greatly from tribe to tribe.

After Congress appropriates funding to the IHS, the funds are allocated to Areas, Service Units, and tribes using complicated formulas that incorporate such factors as number of users, geographic location, cost of delivering services, historic funding levels, and decisions by tribes to withdraw their shares from the Headquarters operations. Thus, the per capita expenditures vary from Area to Area. Mather (1998) found the per capita expenditure through the IHS in the Alaska Area to be $3,300 in fiscal year 1997, while the Albuquerque Area was $1,447, the Bemijdi Area was $1,272, the Oklahoma Area was $997, and California was $745. The reported expenditures vary in part by whether or not third-party income is reported through the IHS accounting system and the effectiveness of different Areas in collecting Medicaid and Medicare. Since Medicaid eligibility rules and benefits vary from state to state, the opportunities to collect Medicaid also vary from state to state.

The bottom line is that the level of funding determines the level of services. Some people believe that a minimum benefit package would assure that all people who are eligible for the IHS receive the same minimum amount of services. Also, a defined benefit package could be used to establish a benchmark funding level by comparing the cost of providing that benefit package with the cost of providing a similar benefit package in the private sector or another public program. This was the approach used by the LNF Workgroup.

While the concept of a defined benefit package has a great deal of appeal, particularly for those in Areas with lower amounts of per capita funding, it also faces significant obstacles. For a defined benefit package to work, the necessary funding would have to be guaranteed, thereby creating an entitlement program, which Congress so far has been unwilling to do. Without an entitlement, the result could be a redistribution of funding between the Areas. Because the entire system is already under funded, no tribe is willing to sacrifice their funding. Also, a defined benefit package could be construed as an intrusion on tribal sovereignty. Tribes want to reserve the power to make decisions about what services to provide rather than being confined to providing a benefit package that is defined by the federal government.

An entitlement with a defined benefit does not necessarily guarantee that services would be available in tribal communities. For example, Medicaid and Medicare cost controls have led to the closure of many rural hospitals across the country. A defined benefit package would have to include standards for accessibility of services. In urban areas, it is expected that a patient would not have to drive more than 30 minutes to a hospital. However, very few AI/AN who live outside urban areas can access hospitals within 30 miles of their residence. In Alaska where there are few roads, IHS beneficiaries usually have to take an airplane to the hospital. It is more cost effective for the IHS to fund patient transportation in Alaska than to build hospitals in every village. Yet, the extraordinary costs of Alaska Native patient transportation are difficult to handle in any comparison to costs of defined benefit packages.

PUBLIC HEALTH FUNCTIONS

Because the IHS was developed in a public health context rather than using a medical model, the IHS budget and programs contain items that are not usually part of insurance programs or managed care plans. These include environmental programs, such as construction of water and sewer systems and providing rabies vaccinations to dogs. When trying to compare IHS programs to other health systems, it is fairly easy to factor out the cost of environmental health programs.

It is much more difficult to take into account the cost of community health programs that are part of the IHS system, such as public health nurses, Community Health Representatives who provide outreach and transportation services, and community health educators. Typically, these types of programs are provided by local governments, such as city or county health departments. In Indian Country, however, they are provided by tribal health departments with funding from the IHS. Again, it is possible to isolate these costs and factor them out of any comparisons with the costs of managed care plans. But, tribes operate on more of a community model rather than the private-sector-medicine model, which tends to treat the individual. So, as tribes assume more control over their health programs, they may tend to shift resources into prevention and community-based activities (Dixon et al 1998). The line between medical care and public health is somewhat blurred in the Indian health system; public health nurses may be providing prenatal care, immunizations, and case management. These types of activities could be considered part of a typical benefit package for a medical plan. In addition, public health and preventive services may reduce the need for other services, but this benefit is difficult to quantify.

CONSTRUCTION OF MEDICAL FACILITIES

An even more vexing problem is facilities funding. The cost of medical services paid by Medicaid, Medicare, and virtually every other third party payer includes facilities funding through debt funding and depreciation. Every private medical provider considers their facility as part of the cost of doing business and builds this cost into charges for their services. Every responsible medical business either finances new construction through loans that are paid with income from services, or they set aside a portion of their income for a facilities replacement fund, or both. This is not true for the IHS.[16]

The federal government funds IHS facilities in a capital appropriation that is separate from the appropriation to cover operating costs. While there are 558 federally recognized tribes in the country, Congress only funds up to 10 new facilities per year. As a result, most of the IHS clinics are old and outdated. There is no mechanism for the IHS to divert a portion of its operating funds or its income from third-party payers to major facilities expansion, remodeling, or replacement. Instead, the IHS and tribes apply to have construction projects placed on a priority list that is sent to Congress. Just as Congress has consistently under-funded the IHS appropriations for operating costs, so too has Congress been reluctant to provide the American Indian and Alaska Native people with adequate health care facilities.

---

[16] However, Federally Qualified Health Centers (FQHCs) may use facilities costs to establish their rates for billing Medicare and Medicaid. Before the FQHC rate was phased out by the Balanced Budget Act of 1997, this option was available to tribes and urban Indian clinics.

INDIAN HEALTH CARE IMPROVEMENT FUND

The Indian Health Care Improvement Fund (IHCIF) was created in the Indian Health Care Improvement Act (P.L. 93-437) to address inequities in funding between service units in the IHS. It is proposed that the LNF formula will be used to distribute these funds. The LNF analysis showed that in 2000, the IHS average funding for personal medical services was only 60 percent of the federal benchmark; the amount of funding for some operating units was only 30 percent of the need. The lowest funded Area was Oklahoma with an average of $856 per person, compared to the $2,980 needed to assure benefits equivalent to those in a mainstream health plan.

According to the LNF calculations, it would take $266 million to raise operating units that were below the IHS average up to the 60 percent level. In the FY2000 budget, $10 million was appropriated to raise those below the average 3.5 percent closer to the IHS average. Congress appropriated an additional $30 million for the IHCIF in FY2001. The LNF methodology is being refined and is gaining acceptance from the tribes and Congress as a way to quantify funding needed to reduce disparities in personal medical care.

To complement the medical model inherent in the LNF methodology, the IHS is forming a workgroup to consider a formula to assess the needs for wraparound services, such as community health nursing, community health representatives (CHRs), and patient transportation, that are a part of the public health mission of the IHS but not included in the LNF formula.

HONORING THE FEDERAL TRUST RESPONSIBILITY

While comparisons may be imperfect, every attempt to compare the level of per capita funding for IHS with other health systems in the United States shows that the American Indian and Alaska Native people are not getting a comparable level of funding for health services. Regardless of the methods used and the estimated amount of funding needed to close the gap, the Administration and Congress have never come close to addressing the identified funding needs. A more elegant method of demonstrating comparative funding levels is not likely to produce better results from Congress if there is a lack of commitment to honor the federal trust responsibility.

Many tribal leaders are worried that the changing role of the IHS as a funding agency, without the bricks and mortar of federally owned and operated hospitals and clinics, makes it easier for Congress to not only reduce, but also eliminate, funding for Indian health. The fear of termination of tribal health benefits is a very real concern for tribal leaders, particularly those who have lived through previous eras of termination.

Congress has established clear goals of tribal empowerment in the Indian Self-Determination Act. It has also declared that the health status of Indian people should be "raised to the highest possible level" through the Indian

Health Care Improvement Act. These two goals have been the foundation for Congressional policies governing Indian health care for the past 3 decades. While large strides have been made, progress has stagnated in the past decade. Despite the demonstrated need for additional support, in the 1990s Congress reduced the per capita appropriations for the Indian Health Service. Tribes have been forced to develop other funding sources and to use revenues from new economic development to keep pace with the need for health services and pay for necessary administrative costs.

American Indians and Alaska Natives are struggling to maintain their culturally distinct institutions and to improve the quality of life for tribal members. Congress must honor the federal trust responsibility and provide substantially greater appropriations to the Indian Health Service to fulfill that responsibility. Only then can progress resume in raising the health status of our country's First Americans to the level that others enjoy as citizens of the country that has the highest standard of living in the world.

REFERENCES

Cox D, Langwell K, Topoleski C, Green JH. *Sources of Financing and the Level of Health Spending for Native Americans*. Menlo Park, CA: The Henry J. Kaiser Family Foundation; 1999.

Dixon M. *Indian Health in Nine State Medicaid Managed Care Programs*. Denver, CO: National Indian Health Board; 1998a.

Dixon M. *Managed Care in American Indian and Alaska Native Communities*. Washington, D.C: American Public Health Association; 1998b.

Dixon M, Shelton BL, Roubideaux Y, Mather D, Smith CM. *Tribal Perspectives on Indian Self-Determination and Self-Governance in Health Care Management. Vol 4*. Denver, CO: National Indian Health Board; 1998.

Jorgensen JG. Comment: Recent Twists and Turns in American Indian Health Care. *American Journal of Public Health*. 1996; 86:10:1362-1364.

I & M Technologies Inc. and Center for Health Policies Studies. *Final Report: Level of Need Funded Cost Model*. April 30, 1999.

Indian Health Design Team. *Design for a New IHS: Final Recommendations of the Indian Health Design Team, Report Number II*. Rockville, MD: Indian Health Service; 1997.

Indian Health Service, U.S. Department of Health and Human Services. *Baseline Measures Workgroup Final Report*. Rockville, MD: Indian Health

Service; 1996.

Kalt, JP. *Statement Before the National Gambling Impact Study Commission, March 16, 1998.* Cambridge, MA: Harvard Project on American Indian Economic Development, Harvard University; 1998.

Kunitz, SJ. The History and Politics of U.S. Health Care Policy for American Indians and Alaska Natives. *American Journal of Public Health.* 1996; 86:10: 1464–1473.

LNF Workgroup. *Level of Need Funded Study (LNF Workgroup Report II).* Rockville, MD: Indian Health Service; 1999.

Mather D. IHS Financial Trends during Self-governance (Title III) Compacting, FY 93 to F 97. In: Dixon M, Shelton BL, Roubideaux Y, Mather D, Smith CM. *Tribal Perspectives on Indian Self-Determination and Self-Governance in Health Care Management. Vol 4.* Denver, CO: National Indian Health Board; 1998.

National Indian Health Board and American Indian Technical Services. *Evaluation Report: The Indian Health Service's Implementation of the Indian Self Determination Process.* Rockville, MD: Indian Health Service; 1984.

Rhoades ER. Editorial: Changing Paradigms and Their Effect on American Indian and Alaska Native Health. *Annals of Epidemiolog.* 1997:7; 227–228.

Rhoades ER. Reflections on a Decade as the Director of the IHS. *The IHS Primary Care Provider.* 1997; 22:1:1–4.

Roubideaux Y. Impact on the Quality of Care" In: Dixon M, Shelton BL, Roubideaux Y, Mather D, Smith CM. *Tribal Perspectives on Indian Self-Determination and Self-Governance in Health Care Management. Vol 4.* Denver, CO: National Indian Health Board; 1998a.

Roubideaux Y. *Current Issues in Indian Health Policy.* Tucson, AZ: Udall Center for Studies in Public Policy, University of Arizona; 1998b.

Schneider A, Martinez J. *Native Americans and Medicaid: Coverage and Financing Issues.* Washington, D.C.: The Center on Budget and Policy Priorities for the Kaiser Commission on the Future of Medicaid, The Henry J. Kaiser Family Foundation; 1997.

Sizemore, JM. *Determining the True Cost of Contracting Federal Programs for*

Indian Tribes. Second Edition. Portland, OR: Northwest Portland Area Indian Health Board and the Affiliated Tribes of Northwest Indians; 1997.

United States Department of Health and Human Services. *Bridging the Gap: Report on the Task Force on Parity of Indian Health Services*; 1986.

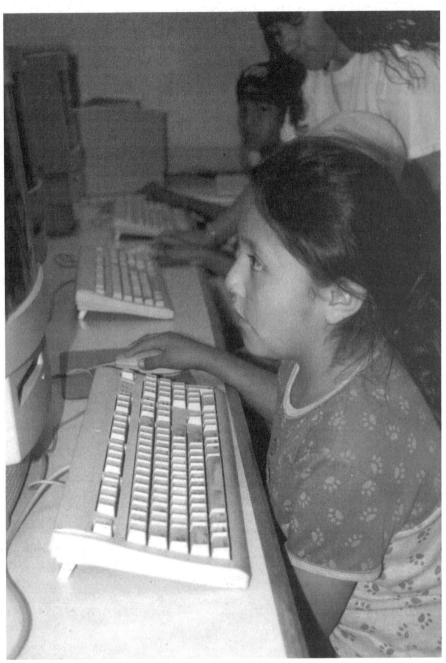

PHOTO BY ALEJANDRO LOPEZ AND ARIE PILZ
COURTESY OF THE NATIONAL INDIAN YOUTH LEADERSHIP PROJECT

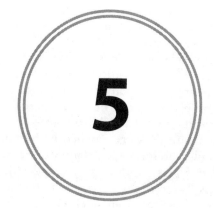

CHALLENGES IN SERVING THE GROWING POPULATION OF URBAN INDIANS

Ralph Forquera

INTRODUCTION

Throughout the 20th century, there was a steady migration of American Indians and Alaska Natives (AI/AN) to American cities. The 1990 Census found that more than 56 percent of the nearly 2 million Americans self-identifying as AI/AN were living in major metropolitan cities.[1] However, little attention has been given to the health and social welfare of urban Indians. Efforts to address their health care needs are fragmented and lack adequate resources.

This chapter will describe the factors that have influenced this shift in residency and the political questions addressed by these changes. We will also describe the evolution of the federal government's response to dealing with the health of urban Indians. The paper will conclude with a list of challenges that continue to hinder a systematic and rational approach to urban Indian health care.

WHO ARE URBAN INDIANS?

Urban Indians are members of, or descendants of members of, one of the many Indian tribes, bands, or organized groups of aboriginal inhabitants of the Americas who now live in American cities. A significant portion of these indi-

---

[1] U.S. Bureau of the Census, 1990 report update. Approximately 62 percent of self-identified AI/AN lived off-reservation, 58 percent lived in major metropolitan service areas (MSAs) with populations in excess of 50,000.

viduals are directly linked to the forcible relocation efforts of the ill-fated Termination and Relocation policies of the 1950s.

In 1890, nearly all of the 240,000 American Indian people who survived the wars and disease caused by the European occupation of North America were living on reservations (Sandefer et al 1996). Reservations were lands set aside by the federal government to house Indians and to provide protection from presumed hostility for white settlers. As the threat of these hostilities diminished, federal military supervision of Indian lands was also reduced giving Indians greater freedom of movement, but few chose to venture away from their home reservations until the United States entered World War I. Young Indian men joined the military in large numbers both to prove their loyalty to the United States as well as to fulfill their warrior spirit muted by the reservation experience. Others sought work in the war industries, leaving the reservation to acquire job skills and trades. Exposure to the urban lifestyles agreed with many Indians who chose to remain in cities after the war.

In 1940, 30 percent of AI/AN were now living in urban areas (U.S. Bureau of the Census, 1940). The advent of World War II brought a second wave of AI/AN into cities. After the war, those returning to their reservations found poverty rampant and housing scarce. Tribal leaders, highly critical of the paternalistic practices of the Bureau of Indian Affairs' (BIA), flooded Congress with letters expressing their discontent. Realizing that there was a housing shortage on reservations, and aware of the rising dissatisfaction with the BIA, Congress proposed a radical shift in Indian policy by enacting House Concurrent Resolution-108 in June of 1953. The non-binding resolution expressed "a sense of Congress" that, "as quickly as practical," federal supervision of Indian tribes by the BIA be ceased (Cohen and Felix 1982).

Many in Congress believed at that time that AI/AN should be assimilated into the mainstream of American society. AI/AN had proven their loyalty in war and had demonstrated their ability to contribute to the broader society in their work in the private sector. Now, Congress felt it was time to end the historic "oppression" of Indians resulting from the BIA's supervision.

HCR-108 set about a series of bills designed to facilitate assimilation. Between 1954 and 1961, 109 Indian tribes had their federal recognition discontinued affecting more than 36,000 people (Olsen et al 1984). The loss of federal recognition left individual tribes subject to state and local taxation and ended their eligibility for federal benefits available only to federally recognized tribe members. To ease the burden of this change, Congress established a relocation program offering individual Indians and entire families assistance in moving to cities. Eight cities were originally chosen as relocation centers.[2]

The effects of termination were devastating to the tribes, and relocation had the effect of exchanging reservation for urban poverty. Relocation centers never received the level of funding from Congress needed to provide proper aid

---

[2] There were eight cities originally designated as relocation centers under the Bureau of Indian Affairs relocation program in the 1950s: Tulsa, Oklahoma City, Los Angeles, San Francisco, Minneapolis, Dallas, Seattle, and Chicago. From Sandefer et al 1996, page 38.

for Indians. Now relocated, Indians found themselves without a reservation to which they could return. Families and communities were disrupted. Feelings of betrayal, anguish, anger, and depression ensued.

In many cities, the Indian bar became the center for socialization; alcohol became a common denominator for retaining an Indian identity. The vision of the drunken Indian, while a negative stereotype to mainstream America, was an image that meant to Indians that they were still "Indians."

Relocation and termination was declared a failure early in the 1960s, and the evolving civil rights movement drew attention to the plight of ethnic-minorities in America including Indians both on- and off-reservation. The 1970 census found that 45 percent of Indians were now living in cities (U.S. Bureau of Census, 1970); many remained in poverty, stripped of their identity, and without financial or emotional support.

In 1970, President Richard Nixon issued the first ever Presidential Indian Policy statement.[3] In the text, Nixon recognized the effect termination had had on Indians declaring that the government shared a responsibility to non-reservation Indians because of the termination and relocation policies. But unlike Indians living on reservations, many urban Indians no longer possessed a direct connection with an Indian tribe or their membership was to a tribe that was no longer recognized by Congress. Thus, a different approach would be required to address off-reservation Indian needs.

THE EVOLUTION OF URBAN INDIAN HEALTH

In 1955, the federal responsibility for Indian health was shifted to the Department of Health, Education, and Welfare. This change provided for the creation of the Indian Health Service, which was developed as a health care delivery system for AI/AN that used government employees as providers and administrators. Hospitals and clinics were built on reservations, and access to direct health care improved for many reservation Indians.

The development of the Indian Health Service bypassed urban Indians entirely until just over two decades ago. Fortunately, Congress became aware of the plight of urban Indians during the tumultuous 1960s. The first recorded Congressional acknowledgment of urban Indian health needs came in 1967 when Congress added funding to the annual Indian Health Service budget to establish a health clinic in Rapid City, South Dakota.[4] Indians from surround-ing reservations often gathered in Rapid City where alcohol use, accidents, and violence became a problem for local officials. In 1972, Congress again author-ized funds for a study in Minneapolis, Minnesota on ways to improve access to health care for urban Indians. The study found that by providing information and referral services to urban Indians, access to care improved. (Senate Report

---

[3] In President Richard Nixon's Special Message to the Congress on Indian Affairs, issued July 8, 1970, Section 7 of the message discusses "Helping Urban Indians." The message acknowledges the failure of past Indian policies and the effect that had on the urbanization of AI/AN.

[4] The Report of the Senate Committee on Interior and Insular Affairs to S-522, section on Federal Policy and Urban Indian Health Care, May 13, 1975, page 136.

to S-522, page 137) This model became the foundation for efforts to improve health care for this population.

During this same time, Indian leaders and non-Indian advocates began to organize health services in several cities using volunteer doctors and nurses. Several of these "free clinics" incorporated as community clinics and received funds from local and national poverty programs.

In Seattle, Washington, a group approached Senator Henry "Scoop" Jackson, the chair of the Senate Appropriations Committee, seeking help for urban Indians. Jackson had recently accepted an appointment to the Interior Committee, which had oversight on Indian issues. There he met Forrest Gerard, a Blackfeet from Montana and an astute political operative. Gerard, realizing that support for legislation to help urban Indians would not get sufficient support, contacted Dr. Emory Johnson, the enigmatic director of the Indian Health Service. Together Gerard and Johnson crafted a bill that would change the direction of Indian health, expand access to such Jackson-sponsored initiatives as the National Health Service Corps, and create a distinct program for urban Indians.[5]

TITLE V: URBAN INDIAN HEALTH

Jackson introduced S. 522 in 1975, which eventually became the Indian Health Care Improvement Act (P.L. 94-437). Title V of the bill established a discrete program for urban Indians modeled after the successful Neighborhood Health Center initiative that had evolved out of the Great Society programs of President Lyndon Johnson. Instead of expanding the role of existing Indian health services into cities, Congress set up a program whereby local Indian groups were encouraged to form non-profit corporations that would then contract with the Indian Health Service. Like the Neighborhood Health Centers, and in keeping with President Nixon's call for Indian self-determination, the governance of these local non-profits required a Board of Directors, the majority of which were American Indians, to assure "maximum participation of Indian people."[6]

Initially, contracts were designed to help Indian communities form information and referral networks; such networks had proved most effective in improving access to health services for Indians from the Minneapolis study. But in those cities where Indian community clinics had already formed, funds were also used to enhance or expand clinical services.

The first direct Indian Health Service funding for Title V programs came in 1979. Figure 5.1 shows a history of urban Indian health funding in com-

---

[5] In Dr. Abraham Bergman's interviews in "A Political History of the Indian Health Service", *The Milbank Quarterly*, Vol. 77, No. 4, 1999, Bergman describes how Gerard and Dr. Johnson worked to draft S. 522 which became the Indian Health Care Improvement Act, P.L. 94-437.

[6] In his Special Message to the Congress on Indian Affairs, President Nixon, in establishing a call for Indian self-determination, wanted policy to establish ways to assure "maximum participation of Indian people." This approach was codified in P.L. 94-437 by requiring that the Board of Directors for a Title V, urban Indian health program, have a majority of its members of Indian heritage.

Year	Total IHS	Total Urban	% of IHS Budget
1979	492,193	7,270	1.48%
1980	546,569	8,000	1.46%
1981	606,709	8,900	1.47%
1982	599,645*	8,160	1.36%
1983	679,216	7,385	1.08%
1984	778,812	9,000	1.15%
1985	890,567	9,800	1.10%
1986	820,979	9,644	1.17%
1987	867,704	9,000	1.00%
1988	943,297	9,624	1.02%
1989	1,020,106	9,962	0.09%
1990	1,178,337	13,049	1.11%
1991	1,353,167	15,687	1.16%
1992	1,431,603	17,195	1.20%
1993	1,524,992	20,965	1.37%
1994	1,646,088	22,834	1.39%
1995	1,707,092	23,349	1.37%
1996	1,760,842	23,360	1.33%
1997	2,057,000	24,800	1.20%
1998	2,098,612	25,379	1.20%
1999	2,118,349	26,382	1.25%

* Congress adjusted the IHS budget excluding some reimburseable positions that had been previously counted.

FIGURE 5.1 COMPARISON OF URBAN INDIAN FUNDING TO TOTAL INDIAN HEALTH SERVICE FUNDING — 1979 — 1999 (IN THOUSANDS)*
SOURCES: INDIAN HEALTH SERVICE, HEALTH SERVICE APPROPRIATION HISTORY, 1983 –1999, MARCH 12, 1999; INDIAN HEALTH SERVICE, HISTORY OF APPROPRIATIONS 1911– 1982, JANUARY 9, 1982

MSA	1990	Reservation	1990
Tulsa, OK	48,348	Navajo, AZ	143, 405
Oklahoma City, OK	46,111	Pine Ridge, SD	11,182
Los Angeles/Long Beach, CA	43,638	Fort Apache, AZ	9,825
Phoenix, AZ	38,309	Gila River, AZ	9,116
Seattle/Tacoma, WA	32,980	Papago, AZ	8,480
Riverside/San Bernadino, CA	25,938	Rosebud, SD	8,043
New York City, NY	24,822	San Carlos, AZ	7,110
Minneapolis, MN	23,338	Zuni Pueblo, AZ	7,073
San Diego, CA	21, 509	Hopi, AZ	6,061
San Francisco/Oakland, CA	21, 191	Blackfeet, MT	7,025
Tucson, AZ	20,034	Turtle Mountain, MT	6,772
Dallas/Fort Worth, TX	19,933	Yakima, WA	6,307
Detroit-Ann Arbor, MI	19,331	Osage, MO	6,088
Sacramento, CA	18,164	Fort Peck, MT	5,782
Chicago, IL	16,518	Wind River, WY	5,676

FIGURE 5.2 INDIAN POPULATION DISTRIBUTION 1990 CENSUS METROPOLITAN STATISTICAL AREA/INDIAN RESERVATIONS (IN DESCENDING ORDER)
SOURCE: 1990 CENSUS

parison to the total IHS annual appropriations for the past 20 years. Note that funding for urban services has remained approximately 1.19 percent of the total IHS funding each year while the urban population has grown dramatically.

Figure 5.2 shows a comparison of Indian populations between Metropolitan Statistical Areas (urban) and Indian reservations. Other than the great Navajo Nation, which encompasses a large geographic area, the largest concentrations of Indians are in cities. But unlike reservations, urban Indian populations are highly diverse.

In 1999, there were 34 non-profit, Indian health programs operating 41 sites in 19 states that contract with the Indian Health Service under Title V (Figure 5.3). These 34 programs vary considerably in size and extent of services offered. The more successful programs are located in areas where social programs are broadly supported by local and state governments. Many have been in operation for more than 25 years and have become an integral part of the safety net system. Still others have learned to partner with like institutions to expand services and increase access to needed care. All have evolved with a community focus; thus each program has developed characteristics that are unique to local needs.

DESCRIBING A TYPICAL URBAN INDIAN COMMUNITY

It is difficult to use the term "community" to describe the urban Indian experience. With few exceptions, urban Indians live in a highly fragmented fashion when compared with reservation lifestyles. Urban Indians are often geographically dispersed throughout a metropolitan area. Clusters of Indian families may be found in lower income areas, but in general, Indians can be found throughout the region. Reservation Indians, while sometimes geographically distant from one another, retain a sense of community—a feeling of being a part of the reservation clan. The sense of social isolation seen among some urban Indians may be a major contributor to mental and emotional problems.

Urban Indians are very diverse tribally. For example, a study conducted for the Seattle Indian Health Board found that during the 10-year period from 1989 to 1999, Indians from 238 different federally recognized tribes received health care from this urban Indian provider.[7] This number did not include the approximately two-dozen Indians tribes which are not recognized by the federal or state governments, who also received care.

Urban Indians constitute a wide array of levels of social adaptability and societal integration. For example, many urban Indians have lived most or all of their lives in cities. These individuals have learned to adapt to the social and cultural structure of contemporary urban life. Many have achieved significant levels of success by contemporary standards. Still others may be new residents, new arrivals to the urban environment. Frequently, these individuals lack an

---

[7] In 1999, as part of their tribal registry project, the Northwest Portland Area Indian Health Board conducted a record linkage project for the Seattle Indian Health board. In performing the records review, they listed the number of Indian tribes named in the records. The list included 238 federally recognized tribes.

Area	Program	Location
Aberdeen Area	South Dakota Urban Indian Health, Inc.	Pierre, SD
	Nebraska Urban Indian Health Coalition	Lincoln, NE
Albuquerque Area	Denver Indian Health and Family Services	Denver, CO
	First Nations Community Health Source	Albuquerque, NM
Bemidji Area	Indian Health Board of Minneapolis	Minneapolis, MN
	American Indian Health & Family Services	Detroit, MI
	United Amerindian Health Center, Inc.	Green Bay, WI
	Milwaukee Indian Health Center	Milwaukee, WI
	American Indian Health Services of Chicago	Chicago, IL
	Billings Area Indian Health Board of Billings, Inc.	Billings, MT
	North American Indian Alliance	Butte, MT
	Native American Center, Inc.	Great Falls, MT
	Helena Indian Alliance	Helena, MT
	Missoula Indian Center	Missoula, MT
California Area	Native American Health Center	Oakland, CA
	Sacramento Urban Indian Health Project	Sacramento, CA
	Indian Health Center of Santa Clara	San Jose, CA
	American Indian Health & Services	Santa Barbara, CA
	San Diego American Indian Health Center	San Diego, CA
	United American Indian Involvement	Los Angeles, CA
	Fresno Indian Health Association	Fresno, CA
Nashville Area	American Indian Community House	New York, NY
	North American Indian Center of Boston	Jamaica Plains, MA
Navajo Area	Native Americans for Community Action	Flagstaff, AZ
Oklahoma Area	Dallas Inter-Tribal Center	Dallas, TX
	Oklahoma City Indian Clinic	Oklahoma City, OK
	Indian Health Care Resource Center	Tulsa, OK
	Hunter Health Clinic	Wichita, KS
Phoenix Area	Nevada Urban Indians	Reno, NV
	Native American Community Health Center	Phoenix, AZ
	Indian Health Care Clinic	Salt Lake City, UT
Portland Area	Seattle Indian Health Board	Seattle, WA
	N.A.T.I.V.E. Project	Spokane, WA
	NARA of the NW, Inc.	Portland, OR
Tucson Area	Inter-Tribal Health Care Center	Tucson, AZ

FIGURE 5.3 URBAN INDIAN HEALTH CONTRACTORS BY INDIAN HEALTH SERVICE AREAS—1999

understanding of the different aspects of urban life.

Interestingly, the government's desire to assimilate Indians into the mainstream society has not fully transpired even today. Those who directly experienced the effects of relocation and termination may live in the city, but their acceptance of urban life may be colored by this experience. Most urban Indians remain connected to Indian cultural practices and may frequent pow wows and other social events as a way of maintaining their Indian cultural ties. Others move frequently between cities and their home reservations. This persistence in holding on to one's Indian heritage, despite federal policy and government intervention in the lives of Indian tribes and families, is a factor that also may affect the health of many urban Indians.

Racial discrimination continues to be a factor experienced by urban Indians today. The attitude appears to work both ways, however. Some urban Indians, particularly those mistreated by people from other races, may harbor resentments causing refusal by those affected to participate in services and activities for fear of reprisal. Urban Indians may indirectly experience the backlash against tribes that have turned to gaming or other activities used for economic development purposes on reservations. Those who characterize these activities in a moral context may inappropriately exert their displeasure on urban Indians who have little or no association with tribal business ventures. This type of broad-brush moralization by non-Indians serves to reinforce the biases of Indians against mainstream America whose history of mistreatment of Indians remains clearly etched in their minds.

Although many urban Indians may no longer be directly affiliated with an Indian tribe, their history, culture, and beliefs are derived from this tribal world-view. The majority of urban Indians continue to think and act from a tribal perspective having been removed from this physical experience for only a relatively short period of time. Efforts to dissolve the tribal perspective, assimilating Indians into the independent, individualistic ideals of the American culture, remains a struggle for Indian people regardless of their tribe or their place of residency. The contest to maintain one's "Indianness" in a society that prioritizes the individual over the collective is a challenge that will continue to thwart efforts to address health disparities that affect Indian people.

THE LACK OF DATA AND DEFINING HEALTH DISPARITIES

Title V established a discrete program within the Indian Health Service for urban Indians. Although enacted in 1976, the Indian Health Care Improvement Act did not provide for a method of surveillance to define and track the health status of urban Indians. The fact that urban Indian health services differed from the tribal and IHS approaches both in contracting and in political importance has lead to few efforts to aid urban Indians in needs assessment in a way that allows for comparison with national standards; in fact, little is known about the health status of urban Indians. Only one population-based study has been published describing the health status of this group (Grossman, et al 1994).

Several urban programs have conducted needs-assessment surveys or participated in health risk appraisals often in conjunction with local initiatives. However, these studies are specific to a given area and are not suitable for an understanding of the urban Indians' health conditions on a national basis.

The lack of national data on the health of urban Indians places service providers at a significant disadvantage in advocating for health care resources. Although urban Indian health programs have been around for 20 years or more, it was not until the past 5 or 6 years that urban Indians gained recognition by high-ranking public officials, and the status of urban Indian health became a visible problem.

In 1994, the Assistant Secretary for Health, Dr. Philip Lee, conducted a series of regional consultations to learn about health problems facing Indian people including those living in cities. His efforts were enhanced with the selection of Dr. Michael H. Trujillo as Director for the Indian Health Service. Dr. Trujillo had worked for the Milwaukee urban program and was familiar with the challenges in caring for the health needs of urban Indians. Both of these high-ranking public officials drew attention to the problems faced by urban Indians, which opened doors to other public and private policy and financing groups.

As concern grew over the continuing gap in health disparities, particularly among American minorities, the lack of a national initiative to define health problems in urban Indians became increasingly acute. Recently, the Seattle Indian Health Board, a Title V contractor, was awarded a grant to initiate an urban Indian epidemiology center to begin to correct the information deficiency. However, until a uniform, on-going data collection system can be created, defining and comparing health disparities for urban Indians will remain problematic.

URBAN INDIAN HEALTH PROGRAMS AS SAFETY NET PROVIDERS

The health insurance crisis continues to plague the nation, and reliance on private managed care systems has not resolved the problem. As more and more Americans of all races and ethnicities are living without health insurance, the need for a safety net system has drawn considerable attention among health policy experts.

Like other community health centers, urban Indian health programs serve a vital role in assuring access to primary medical care for low-income urban Indians. Many Title V programs now offer an array of direct health care services, and those that do not provide on-site care often form partnerships with hospitals, public health clinics, or non-Indian community clinics to facilitate care. In some regions where tribal and IHS facilities may be close at hand, urban programs have served as advocates and case managers, improving access for Indians in need.

Title V urban Indian programs have been included under the umbrella of publicly financed health programs eligible for Federally Qualified Health Center status. As FQHCs, urban programs are eligible to receive cost-based reimbursement for Medicare and Medicaid services offered. They are also eligible to be providers under the Children's Health Insurance Program (CHIP). Access to these revenue streams helps expand the financial base of urban Indian programs, allowing for expanded services.

URBAN INDIAN VS. TRIBAL HEALTH

The tribal health care system is based on the IHS, which is a comprehensive public health model created more than 40 years ago. The model includes a broad array of direct health care, including funding for specialty and hospital care, and certain public health services needed to address environmental concerns.

The urban Indian health model was initially defined as a way to improve access to health care for tribal members living away from the reservation. As noted previously, the 1972 study in Minneapolis demonstrated the value of providing information and referral assistance to urban Indians. As time passed, and circumstances permitted, urban Indian programs evolved into direct care programs. But unlike the reservation-based tribal programs, urban Indian health is wholly dependent on the broader health care community. There are no urban Indian hospitals, and very few urban programs offer more than just general primary care services. A few urban programs offer dental care, for example, however, most urban clinics have secured funding through small grants for substance abuse and mental health services.

Urban Indian health programs and their health providers are required to be state licensed. However, these requirements cannot be imposed on tribal or IHS facilities located on reservations. Non-Indian contracts and grants place additional restrictions on services or prioritize health problems that may or may not be of greatest need in a given community.

Urban Indian health programs are also subject to all federal and state anti-discrimination laws that require services to be open to anyone seeking assistance. This differs from IHS and tribal clinics, which only offer their services to members of federally recognized tribes.

Urban Indian clinics must also charge for services. Most direct medical and dental care is offered using a sliding-fee schedule; publicly-sponsored programs for the uninsured and indigent require the application of a sliding-fee schedule as a condition of receiving funds. Some programs require a minimum fee for services, and others that contract with health insurers and managed care plans may be required to accept co-payments or other cost-sharing arrangements. Services offered at IHS and tribal clinics are normally offered at no cost to the patient. This policy appears to be changing as individual tribes under self-governance compacts with the IHS are exploring financing options to augment their annual IHS funding.

ACCESS

A Kaiser Commission on Medicaid and the Uninsured Report found that while many American Indians and Alaska Natives are eligible for public assistance programs such as Medicaid, the number who actually enroll to receive the benefits are small (Kaiser Commission, 2000). Numerous factors appear to contribute to this finding including a lack of awareness about the program, the difficulty in the enrollment process itself, and a general reluctance of Indian people to use non-Indian, government sponsored resources. For urban Indians, the lack of health insurance is a serious obstacle to receiving comprehensive health care assistance. Since urban programs provide only primary care services, access to specialty and hospital care for the uninsured is increasingly limited.

Changes in the health industry and the expansion of managed care as a preferred approach to insurance has added barriers to care through both written and unwritten policies for providers. Mergers and acquisitions of medical groups and hospitals have also changed the historic relationships among service providers for the uninsured and indigent. Access to specialty consultation in particular is a growing problem for urban Indian health programs.

As the cost of health care continues to rise, and as health insurance premiums rise to meet these costs, larger segments of the urban Indian community are without health insurance. This is particularly true for dependent family members because the escalation in cost for employer-sponsored insurance has prompted employers to shift dependent coverage costs to the employee, forcing those with lower salaries to leave their dependents without insurance protection.

A particular problem for urban Indian health systems has to do with Indians who have recently left the reservations. Many of these individuals assume that services at urban Indian health programs are similar to those offered at IHS or tribal sites on reservations; most are surprised to learn that fees are charged for care. This misunderstanding can often become a barrier to continued care.

URBAN INDIANS ARE STILL INDIANS

Throughout the past five centuries, efforts to destroy Indian cultures and exterminate Indian people have failed. European colonization has altered, but not eliminated Indians from the Americas. The standing of Indian tribes as sovereign nations with self-governance authority remains a symbol of the tenacity and strength of the Indian ideals.

American citizenship was bestowed on all Indians in 1924(8 U.S.C.A., Section 1401b). American Indians born in the United States are now citizens by birth. Likewise, they are also citizens of the state within which they reside by virtue of the 14th amendment to the Constitution, which stipulates that state citizenship is derived from national citizenship (U.S. Constitution, amendment XIV). Thus, Indians are entitled to the same rights and bear the same responsibilities as all other citizens. Most Indians are also members of an Indian tribe, which is a political body that exercises considerable power of self-governance.

There are currently 558 Indian tribes and Alaskan Native villages that are recognized by the Federal government.[8] These tribes are granted certain benefits that are allocated in recognition of the federal trust responsibility to Indians by virtue of treaties, Supreme Court decisions, legislation, and the U. S. Constitution. In addition, there are approximately another 150 Indian groups

---

[8] The Department of the Interior, Bureau of Indian Affairs publishes a yearly list of tribal entities recognized by the federal government pursuant to Section 104 of P.L. 103-454: 108 Stat. 4792. In the Federal Register 65, No. 49 (March 13, 2000), 558 Indian tribes and Alaska villages were listed.

that have organized as tribes.[9] Many are tribes that were terminated during the 1950s. Several of these groups have received recognition from individual state legislatures, and most are awaiting federal acknowledgement. Congress has the authority to reestablish the federal–tribal relationship with a terminated tribe at any time. Congress' authority extends to all Indian communities in the United States including terminated and non-federally recognized tribes (*United States v. Candelaria*, 271 U.S. 432, 439 (1926); *United States v. Sandavol*, 231 U.S. 28, 45-46 (1913)).

Not all Indian tribal members share equal standing in Indian Country. Since each tribe has the authority to determine membership, tribes may periodically change their membership requirements. Tribes are political entities, and as such membership in a tribe is a political distinction, and not necessarily an ethnic designation; because tribal membership is political and not necessarily racial, benefits afforded a tribe must be extended to any tribal member regardless of their ethnicity.

Intermarriage between whites and Indians in the United States has a long history. Prior to the removal of Indians to western areas in the mid-1830s (R.S. Section 2114, Act of May 28, 1830. C. 148, 4 Stat. 12.), it was believed that intermarriage facilitated good relations between Indians and whites. Early French trappers and hunters often took Indian wives. There were, in fact, some legal attempts to promote intermarriage. For example, in 1784, a bill was presented to the Virginia legislature providing that "every white man who married an Indian woman should be paid ten pounds, and five for each child born of such marriage."[10] If a white woman married an Indian man, the white woman was also entitled to "ten pounds with which the county court should buy them livestock."

Early federal guidelines usually considered one-quarter Indian blood as a minimum standard for benefits. However, contemporary tribal definitions may only require a demonstration of Indian decendency without a blood quantum factor in response to this history of intermarriage and the continuation of this practice today.

The definition of "urban Indian" in P.L. 94-437 expands the criteria for eligibility for Indian health care (25 U.S.C.A., Section 1601 (f).). In many respects, this legislation recognizes the ethnic and political nature of Indian affairs, attempting to rectify these confusing and potentially conflicting factors. Thus, for purposes of receiving health care from an urban Indian health contractor, strict guidelines are not required to be viewed as "Indian."

---

[9] National Archives web site. National Archives & Records Administration, American Indian History and Related Issues, Indian of America, List of Federally Non-Recognized Tribes compiled by Professor Troy Johnson, California State University, Long Beach.

[10] Neither the Virginia bill nor an attempt in 1824 by William H. Crawford who advocated for similar legislation before the U.S. Congress ever became law. However, the practice may well have been used to support this idea. Sandefer 1996, page 211.

SUMMARY

The migration of Indian people to American cities is a fact clearly supported by census figures. While fewer than 2 million Americans self-identified as "Indian" in the 1990 census, over 8 million Americans acknowledged Indian heritage.[11] This figure appears to support the premise that factors like intermarriage, relocation, and multi-generational city life have distanced many people from the political realities that shroud Indian affairs today. As a result, many Americans of Indian heritage may choose to claim themselves as racially Indian consistent with the census findings.

As is frequently expressed when addressing Indian issues, Indians are the beneficiaries of certain resources and programs allocated through their tribes as a result of the special trust relationship created by the U. S. Constitution and enhanced and clarified through Supreme Court decisions, legislation, Executive Orders, and treaties. Indian people are the expected recipients of these benefits, yet historic and political events have fragmented the Indian world leaving out a potentially large number of AI/AN in urban areas. Despite the fact that the federal government accepts some obligation in facilitating access to health care for urban Indians, a significant gap remains in information dissemination and in the lack of a coordinated effort in addressing the health problems of urban AI/AN.

Urban Indian health is faced with significant challenges. Congress continues to allocate just over 1 percent of the federal annual appropriation for Indian health to serve this growing population. Health care costs, particularly in cities, continue to rise at rates that far exceed government sponsorship. Changes in health care financing, particularly the shift to managed care, add new barriers for those who lack health insurance. Social, cultural, and historic factors remain obstacles in engaging and involving Indian people in the benefits western medicine has to offer. The lack of a national uniform data collection and reporting system prohibits urban Indian health programs from accurately describing their needs or comparing the intensity of problems with other affected groups.

Major steps have occurred in the past half-decade to raise the level of awareness to the plight of urban Indians. But raising the health status of this group to parity with mainstream Americans will require a long-term investment.

REFERENCES

Cohen FS. *The Handbook of Federal Indian Law*, 1982 Edition. William S. Hein & Co.,Chapter 2, Section E2f, Termination, pages 169 -175.

---

[11] The 1990 Census asked the question "what is this person's ancestry or ethnic origin." To this question, 8,798,000 individuals stated American Indian ancestry indicating a very large pool of "potential" American Indian persons who may or may not choose to identify as American Indian by race. Sandefer 1996 page 86.

Grossman D, Krieger J, Sugarman J, Forquera R. Health Status of Urban American Indians and Alaska Natives: A Population-Based Study, *Journal of the American Medical Association*, Volume 271, No. 11: March 16, 1994; p 845–850.

Kaiser Commission on Medicaid and the Uninsured. *Fact Sheet: Health Insurance Coverage and Access to Care Among American Indians and Alaska Natives*. June 2000.

Olsen JS, Wilson R. *Native Americans in the Twentieth Century*. Provo, Utah: Brigham Young University Press; 1984.

Sandefer G; Rindfuss R, Cohen B Eds. *Changing Numbers, Changing Needs — American Indian Demography and Public Health*, Washington, D.C.: National Academy Press; 1996.

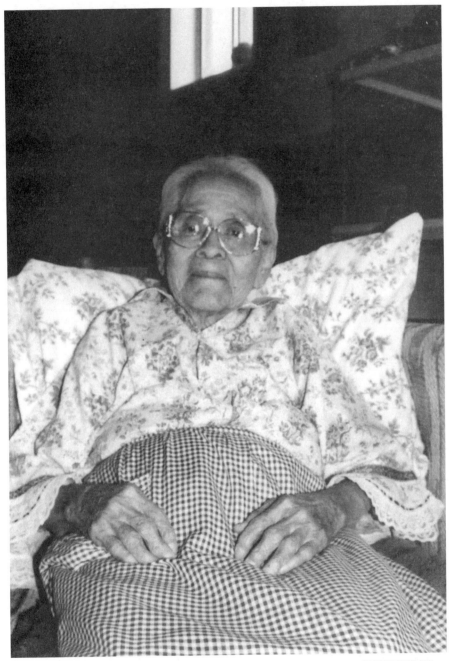

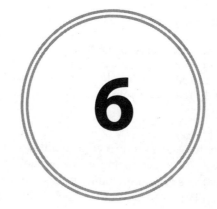

THE ELDER INDIAN POPULATION
AND LONG-TERM CARE
Dave Baldridge

O f the many distinctive values held by America's 556 federally recognized Indian tribes, perhaps none is as universally acknowledged as that of respect for elders. In traditional Indian cultures, elders are viewed as possessors of knowledge, history, and spirituality. Throughout Indian Country, elders and the values they embody are recognized as a legacy to be honored.

Historically, the roles of elders have comprised an important thread in the daily fabric of Indian life. As part of extended families which often included uncles, aunts, grandchildren, other relatives, and clan members, elders served as mentors and counselors, reinforcing a wide range of mores and folkways. Elders also tended crops and gardens, maintained households, and provided day care for young relatives.

Assimilation in the last century began to change the primary roles of Indian family members, including elders. On reservations, once-essential hunting or agricultural skills diminished in value as entire communities became reliant on processed foods. Diets changed dramatically with an influx of commodity and "fast foods." Reservation lifestyles became sedentary. Urban Indians, removed from their extended families, lost contact with tribal socialization and support mechanisms. They began to integrate into new communities and lifestyles.

> Traditional medical values were replaced by contemporary (values). Traditional leaders . . . were replaced by appointed or elected tribal officials. Extended, family-based long-term care was replaced by distant nursing homes. Reservation economics required elders to seek full or part-time employment. Traditionally healthy elders began to experience health problems associated with diabetes and alcoholism. The elder population, once carefully nurtured . . . became instead primary care givers and, frequently, sole financial providers. (Baldridge 1996, p. 185)

Given their former status and prominence in traditional Indian society, both rural and urban elders are experiencing an evolution into unclear and less meaningful roles. At the same time, Indian elders are living longer, and the emergence of chronic diseases creates greater needs for health care, including long-term care.

DEFINING INDIAN ELDERS

The traditional tribal concept of an Indian "elder" as deserving of respect and deference exists without regard for numerical age. It is defined more by the significance of the elder's role in tribal society. Politically, the definition of an elder is most commonly based on eligibility for federal aging programs, which begins at age 55 or 65, depending on the program as shown in Table 6.1.

The 55-and-older definition is commonly used by advocates, and is the minimum age for voting membership in the National Indian Council on Aging

Federal Program	Minimum Age
Older Americans Act, SCSEP*	55
Older Americans Act, Title VI nutrition/other services	50
Social Security/Medicare	65**
IHS Elder Health Care Initiative	55
Medicaid, Old Age Assistance	65
Tribal Aging Programs	Varies

*SCSEP is the Senior Community Service Employment Program.
**Social Security is raising its minimum age for full benefits by two months each year to phase in a minimum age of 67 by the year 2022.

TABLE 6.1 AGE DEFINITIONS OF "ELDER" BY FEDERAL PROGRAM

(NICOA). NICOA believes that although some programmatic age definitions may be required, it is important to remember that to develop a comprehensive continuum of care requires involving people of all ages in advocacy and planning.

Any definition of Indian elders, of course, also depends on the more complex consideration of "who is an Indian." This definition varies widely by tribe and by federal agency. This consideration is of no small importance in Indian Country, where eligibility for care through the Indian health system or membership in a profitable gaming tribe may have financial implications. Many tribes use a minimum blood quantum as the criterion for tribal membership. Upon request, the Bureau of Indian Affairs issues Certificates of Degree of Indian Blood (CDIB) cards to Indians, documenting degree of Indian blood.

Some tribes, such as the Cherokee Nation, base tribal membership on proof of ancestry as recorded by public documents in the 1800s and early 1900s. Thus, people may be members of the Cherokee Nation even though they may have such small percentages of Indian blood that they would be ineligible for membership in a tribe that used a blood quantum approach.

As we seek to understand the health problems of American Indian/Alaska Native elders and to propose systemic improvements to better serve their needs, it should also be noted that data sets and policy approaches are derived from sources that use different definitions of American Indian. Indian Health Service eligibility depends on enrollment in a federally recognized tribe, accepting the different tribal definitions. The U.S. Census and most federal programs identify Indians by self-report, regardless of tribal membership. National organizations that provide leadership on American Indian issues differ in their membership requirements: the National Indian Council on Aging (NICOA) requires that its voting members be from a federally recognized tribe, but the National Congress of American Indians (NCAI) accepts tribes that have been recognized by individual states but not by the federal government.

DEMOGRAPHICS

In 2000 there were approximately 259,000 American Indians and Alaska Natives (AI/AN) age 55 and older, according to the U.S. Census Bureau projections, although many advocates feel that undercounting and misclassification result in significant inaccuracies (Bureau of the Census 2000). These elders are diverse members of the 556 federally recognized tribes:

> They live on treaty-based reservations, executive order reservations, state-created reservations, or . . . with bands of Indians who do not have federal recognition . . . . They speak more

than (est.) 150 different languages. Eighty percent live west
of the Mississippi, divided more or less evenly between reservation and urban residences. More than five thousand elders
live in Los Angeles. They live diversely–in Arizona hogans
miles from the nearest paved roads, and in Oklahoma HUD
housing projects. (Baldridge 1996, p. 185)

The Administration on Aging reports that Indian elders reside in each of the 50
states and the District of Columbia. Almost half of AI/AN elders live in three
states: Oklahoma, California, and Arizona. Other states with substantial numbers include New Mexico, North Carolina, Alaska, New York, Texas,
Washington, and Michigan (National Committee to Preserve Social Security
and Medicare 1999). AI/AN elders are the most rural of all ethnic elderly.
Widely dispersed geographically, about half of elders live in rural areas. They
often live in small reservation communities, miles from the nearest health care
facility.

Indian elders live in poverty more often than other elders in our country.
According to the 1990 Census, 27 percent of American Indians 65 to 74 years
old lived below the poverty level, compared to 10 percent of the U.S. All Races
population and 8 percent of Whites. As AI/ANs live longer, their poverty rates
are double those of other elderly people. One-third of AI/AN elders older than
75 live in poverty, compared to 17 percent for All Races, and 15 percent for
Whites (Indian Health Service 1996). While 14 percent of AI/AN elderly in
urban areas are in poverty, in non-metropolitan areas the proportion is even
larger at 24 percent (U.S. Dept. of Commerce 1993). The median income for
AI/AN males aged 65 or over is $9,967, as compared to $14,775 for White
males. For women in this age group, the median income is $6,004 for AI/AN
and $8,297 for whites (Bacon 1993).

Poverty on Indian reservations involves more than income. It is also reflected in substandard, overcrowded housing:

Homes are generally considered crowded if they contain more
than one person per room. Nationally, 5 percent of all households were crowded in 1990. This percentage was much
lower than the approximately 20 percent back in 1940 . . ..
But the national conditions of a half-century ago were nothing
compared to what American Indian households on reservations face today. In 1990, an astounding *one-third* of them
were crowded! (Bureau of the Census 1994, p.4)

Several sources describe the inadequacy of AI/AN housing. The 1980 Census
reported that 16 percent of reservation homes lacked electricity, 17 percent
had no refrigerators, 21 percent had no indoor toilets, and 50 percent had no

telephones. A 1981 White House Conference on Aging report added that 26 percent of AI/AN homes were built prior to 1939, 26 percent had no indoor plumbing at all, and only 50 percent had complete bathrooms indoors. And an unpublished 1988 NICOA study described the living conditions of AI/AN elders, revealing that 69 percent of elders' homes had more than three persons co-resident; 49 percent had areas with no floor covering; 42 percent had broken windows, 35 percent had broken doors, 47 percent had no heat other than wood stoves or fireplaces, and 75 percent had no telephones.

Dismal reservation economies and lack of education have contributed to Indian elder poverty. Lack of employment undoubtedly contributes to the low rates of AI/AN participation in Social Security. Since Social Security creates eligibility for Medicare, this also results in lower participation in Medicare. Furthermore, the pattern of low employment that starts early in life in AI/AN communities continues into the older ages. In 1990, 15 percent of AI/AN males age 65 to 69 participated in the labor force, compared to 28 percent of their White counterparts. Less than 9 percent of AI/AN males age 70 and older participated in the labor force in 1990 (National Committee to Preserve Social Security and Medicare 1999).

Nearly 10 percent of all AI/AN elderly have no formal education and only about 27 percent have graduated from high school (Bacon 1993). An estimated 150 Indian languages are spoken today, many of which serve as primary languages in elder households. Because English is often their second language and their education is limited, many AI/AN elders are not proficient in reading, writing, speaking, or understanding spoken English. AI/AN elders indicate that they frequently don't understand explanations of their eligibility for federal benefits, for example. This perception is substantiated by the Health Care Financing Administration (HCFA 1996) statistics indicating that 157,000 Indians who are eligible for Medicaid are not receiving those benefits.

HEALTH AND DISABILITY STATUS

Despite provisions in the 1921 Snyder Act that define the federal trust responsibility to American Indians to include health care, Indian elders suffer poorer health than any comparable population in America. When compared to the U.S. All Races population, Indians are 5.8 times more likely to die of alcoholism, 4.8 times more likely to die of tuberculosis, 2.3 times more likely to die of diabetes, and 2.1 times more likely to die in accidents (Indian Health Service 1997a). Table 6.4 gives the leading causes of death for American Indians and Alaska Natives older than 65 years of age.

Even though AI/AN elder life expectancy has improved dramatically in recent years, longevity has been accompanied by relatively high rates of chronic illness (John 1994). Of all the health conditions affecting Indian elders, Indian country's ongoing epidemic of type 2 diabetes is the most dramatic. Since at least the 1980s, this epidemic has exploded, not only in Indian

Sources of Income	American Indian & Alaska Native	U.S. White Population
Social Security	30.3%	25.0%
Earnings	36.4%	34.1%
Asset Income	9.2%	23.9%
Pension	15.4%	14.6%
Public Assistance	5.4%	1.0%
Other	3.3%	1.4%

TABLE 6.2 INCOME SOURCES FOR AMERICAN INDIANS AND ALASKA NATIVES OLDER THAN 60 YEARS OF AGE, BY PERCENT OF INCOME IN 1989
SOURCE: NATIONAL COMMITTEE TO PRESERVE SOCIAL SECURITY AND MEDICARE (1999)

Population Group	Percent Eligible for Medicaid Who are Receiving Medicaid
Hispanics	91%
Whites	87%
Asian/Pacific Islanders	83%
African Americans	82%
American Indians	65%
U.S. Total Population	88%

TABLE 6.3 ACCESS TO MEDICAID BENEFITS
SOURCE: HEALTH CARE FINANCING ADMINISTRATION MEDICAID STATISTICS 1996

Country, but in communities of color throughout the world. Among the Pima people in Arizona, who have the highest known rates of diabetes in the world, 80 percent of tribal members over age 55 have diabetes (Sevilla 1999). The IHS 1998 Diabetes Audit shows that 48 percent of Indians with diabetes are older than 55 and 22 percent are older than 65. Nationally, more than one in five Indian elders have diabetes.

In a growing number of Indian communities, more than 50 percent of the population over age 50 has the disease. It accounts for one of every three elder visits to clinics (Kelly Acton, M.D., Director, IHS Diabetes Program, personal communication, April 7, 2000). Obesity, poor nutrition, lack of public health education, and lack of access to regular medical care all contribute to the difficulties Indian elders—and their family caregivers—experience as they try to deal with this disease.

Cause of Death	AI/AN		U.S. All Races	U.S. White	Ratio of AI/AN rate to U.S. rate for:	
	Number	Rate	Rate	Rate	All Races	White
All Causes	10,709	4,790.8	5,047.7	5,036.6	0.9	1.0
Diseases of the heart	3,439	1,538.5	1,891.0	1,895.6	0.8	0.8
Malignant neoplasms	2,081	931.0	1,133.7	1,123.4	0.8	0.8
Cerebrovascular diseases	727	325.2	401.4	397.4	0.8	0.8
Diabetes mellitus	698	312.3	123.6	114.5	2.5	2.7
Pneumonia, influenza	592	264.8	225.3	228.4	1.2	1.2
COPD and allied conditions	454	203.1	263.7	275.6	0.8	0.7
Accidents	316	141.9	84.8	84.7	1.7	1.7
Nephritis, nephrotic syndrome, nephrosis	225	100.7	60.2	56.2	1.7	1.8
Chronic liver disease, cirrhosis	167	74.7	31.5	32.0	2.4	2.3

TABLE 6.4 LEADING CAUSES OF DEATH FOR AMERICAN INDIANS AND ALASKA NATIVES OLDER THAN 65 YEARS, COMPARING MORTALITY RATES WITH OTHER U.S. POPULATIONS, 1993 *(Rates per 100,000 population. AI/AN numbers and rates are adjusted for miscoding of Indian identify on death certificates.)*
SOURCE: INDIAN HEALTH SERVICE. 1997 TRENDS IN INDIAN HEALTH, TABLE 4.7, P. 61

Diabetes and other chronic illnesses result in functional impairments among American Indian elders. The majority of Indian elders, 73 percent of those aged 55 and over, report limitations in their ability to carry out the basic activities of daily living (NICOA 1981).

According to the U.S. Dept. of Education (1987), the prevalence of disability among American Indians is among the highest of any ethnic group in the nation. Advocates say that similar studies have found that disabled American Indians experience higher rates and greater severity of secondary conditions than other groups. The American Indian Disability Legislation Project (AIDLP) estimates that about one-fourth of America's AI/AN population is disabled (Fowler, et al 1996). In a 1995 survey of 143 tribal governments, the AIDLP identified the following types and rates of disability for American Indians in the lower 48 states: 29 percent with diabetes; 22 percent with emotional problems, and 11 percent who were slow to learn. In survey results from Alaska, emotional problems ranked first (31 percent), followed by slow to learn (17 percent), hearing impaired (15 percent), and diabetes (12 percent).

The *NICOA Report: Health and Long-Term Care for Indian Elders* (John and Baldridge 1996) noted distinct gender differences in disabilities for Indian elders. Among male Indians older than 65, approximately 27 percent reported mobility or self-care limitations, compared to 32 percent for females. Indian elders reported the highest level of work disability among five racial groups, 44 percent compared to only 29 percent of their non-Hispanic White age peers. Among American Indians between the ages of 65 and 74, a total of 21 percent of men and 23 percent of women reported either a mobility or self-care limitation. In the 75 and over age group, 33 percent of men and 41 percent of women reported these limitations (National Committee to Preserve Social Security and Medicare 1999).

ELDER ABUSE AND VICTIMIZATION

Caught in a vicious cycle of poverty and rural isolation, disease and disability, Indian elders often suffer the secondary effects of these problems, including alcoholism (both their own and that of others), domestic violence, and crime. Baldridge and Brown (1988) concluded that studies on American Indian elder abuse confirm a national pattern that "most elder abuse is related to the many problems of elderly people being cared for at home by informal caregivers." Elder abuse can be physical, emotional, or financial, and may include neglect.

Not only is institutional care generally unavailable in Indian Country, few community-based programs are in place. Not surprisingly, the burden of long-term care falls to families, whose traditional tribal values include familial obligations and interdependence (Red Horse study as cited in Hennessy and John 1996). However, family members often undertake extremely demanding tasks in caring for and preventing the institutional placement of an elderly relative (Manson 1989). Care giving often takes individuals out of the workforce and creates a greater strain on family finances.

One study suggests that Indian and white caregivers differ in their perceptions of care giving. American Indians perceived themselves as having less control over the situation and placed more emphasis on the positive aspects of managing an elder's long-term care (Strong study as cited by Hennessy and John 1995). Strong characterized Indian caregivers' coping strategy as one of "passive forbearance," of accepting and adapting to the care giving situation rather than trying to actively control it. Other researchers identified sources of perceived burden among caregivers in five New Mexico tribes, including competing responsibilities and negative effects on family relationships and on personal health and well-being:

> These burdens were often produced or exacerbated by conditions encountered . . . such as lack of indoor plumbing, the need to chop and haul wood, or lack of availability or access to comprehensive services. (Hennessy and John 1995, p. 5)

Finding Indian caregivers to be more proactive, and even resentful about the lack of services available to them, Hennessy and John also found that care giving families sometimes coped by taking advantage of available IHS facilities for (unauthorized) respite care.

A study of Navajo elderly found a number of caregiver factors associated with elder abuse, including the suddenness of becoming dependent and families "having care giving responsibilities thrust upon them for which they were unprepared" (Brown et al 1990).

In 1998, the National Indian Council on Aging conducted an informal survey of 189 elders in five states, soliciting comments about the perceived impact of Welfare Reform legislation. More than four out of five elder respondents (81percent) thought that "some elders are worried about being abused." Among respondents, 86 percent indicated that elders should not be asked to care for young children for extended periods of time. Furthermore, if it was difficult for an elder to take care of young children, 77 percent felt that asking them to do so would be "abusive or wrong."

However, elders do not always perceive abuse. Elder victims of financial exploitation believe that "giving money to family members in need was a cultural duty. They insisted that it was their responsibility to share financial resources with family members even though they were often severely deprived as a result" (Brown, et al 1990).

The Final Report from NICOA's 1998 national aging conference, *American Voices: Indian Elders Speak*, included comments from elders that "violence, gang activity, and undisciplined children are real threats to elders on the reservations." Elders asked for "Abused Elderly Protection Teams" and for advocates to alert tribal leaders about grants designed to reduce youth and gang violence. Elders' concerns about crime appear to be substantiated by statistics. The Department of Justice (1998) cites some disturbing statistics:

- Violent crime is rising significantly in Indian Country—in sharp contrast to national trends;

- A 1995 Bureau of Indian Affairs study showed 375 gangs with some 4,650 gang members in or near Indian Country;

- The homicide rate for Indian males is almost three times higher than the rate for white males. In 1996 the Navajo Nation's homicide rate would have placed it among the nation's top 20 most violent cities.

Community and family violence is distressing for elders, particularly since the concepts of intra-tribal crime and familial abuse are so foreign to their beliefs.

ACCESS TO HEALTH CARE

The IHS reports that people over age 64 comprise 5.6 percent of the user population and consume 10.7 percent of ambulatory medical clinical services, 14.4 percent of inpatient discharges, and 21.7 percent of inpatient days (IHS 1996). The report notes that Indian elders receive health services at lower rates than their counterparts in the general population. For example, the IHS hospital discharge rate of 182.9 discharges per 1,000 population is 46 percent less than the U.S. rate of 341.6.

Indian elders generally face the same barriers to access as others who live in poverty, including lack of transportation, low levels of education, and an obvious lack of resources. Housing conditions are often so dismal that home health care becomes nearly impossible. For example, home dialysis is not possible without running water, electricity, and a telephone.

In addition, AI/AN elders living on reservations and in Alaska Native villages face rural access problems, including a lack of services and a shortage of jobs that provide health and retirement benefits. Distinctive cultural issues compound both the problems of poverty and of rural access to care; these cultural barriers often include limited proficiency in English, although cultural factors extend beyond language and the need for translators. Often Western medical providers are ignorant about tribal social and family structure, cultural beliefs about health and illness, traditional Indian medicine, and appropriate and respectful ways of interacting with elders.

In many ways, the problems that Indian elders face in accessing care are no different from the access issues experienced by other members of their tribes. The problems are pervasive and cannot be solved by isolating elder issues in order to address them. If an elder has little education, it may be indicative that the tribe may not have adequate schools. If the elder cannot find a job, the tribe may not be able to attract viable employers to the reservation. If the elder cannot afford a car, neither can the tribe provide regular public transportation or safe roads.

Lack of alternate medical resources, whether private insurance or public programs, may limit AI/AN access to specialty medical- and long-term care, including eyeglasses, hearing aids, or other assistive devices and durable medical equipment that are not included as part of IHS health benefits.

Furthermore, there are psychological barriers to accessing health care. Joyce Dugan, former principal chief of the Eastern Band of Cherokees, expresses dismay about Indian country's apparent acceptance of diabetes:

> My concern is that we as a people are beginning to accept the disease as our fate, that (we think) we can't do anything about it. We have come to believe that it is not a matter of whether we will get the disease but when we will get it." (Joyce

Dugan, former chief, Eastern Band of Cherokee Indians, personal communication, October 9, 1999)

A long history of disease and disability can make people feel resigned to their fate rather than proactive in prevention, early detection, and treatment of their health conditions.

Ironically, of all the epidemics that have ravaged Indian country over the past three hundred years, diabetes is unique in that the patient generally can manage it. Rather than resignation and hopelessness, diabetes presents opportunities to live a healthy life through daily regulation of diet, exercise, and (sometimes) insulin. However, most people cannot do this alone. New money for diabetes prevention, education, and treatment appropriated by Congress in the Balanced Budget Act of 1997 is just beginning to help tribes develop prevention programs. The expense of public health education about the dangers of obesity, for example, are miniscule when compared to the costs of dialysis—to the patient, the tribe, the provider, and the insurer (Medicare covers the cost of dialysis treatment for End Stage Renal Disease (ESRD)). Diabetes in Indian elders demands a continuum of care that includes prevention, clinical treatment, and intensive home-based long-term care.

Most Indian elders who require nursing home care would meet Medicaid eligibility standards. The reality, however, is that most elders needing nursing home care must either go to an off-reservation nursing home that is typically a long distance away in an unfamiliar or uncomfortable setting, or forego the needed level of care. Mainstream health care providers, especially long-term care providers, historically have found the rural isolation and small numbers of American Indian and Alaska Native communities to be insurmountable barriers to establishing profitable health or long-term care programs. Even those communities where long-term care services are available, the lack of private or public third-party payers makes such services virtually unobtainable. The high costs of these services make them financially out-of-reach for most people of limited means, including the AI/AN population. Third-party payers make it more economically feasible to provide long-term care services in a particular area. However, this may not be sufficient incentive to operate long-term care services in remote reservation areas.

The small body of research available indicates that most long-term care in Indian communities is provided by family members, with little or no support from national, state, or even community-based programs. Nevertheless, the I/T/U system offers a network of Public Health nurses and Community Health Representatives (CHRs) who serve as the primary interface between the AI/AN elder and the health care delivery system.

RATIONING CARE

Having lived most or all of their lives as IHS clients, Indian elders have long become accustomed to rationed health care and the absence of geriatric services; perhaps foremost among potential health services that the IHS has not provided to Indians is long-term care.

The IHS' historical failure to provide long-term care is based in part upon the limited resources that have affected the agency's priorities for health care spending. From the time that the U.S. Public Health Service assumed responsibility for Indian health, a high priority was given to maternal and child health because the Indian population was characterized by: (1) very high birth rates; (2) high rates of maternal/infant mortality; and (3) life spans that (30 years ago) were 18 years less than the national average. Two of the agency's foremost achievements over the past two decades have been a 90 percent reduction in maternal/infant mortality since 1955 and an increase in Indian life expectancy from 61 to 72 years between 1972 and 1994 (IHS 1997).

The prohibitive costs of providing institutional long-term care doubtless weighed heavily in the decision by the IHS to exclude this service. This was further justified by interpretations of legislation authorizing the IHS to engage in various activities.

> Historically, IHS solicitors have argued that the agency 'is not authorized' to provide long-term care, and that authority for institutional care was retained by the BIA when the Transfer Act of 1954 charged IHS with the responsibility for Indian health care. (John and Baldridge 1996, p.9)

However, this interpretation was never construed to prevent the IHS from providing all services in the long-term care continuum.

Perhaps the foremost factor contributing to the absence of long-term care in the IHS program was that, until the mid-1990s, demands for long-term care by tribes were few. Long-term care seldom ranked among top ten priorities presented annually to IHS leadership by either tribal leaders or IHS Area directors. If the IHS has been shortsighted regarding the growing need for long-term care, it appears in retrospect that Indian Country's leadership may have been responsible as well.

Having conquered some of the most fundamental public health challenges of maternal and child health and infectious disease, a new look at the epidemiology of American Indians and Alaska Natives suggested the emergence of chronic diseases and a growing elderly population:

> In part, the interest in long-term care for American Indian elders has been aroused because this group constitutes one of the

fastest growing and neediest subpopulations in the United States. Moreover, it is estimated that by the end of the century, the number of American Indians aged 75 years and older— some 42,473 by the 1990 census—will at least double. (Manson study as cited by Hennessy and John 1996, p. 275)

However, the lack of funding, lack of demand from tribes, and lack of advocacy for and by elders meant that IHS was not addressing long-term care:

> The IHS does not actively recruit geriatricians or provide geriatric training . . ... does not provide community-based long-term care programs or home-delivered long-term health care services, nor does the agency operate nursing homes or any other long-term care residential facilities. For the most part, no federally funded long-term care is available in Indian Country. Not only is geriatric care absent from the IHS infrastructure, the agency has resisted assuming the lead in coordinating the currently fragmented and incomplete community-based services available through . . . other federal agencies. (John and Baldridge 1996, p.9)

Indian elder advocates began to question the IHS interpretation of the statute. Recognizing that the IHS may be legally prevented from building hospitals or facilities to provide primarily domiciliary care, Spencer and Funk nevertheless contended that:

> . . . the provisions do not preclude the IHS from providing technical assistance and medical support to tribal home and community care programs and facilities, including skilled nursing homes. Nor is the IHS prevented from providing formal home health care programs or geriatric training for its staff. (Spencer and Funk 1995, p. 5)

The demand for greater IHS involvement in long-term care has not resulted in additional Congressional appropriations to meet this need.

However, significant structural changes were being implemented in the Indian health care delivery system—changes that would alter the course of Indian health care delivery throughout the nation. Beginning work in 1993, a national Indian Health Design Team issued its Final Report in 1998, confirming a process that was already underway— a major shift of authorities and responsibilities from the IHS to tribes. Under Public Law 93-638 (Indian Self-Determination and Educational Reform Act), Indian tribes were assuming responsibility for the provision of health care to their members.

Decentralization of Indian health care delivery in the 1990s meant that individual tribes would soon be providing all or most of their own long-term care.

Presently, however, because the IHS has never taken the lead in long-term care services, tribes currently have little assurance that eligibility, funding, or reimbursement mechanisms are in place. Tribes have had to develop their own relationships with the Health Care Financing Administration (HCFA) and states to negotiate regulations and funding mechanisms for long-term care facilities.

TRIBALLY-OPERATED NURSING HOMES

Tribes face especially daunting challenges related to building, owning, and operating nursing homes. Nationally, only 12 reservation-based nursing homes existed in 1993 (see Table 6.5). These nursing homes are located in only 10 of the 34 states with tribes.

A pivotal issue in the decision to build and operate a tribal nursing home is how to finance the care provided within the facility. Since few Indian elders can pay for the high cost of nursing home care themselves, financial support is needed from the tribe's own resources or from third-party payment sources. Several nursing homes in Indian Country remain in operation today only because tribes heavily subsidize them; however, most tribes do not have the resources to do this. The most likely payment source is Medicaid.

States are responsible for certifying and licensing nursing homes for purposes of Medicaid payment, but obtaining state certification and licensing is often viewed by tribes as an intrusion on their sovereignty. Furthermore, a history of adversarial relationships between tribes and states often makes it difficult for tribes to establish nursing homes, because the decision to seek Medicaid certification requires significant interaction with state government. Moreover, Medicaid-certified nursing homes must meet stringent standards under both state and federal law. The cost of building a facility or converting a building from another use requires significant construction costs to meet Medicaid standards. The debt load on the financing of mortgages for nursing homes can be extremely burdensome for long periods of time.

Still another challenge to tribes running their own nursing homes is the ability to attract, train, and retain qualified staff that meets state and federal standards. Nursing homes are especially labor-intensive enterprises. While finding certified nurse assistants to provide most of the daily hands-on care in nursing home might be seen as a challenge, it is also an opportunity for tribal employment. However, there may be a need to coordinate with tribal colleges to provide the necessary training, and not every tribe has tribal colleges or other training facilities available.

Most tribes desiring to operate their own nursing homes want to make their facilities culturally attractive to their elders. However, tribes must also decide whether to make the facility available to other tribes and the larger non-

Facility Name	State	Tribe(s) Operating The Facility	Number of Beds
Chinle	AZ	Navajo	79
Blackfeet	MT	Blackfeet	49
Oneida	WI	Oneida	50
Toyei	AZ	Navajo	64
Carl T. Curtis	NE	Omaha	25
White River	AZ	Apache	10
Laguna Rainbow	NM	Laguna	25
Colville	WA	Colville	52
Morning Star Manor	WY	Shoshone, Arapahoe	50
Choctaw Residential Center	MS	Mississippi Band of Choctaw Indians	120
Kotzebue Senior Citizens Cultural Center	AK	Eskimo	9
Jourdain/Perpich Extended Care Facility	MN	Red Lake Chippewa	47

TABLE 6.5 TRIBALLY-OPERATED NURSING HOMES IN THE UNITED STATES IN 1993

Indian community. Opening the facility to the broader community may be essential for financial viability, since there are often not enough Indian elders in need of nursing home care to maintain an adequate occupancy rate. Furthermore, some non-Indian patients may have more comprehensive insurance coverage that will help to absorb the costs of caring for AI/AN patients who do not have alternate resources.

FINANCING LONG-TERM CARE

The provision of long-term care in the United States can be characterized by two overall patterns. First, most care for people of all ages with chronic illnesses and significant disabilities that limit one's independence is provided on an informal basis by family members. It is estimated that as much as 80 percent of all long-term care services are provided by informal caregivers, most typically spouses and adult children. Second, for those who obtain formal, paid, long-term care, the primary source of such care has been in the institutional setting, usually a nursing home.

These two patterns have been driven primarily by availability and cost considerations. Over the past four decades, the principle source of payment for long-term care-related services has been through the federal Medicare and Medicaid programs. Medicare and Medicaid accounted for 57 percent of all nursing home expenditures in the nation in 1994 (HCFA 1998). Despite their overall scope, coverage for long-term care services under either program is quite limited and for the most part has emphasized payment for stays in nursing homes ("nursing facilities").

MEDICAID

Medicaid is the most important source of coverage and subsequent payment of services for individuals with chronic illnesses and long-term significant disabilities. Medicaid is the major public payment source for nursing home care in the U.S., paying more than 50 percent of nursing home costs and covering 68 percent of nursing home residents (HCFA 1999a).

While Medicaid was enacted into law in 1965 to be the nation's health care program for the poor, the single largest category of expenditure within Medicaid is for nursing home care. This is due to two key elements of Medicaid policy: first, Medicaid has always recognized nursing home care as a covered service; second, Medicaid policy allows individual beneficiaries to "spend down" their personal income and assets to qualify for Medicaid coverage, thus opening the door to a beneficiary population whose income would otherwise not meet traditional poverty thresholds.

The majority of Americans who need long-term care for chronic illnesses and disabilities have had access to Medicaid coverage in a nursing home, provided their impairment levels were great enough and their income and assets were limited enough to meet Medicaid standards. Under Medicaid, the individual's income is first applied to the nursing home's cost and then Medicaid provides payment to the facility for the difference between the amount the individual pays and the facility's Medicaid-approved rate.

Medicaid is an increasingly important source of payment for long-term care services provided in settings other than nursing facilities. Unlike Medicare, which is a federal program, Medicaid is a shared responsibility between the federal government and individual states. While federal Medicaid law establishes national minimum standards, states have some latitude to determine the services they wish to provide beyond federal requirements. As states have become increasingly concerned about their expenditure patterns for nursing facility care and more sensitive to public demands for covering care in less institutional settings, there has been growth in coverage for care in non-nursing facility settings.

As of 1997, 31 states were exercising their option under Medicaid law to provide "personal care" services to eligible individuals. Examples of such services that help impaired individuals to remain at home include bathing, dressing, toileting, personal hygiene, and light housekeeping. Moreover, most states now provide some form of home and community-based care, such as personal care, meal preparation, adult day health, and respite care, to frail elders and other disabled Medicaid recipients through Medicaid "waivers" granted by the federal government for home and community based services (HCBS).

Requirements governing state use of Medicaid HCBS waivers are stringent. States must assure the federal government that, on an average per capita basis, the cost of providing home and community-based services will not exceed the cost of care for an identical population in an institutional setting. While the use of Medicaid waivers and the personal care option vary considerably from state-to-state, every state has at least one HCBS waiver in operation (Health Care Financing Administration 1999).[1]

[1] Technically, Arizona does not have a HCBS waiver, but another form of Medicaid waiver that allows the state to provide the equivalent of HCBS.

Indian Country has not benefited from Medicaid's long-term care funding in the same way that the general population has, despite the disproportionate level of eligibility among Indian elders. This is not only because there are few nursing homes in Indian country due to federal and state Medicaid requirements and reimbursement levels, but because there are also state certification hurdles that make it exceptionally difficult for tribes to open and sustain a nursing facility. Similar barriers exist with regard to tribes starting up and maintaining various home and community-based long-term care services, such as personal care, respite services, and adult day care.

In addition to complicated rules governing nursing care, tribes face an equal number of problems trying to secure Medicaid funding for home- and community-based long-term care services. Under Medicaid, the state may not cover the services offered or needed by the tribe. If they do, the requirements for operating such services may be too difficult for a tribe to meet. The state's Medicaid waiver services may not include the tribe, or the number of individuals approved for services under the state's waiver may be too few to make it economically or geographically feasible for services to reach tribal communities.

MEDICARE

Unlike Medicaid, Medicare is a solely federal program. Coverage for long-term care services under Medicare is much more limited than under Medicaid. In general, Medicare does not provide coverage for long-term care; rather, Medicare services are generally linked to acute illnesses and short-term "spells of illness." Medicare does not cover custodial care, such as help with bathing, dressing, toileting, and eating at home or in a nursing home. The nursing home care provided under Medicare is for "skilled" or rehabilitative care only, provided in a Medicare-certified skilled nursing facility (SNF). SNF coverage requires that the Medicare beneficiary must first have been an in-patient in a hospital prior to admission to the SNF. Medicare covers up to 100 days of SNF care per benefit period as long as the beneficiary needs skilled nursing or rehabilitation services (e.g., physical therapy) on a "daily" basis, as defined by Medicare policy. The cost of SNF care is very steep. Medicare covers the first 20 days of SNF care completely. From days 21-100 the beneficiary is responsible for a daily coinsurance of $96.00 in 1999. Coverage for the SNF benefit is provided under Part A of Medicare.

Medicare also covers home health care; but as with the SNF benefit, the requirements for beneficiaries are stringent. To receive Medicare home health care, the individual must be homebound and need skilled nursing care or therapy (e.g., speech, physical) on a part-time or intermittent basis only. Intermittent means "fewer than seven days per week or daily for a finite and predictable time." Part-time is defined as "fewer than eight hours per day for periods of 21 days or less" (Medicare Rights Center 1999). Moreover, beneficiaries must have a home health plan-of-care signed by a physician. Perhaps the most difficult requirement for tribes is that the care must be provided by a certified home health agency. Medicare Part A covers the first 100 days of home health care and days beyond 100 are covered under Part B of Medicare.

Access to Medicare's SNF and home health care benefits are even more limited for Indian elders than Medicaid's nursing facility and other home and community-based services. Few Indian owned or operated Medicare-certified home health agencies (HHAs) and SNFs exist, due in large part to the staffing and administrative requirements. The cost of SNF care beyond the first 20 days of a benefit period is far beyond the reach of most Indian elders. There are federal and state programs to assist low-income Medicare beneficiaries with their Medicare-related co-insurance and other out-of-pocket expenses, such as the Qualified Medicare Beneficiary (QMB) program, but there has not been significant outreach to inform people in Indian Country about this type of assistance. HAs and SNFs that are not tribally operated are not frequently accessed by Indian elders for various reasons, including geographic and cultural barriers.

LONG-TERM CARE INSURANCE AND OTHER SOURCES OF FUNDING

The annual cost of nursing home care now averages about $40,000 and often greatly exceeds that amount. Out-of-pocket costs for services not covered by Medicaid or Medicare are prohibitively expensive, whether in nursing homes, assisted living facilities, or home-like settings (such as respite care or in-home care). Few sources of payment or coverage for long-term care services exist, other than Medicaid and Medicare.

Private insurance policies to cover long-term care have grown significantly over the past few years, but a very small percentage of the general population has this coverage. Moreover, the cost of private long-term care insurance makes it an unobtainable option for the vast majority of Indian elders even if they desired to have such coverage. Many AI/AN elders have cannot afford the premiums and co-pays to add Part B to their Medicare coverage, and the additional costs of wrap-around coverage and long term care coverage are beyond their ability to pay.

FEDERALLY FUNDED PROGRAMS PROVIDING COMMUNITY SERVICES

Title VI of the Older Americans Act (OAA) provides the cornerstone of home-based and community services for reservation-based Indian elders. Nationally, some 228 Title VI sites provide communal and home-delivered meals, socialization, information/referral, and limited transportation for elders. Title VI sites operate in Indian Country under a "separate but parallel" mandate similar to the mainstream federal program, Title III, which provides services through State Units and Area Agencies on Aging. However, the Indian programs authorized in Title VI are severely under-funded. Title VI programs are almost always supplemented by tribal funding, but they are often able to provide little more than a single communal meal on weekdays. Title VI directors who are employed by tribes receive little training in nutrition or program management. On an average, they have a high school education and three years of experience in the program. Yet, these underpaid, overworked and overstressed Title VI directors play critical roles in many elders' lives.

As a rule, Indian elders have learned to expect little from the outside world, so they are heavily reliant on the formal and informal support systems available to them through their communities and families. The support systems that affect Indian elders and the disabled with the greatest frequency and effectiveness have some common characteristics: (1) they are available to the elder in his/her preferred setting (home and/or community); (2) they are provided by someone the elder knows and trusts, almost always by another Indian community member; (3) they are provided within a system or program that the elder knows and trusts, generally the I/T/U system and/or the Title VI program; and (4) to the extent possible, the elder's family is involved (Baldridge and Garrett 1999).

ADVOCACY

American Indian and Alaska Native (AI/AN) elders arguably present the greatest challenge to health policymakers and providers both within and outside of the Indian health care delivery system. Regardless of their rural or urban residence, Indian elders are seemingly invisible to policymakers and providers, and their long-term care needs continue to be ignored by both mainstream and Indian health care delivery systems. Urban elders do not live in large enough community groups to organize a neighborhood advocacy system. With few advocates and little access to the Indian health care delivery system, their needs are seldom considered in the formation of public health policy. Rural elders, frequently living in poverty behind a "reservation curtain," rarely gain the attention of the American public. Elders have more health care needs than any other age group of American Indians and Alaska Natives, yet they have the most difficulty accessing needed services.

NICOA believes that the foremost Indian long-term care issue can be simply stated: It is time for all concerned parties to work toward a single, accessible, culturally-sensitive continuum of care—one which will allow older Indians and Alaska Natives to live out their lives in their own homes and communities. The goal of most long-term care advocates is the seamless integration of elder services into the Indian health care delivery system and traditional community-based systems. In addition to specialized programs for geriatric and long-term care, elders need better access to services overall and sources of funding. Nor should it be forgotten that the burden of long-term care usually falls on younger family members, and that they need support as well. The lack of reimbursement to family members for home care, lack of day care for young children, and the unavailability of respite care all represent legitimate long-term care issues in Indian Country.

ADVOCACY WITHIN TRIBES

Indian tribes, because of their sovereign governmental status, are exempt from the regulations of the Americans with Disabilities Act (ADA). Consequently, tribal governments seemingly have little impetus, other than advocacy by the disabled Indian community, to provide accessible facilities and services. The AIDLP found that only one of 143 tribes surveyed had voluntarily adopted the ADA, and only 13 percent of the tribes had line items in their budgets for disability issues (Fowler, et al 1996). Only 6 percent of individual respondents in the survey felt that their tribal governments were even familiar with major disability legislation.

Education of tribal leaders, community advocates, and AI/AN with disabilities is needed for tribes to deal proactively with this issue, according to LaDonna Fowler of the Montana University Rural Institute on Disabilities. She and others would like to establish a national Indian Technical Assistance Center to provide advocacy and education. She is also advocating for local and regional Offices of Independent Living that would assist both tribes and individuals with referrals and advocacy. The first step is to better identify the magnitude of needs, according to Fowler, "We need a clearer picture of disability in Indian Country. Often, the numbers are vastly underreported and the present health care delivery system does not have a way to accurately (collect them)." (Fowler et al 1996.) Fowler believes that if Indian Country's lack of education and understanding about disability issues could be effectively addressed, a shift from an "institutionalization mentality" toward more effective home- and community-based services might result: She says, "we need to consider the issues of accessibility whenever we build . . . changing our attitudes about people with disabilities and making (home) modifications, providing reasonable accommodations and becoming an inclusive society" (Fowler et al 1996).

ADVOCACY ON A NATIONAL LEVEL

In 1992, the National Indian Council on Aging circulated a 32-page questionnaire about elder concerns to tribes and elder programs across the nation. At NICOA's national Indian aging conference that year, 921 elders from 130 tribes and bands were in attendance and they returned more than 800 responses to the questionnaire on behalf of tribal programs and individual elders.

The conference report, *A National Indian Aging Agenda for the Future*, was endorsed by the National Congress of American Indians, the National Indian Health Board, the Association of American Indian Physicians, and other Inter-Tribal organizations. Containing 112 recommendations, the report became the focus of a 1993 Senate Committee on Indian Affairs staff briefing. This report was updated in 1994 and presented at the NICOA meeting in Spokane, Washington; at that time, 50 additional resolutions were submitted. The evolving document has served as the cornerstone for Indian elder advocacy into the new millennium (John and Baldridge 1996).

This report identifies the top five recommendations of Indian elders, two of which related specifically to long-term care:

- Ensure and provide funding for the Indian Health Service to adopt the full set of recommendations of the Work Group on Aging.[2]

- Ensure the provision of adequate funding and training, under Medicare, Medicaid, Indian Health Service, tribal, or Bureau of Indian Affairs programs, for formal and informal providers of long-term care services to Indian elders. Training should include all phases of geriatrics (NICOA: National Indian Aging Agenda for the Future, 1992).

These recommendations have continued to guide NICOA advocacy efforts.

In 1995, NICOA led a 20-member delegation to the National White House Conference on Aging in Washington, D.C. Among more than 2,000 non-Indian delegates, the small Indian contingent achieved remarkable success, securing nine of its twelve objectives. Attached to language of the final conference report were three Indian long-term care provisions:

- Promote and enhance Indian health services (Indian health service delivery systems, tribal, urban Indian programs) to provide a full range of home and community-based care, including Medicare and Medicaid home and community-based programs.

- Allow the Indian Health Service, tribal, and urban Indian health programs to provide home and community based long-term care, Medicare and Medicaid funding, as well as Indian Health Service funding.

- Allow Indian health programs to have full access to federally assisted programs affecting long-term care. (White House Conference on Aging 1995)

Generally, NICOA delegates to the White House Conference on Aging felt that the event afforded an opportunity to "test the water" of American public opinion. And while the delegation was able to generate significant support from non-Indian constituencies for Indian elder long-term care issues, the final report from the conference unfortunately did not impact legislation.

ADVOCACY WITHIN THE DEPARTMENT OF HEALTH AND HUMAN SERVICES

Also in 1995, the NICOA made a presentation to a meeting on Indian health with senior staff of the U. S. Department of Health and Human Services

---

[2] The Work Group's recommendations relate to long-term care, and in part to IHS' endorsement and support of home and community-based, rather than institutional care.

(DHHS) chaired by Dr. Phil Lee, Assistant Secretary. NICOA's presentation stated:

> Until IHS and tribes can gain the resources they need to provide complete health care services to low-income patients, IHS users will increasingly be pressured to use non-Indian health care services that may be inadequate, inaccessible, or culturally inappropriate. The use of non-IHS medical services may be especially difficult for older Indians who are very likely to have transportation problems and who face language barriers when dealing with non-Indian facilities. (National Indian Council on Aging 1995)

NICOA recommended that the IHS should discuss the potential roles of both the federal government and tribes as Medicare and Medicaid program providers:

> Many tribal and urban programs are too small to operate effective home- or community-based programs without IHS technical and medical support. And the IHS in turn does not have the budget to provide these services without help from Medicare and Medicaid home and community health funding. (National Indian Council on Aging 1995)

Since this meeting in 1995, slow progress has been made toward developing Medicare and Medicaid resources to support long-term care in Indian Country. In May 1999, the National Indian Health Board (NIHB) and the National Congress of American Indians (NCAI) arranged a first-ever meeting between Indian tribes and the DHHS Budget Review Board to consider funding for priority services to Indian Country. Among several Indian elder concerns, NICOA presented the following recommendations about long-term care:

1. Allocate $500,000 for the Health Resources and Services Administration (HRSA) to work with tribes and Indian organizations to develop guidelines for the most appropriate long-term care services for Indian Country.

2. The DHHS should dedicate a portion of its research and development funds, especially from the Health Care Financing Administration (HCFA), Health Resources and Services Administration (HRSA), National Institutes of Health (NIH), and the Administration on Aging (AOA), for grants to help Indian Country plan, develop and deliver culturally-appropriate and effective long-term care services.

3. The Administration should support changes needed to authorize Medicare payments for services provided by Community Health Aides (CHAs) and Community Health Practitioners (CHPs) in Alaska and to allocate funding in the 2001 budget for these payments.

4. The Administration should eliminate the barriers for tribes to be reimbursed by Medicaid and Medicare for home health services, including clarifications in the IHS/HCFA Memorandum of Agreement and changes in the Social Security Act.

Whether or not advocacy such as this will make a difference in the future of long-term care in Indian Country remains to be seen. It is encouraging that elder issues were included with other key Indian health issues at this key juncture. Also, advocacy for long-term care is occurring earlier in the federal funding process and with a broader range of funding decision-makers than in the past.

CHANGING IHS POLICY: HOME AND COMMUNITY-BASED CARE

Acting on the recommendation of its informal 1992 Long-Term Care Work Group, the IHS established an Elder Health Care Initiative (EHCI) in 1996. With only nominal funding, the initiative nevertheless represented a positive step by the agency to acknowledge responsibility for the provision of geriatric care.

That same year the IHS Council of Area and Associate Directors (CAAD) meeting in Bemidji, Minnesota, voted unanimously to expand the agency's definition of long-term care to include home and community-based care.

Currently under the leadership of Bruce Finke, M.D., the IHS EHCI is aggressively and effectively advocating within the agency for long-term care issues. According to Dr. Finke, long-term care strategies employed by federal agencies do not easily translate to Indian Country:

> Classic models of long-term care, which involve institutional service provisions, do not apply well to Indian communities. Indian people consider long-term care to be a family issue and tend to provide it without question. It's difficult for a tribe to interface with federal agencies because the institutional approach just doesn't apply to them. Above all, we've got to keep Indian families involved in the decision-making process. (Bruce Finke, personal communication, December 17, 1999)

REAUTHORIZATION OF THE INDIAN HEALTH CARE IMPROVEMENT ACT

Partnering with NICOA and former Deputy Assistant Secretary for Aging, William F. Benson, the IHS EHCI initiated a Statement of Principles for the inclusion of long-term care provisions in the reauthorization of the Indian Health Care Improvement Act (IHCIA). The statement was based on four concepts:

1. Families and communities must be involved in the care and services for their elders and receive appropriate education and training to fulfill meaningful roles in such care;

2. Services must be available to elders regardless of where they live, whether in urban or rural areas;

3. A full array of treatment, rehabilitation, wellness, health promotion and prevention services must be widely available throughout Indian Country and to Indian elders regardless of their place of residence; and,

4. Services must be anchored in tribally based community values and aspirations.

With support from tribal leaders, several long-term care authorizations appear in the IHCIA draft legislation that went to the 106th Congress in 2000. These include authorization of expenditures for hospice and assisted living, long-term care, and home and community-based services. The proposed legislation would authorize tribes to construct, renovate, or expand long-term care facilities.

CONCLUSION

There is little doubt that American Indian and Alaska Native elders comprise the most difficult-to-serve cohort of the nation's Indian population. Exhibiting high rates of poverty and poor health status, their small numbers and diverse demographics often prevent the delivery of cost-effective (or profitable) services. Even so, it is difficult to understand why, seven decades after the federal government began formally providing Indian health care, long-term care services in Indian Country remain almost non-existent. Particularly in the current era of unparalleled national prosperity—an era in which the United States annually extends many millions of dollars in foreign aid—the lack of basic care provided for the elders of North America's original residents is, in the words of Cherokee former Chief Wilma Mankiller, "an embarrassment." While the nation's Indian population is projected to experience high growth rates over the next few decades, there is no adequate infrastructure in place to meet even existing long-term care needs. The message from Indian elder advocates has remained remarkably consistent over the past decade. The most important goal is to integrate long-term care, especially home and community-based care, into a seamless continuum of health services available to Indians.

The future of long-term care in Indian Country may depend on several factors. National long-term care initiatives for Indians will probably not be implemented unless budgets for the Indian health system are increased substantially; as Indian health budgets fare with Congress, so will Indian long-term care. If Indian Country with its exploding population is to avert a worsening long-term care crisis, proactive planning and service delivery initiatives must begin immediately.

Both the IHS and tribes seemingly have failed to anticipate long-term care needs for what will soon become a substantial cohort of older/disabled Indians. As millions of "Baby Boomers" approach retirement age, it seems probable that the federal government will respond by creating new long-term care initiatives; and tribes will need equal access to these new authorizations and funding streams. As tribes continue to assume control of their health care destinies, they will need to assume critical roles as long-term care advocates.

A widely held concept of traditional Indian people, regardless of tribal affiliation, is that of the Sacred Hoop. The Sacred Hoop represents the wholeness and inter-related nature of all things, both animate and inanimate. When the hoop is broken, our world is incomplete. Because there is no long-term care for Indian elders, the Sacred Hoop of Indian health is broken. Seamless integration of geriatric and long-term care services into Indian health programs is a necessary step if we are to mend the hoop.

ACKNOWLEDGEMENTS

The author extends sincere appreciation to William F. Benson for his substantive contributions to this chapter and his ongoing mentoring regarding long-term care issues in Indian Country. Thanks also to Mario Garrett, Ph.D., for providing data, analyses, and interpretations.

REFERENCES

Bacon C, (ed). *A Portrait of Older Minorities*. Washington, DC: American Association of Retired Persons; 1993.

Baldridge D. Elders. In: Mary B. Davis, ed. *Native America in the Twentieth Century*. New York & London: Garland Publishing, Inc; 1996.

Baldridge D, Brown A. *An American Indian Elder Abuse Monograph*. Oklahoma City, OK: Center of Child Abuse and Neglect, University of Oklahoma; 1998.

Baldridge D, Garrett M. The American Indian and Alaska Native Populations in the States of Washington, Idaho, and Alaska Study. In: *Medicare Beneficiary Grassroots Rights and Protections Outreach Project for Vulnerable Populations*. Baltimore, MD: Health Care Financing Administration; 1999.

Brown A, Fernandez R, Griffith T. *Service Provider Perceptions of Elder Abuse Among the Navajo*. Kayenta, AZ: University of Northern Arizona; 1990.

Bureau of the Census, U.S. Department of Commerce. *Social and Economic Characteristics: United States*. Washington, DC: U.S. Government Printing Office; 1993.

Bureau of the Census, U.S. Department of Commerce. *Census of Population and Housing, 1990; Special Tabulation on Aging (STP 14)*. Washington, DC: U.S. Government Printing Office; 1994a.

Bureau of the Census, U.S. Department of Commerce. *Statistical Brief: Housing of American Indians on Reservations—An Overview*. Washington, DC: U.S. Government Printing Office; 1994b.

Bureau of Census, U.S. Department of Commerce. *Projections of Total Resident Population by 5 year Age Groups, Race and Hispanic Origin with Special Age Categories: Middle Series, 1999-2000*. Washington, DC: U.S. Government Printing Office; 2000.

Fowler L, Dwyer K, Brueckmann S, Seekins T, Clay J, Lopez C. *American Indian Approaches to Disability Policy—Establishing Legal Protections for Tribal Members with Disabilities: Five Case Studies*. Missoula, MT: Research & Training Center on Rural Rehabilitation, Montana Affiliated Rural Institute on Disabilities, University of Montana-Missoula; 1996.

Health Care Financing Administration. *Medicaid Statistics: Program and Financial Statistics, Fiscal Year 1995*. Washington, DC: Medicaid Bureau; 1996. HCFA Pub. No. 10129.

Health Care Financing Administration. *Study of Private Accreditation (Deeming) of Nursing Homes, Regulatory Incentives and Non-Regulatory Initiatives, and Effectiveness of the Survey and Certification System*. Report to Congress Available at www.hcfa.gov. 1998.

Health Care Financing Administration. *Medicaid Stats at a Glance*. Medicaid Consumer Information [On-line]. Available at www.hcfa.gov. 1999a.

Health Care Financing Administration. *Medicaid Long-Term Care Services—Home and Community-Based Services Waivers*. Medicaid Consumer Information [On-line]. Available at www.hcfa.gov. 1999 b.

Hennessy CH, John R. The Interpretation of Burden among Pueblo Indian

Caregivers. *Journal of Aging Studies.* 1995; 9(3): 215-229.

Hennessy CH, John R. American Indian Family Caregivers' Perceptions of Burden and Needed Support Services. *Journal of Applied Gerontology* 1996. 15(3): 275-293

Indian Health Design Team. Design for a New IHS: *Final Recommendations of the Indian Health Design Team, Report Number II.* Rockville, MD: Indian Health Service; 1997.

Indian Health Service, U.S. Department of Health and Human Services. *Indian Health Focus: Elders.* Rockville, MD: Indian Health Service. 1996a.

Indian Health Service, U.S. Department of Health and Human Services. *Regional Differences in Indian Health.* Rockville, MD: Indian Health Service; 1996b.

Indian Health Service, U.S. Department of Health and Human Services. *Regional Differences in Indian Health 1997.* Rockville, MD: Indian Health Service; 1997a.

Indian Health Service, U.S. Department of Health and Human Services. *Trends in Indian Health 1997.* Rockville, MD: Indian Health Service; 1997b.

John R. *Health Research, Service and Policy Priorities of American Indian Elders: An Analysis of Applied Literature, 1980–1990.* Washington, DC: American Association of Retired Persons; 1994.

John R, Baldridge D. *The NICOA Report: Health and Long-Term Care for Indian Elders.* Washington, DC: National Indian Policy Center; 1996.

John R, Hennessy CH, Dyson T, Garrett M. *Toward the Conceptualization and Measurement of Caregiver Burden Among Pueblo Indian Family Caregivers.* In press.

Manson S. Long-Term Care in American Indian Communities: Issues for Planning and Research. *The Gerontologist* 1989; 29:1:38-43.

Medicare Rights Center. *How to Access the Medicare Home Health Benefit.* New York, NY: Medicare Rights Center; 1999.

National Committee to Preserve Social Security and Medicare. *Profiles in Diversity: America's Senior Population.* Washington, DC: National Committee to Preserve Social Security and Medicare; 1999.

National Indian Council on Aging. *American Indian Elderly: A National Profile*. Albuquerque, NM: National Indian Council on Aging; 1981.

National Indian Council on Aging. *Long-term care in Indian Country*. Unpublished manuscript. 1995.

National Indian Council on Aging. *Final Report: American Voices: Indian Elders Speak*. Albuquerque, NM: National Indian Council on Aging; 1998.

National Indian Council on Aging and Philomath Films. *Legacy: America's Indian Elders* [Video]. Albuquerque, NM: National Indian Council on Aging; 1993.

Sevilla G. *A People in Peril: People on the Front Lines of an Epidemic*. *The Arizona Republic* available at http://www.azcentral.com/news/specials/pima/. 1999.

Spencer H, Funk P. Meeting the Health and Independent Living Needs of Older Indians. *Native American Law Digest* 5: 4. 1995.

U.S. Department of Justice. *Report on Crime in Indian Country*. Washington, DC: U.S. Government Printing Office; 1998.

White House Conference on Aging. Final Resolutions (unpublished); 1995.

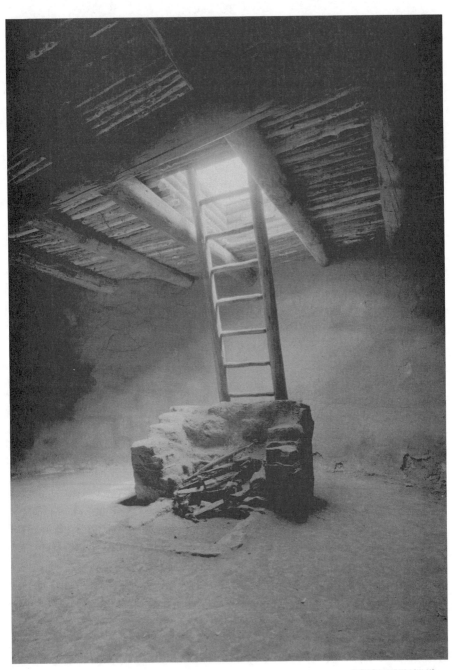

PHOTO BY WALT HOLLOW, MD

Behavioral Health Services For American Indians: Need, Use, and Barriers To Effective Care

Spero M. Manson

This chapter reviews the status of behavioral health services targeted to American Indians, with special emphasis on the need for, utilization of, and barriers to effective care. It begins by briefly describing the different sectors that comprise the local service ecology in these communities, which entails an array of private, tribal, state, and federal programs. This context is critical to appreciating the challenges that face consumers, family members, providers, administrators, and policy-makers in their attempts to reconfigure that care in keeping with local political, fiscal, and cultural realities. The discussion next turns to recent studies that speak directly to unmet service need, patterns of use, and factors affecting service use among Indian people. Observations concerning children are considered first, and then second, those relevant to adults. This chapter closes by highlighting major issues in behavioral health care that demand immediate attention in American Indian/Alaska Native communities, the responses to which will have far-reaching consequences for decades to come. Frankly, these issues do not concern individual provider competencies, particular features of an intervention, or program characteristics; areas often focused upon in the contemporary literature. This is not to deny the importance of such matters. Rather, the pressing questions of the day have to do with matters of availability, access, organization, and financing: do needed services even exist? If so, can people gain entry to them? Who is responsible for their quality and management? How are they best linked and coordinated? What mechanisms can pay for them?

BEHAVIORAL HEALTH SERVICE ECOLOGY IN AI/AN COMMUNITIES

The agency most directly responsible for providing behavioral health services to American Indians is the Indian Health Service (IHS). Specifically, the IHS Mental Health and Social Services Programs Branch, IHS primary health care services, and Alcoholism/Substance Abuse Programs Branch all provide behavioral health services. However, other programs and agencies also play important parts in this effort: namely, the Bureau of Indian Affairs, the Department of Veterans Affairs medical and counseling programs, tribal health programs, urban Indian health programs, state and local service agencies, and traditional healing resources. Together, these services, which are often fragmented, comprise the unique ecology within which American Indian individuals and families seek help for emotional and psychopathological distress.

INDIAN HEALTH SERVICE

MENTAL HEALTH PROGRAMS BRANCH

The mission of the IHS Mental Health and Social Services Programs Branch (MHSSPB) is to provide access for all Indian persons to high quality and culturally appropriate mental health services that are appropriate to the nature and severity of their mental illness (U.S. Department of Health and Human Services 1989). As of April 1995, IHS reported that 251 staff were supported by IHS mental health categorical funds, 198 of whom provide direct care (personal communication, S. Nelson, MHPB, IHS, 1995). On average, then, between 1 and 2 mental health direct treatment personnel are available in each of the 127 IHS Service Units; in actual practice, 80 percent of the service areas have a mental health professional available.

The distribution of mental health resources and staff varies considerably from Area to Area, as does the availability of mental health professionals trained to work with children or adolescents. In fiscal year 1993, the per capita budget for mental health services for all ages in IHS Areas ranged from $6.75 per person in California to $22.00 per person in the Billings and Portland Areas. Only 28 (14 percent) of the 198 direct care professionals were trained to work with children or adolescents, while children ages 19 and younger account for approximately 43 percent of the Indian population. This amounts to an average of 0.44 providers per 10,000 children and adolescents. In 4 of the 12 IHS Areas, there are no child- and/or adolescent-trained mental health professionals.

PRIMARY HEALTH CARE SERVICES

Most of the IHS budget is devoted to the provision of primary acute health care services. Because of the paucity of behavioral health professionals, primary care practitioners may be the principal source of detection and treatment of mental health and substance abuse problems, but the extent of such screening and treatment is not known. On the other hand, this situation is not without problems. In every IHS service area, the ratio of providers to population is well below accepted standards, due to the extensive physical health care needs among Indians, the fact that IHS's financial resources have not increased relative to inflation since 1978, and difficulties in recruiting clinical personnel to IHS service areas (Office of Technology Assessment 1987). Moreover, even if there were a sufficient number of primary care physicians to treat those with behavioral health problems, the delivery of such services by non-psychiatric physicians is a problem in its own right (U.S. Department of Health and Human Services 1987).

ALCOHOLISM/SUBSTANCE ABUSE PROGRAM BRANCH

The Alcoholism/Substance Abuse Program Branch (A/SAPB) of the IHS, originally known as the Office of Alcohol Programs, was established in March 1978. Presently, the IHS funds 309 Indian alcoholism service contracts in Indian reservations and urban communities. The most extensive summary of IHS alcoholism programming efforts can be found in the report by Peake-Raymond and Raymond (1984) that identifies and assesses a series of model projects. This and other reports found that virtually no alcoholism services were designed for Indian adolescents and that there was little coordination or continuity of care among alcoholism, social service, and mental health programs (Alaska Native Health Board 1973, 1976; Charleston, et al 1984).

The A/SAPB is responding to these deficiencies (U.S. Department of Health and Human Services 1985; Indian Health Service 1988). Initiatives made possible through 1986 Omnibus Drug Act funding led to the development of a youth services component that began in fiscal year 1987. The A/SAPB youth services component has three elements: prevention, outpatient treatment, and residential treatment. In fiscal year 1993, a total of 3,249 Indian youth were treated as outpatients, and 522 were treated in residential facilities. Two 24-bed regional adolescent substance abuse treatment centers were providing services by fiscal year 1988. At the present time, there are eight residential treatment facilities in operation in the eight IHS areas. In 1994, IHS reaffirmed its previous commitment by allocating funds to the administration and evaluation of 5 demonstration projects for innovative Indian alcohol and drug abuse prevention programs.

BUREAU OF INDIAN AFFAIRS

The Bureau of Indian Affairs (BIA) was established in 1824 as part of the War Department; it became a part of the U.S. Department of the Interior

(DOI) in 1849, when the DOI was created. The BIA works on a wide range of issues with Indian tribal governments and Alaska Native village communities. It provides educational programs to supplement those provided by public and private schools, and BIA assistance also is available for Indian students attending college, vocational training, adult education, gifted and talented programs, and single-parent programs. Finally, the BIA collaborates with tribal governments to provide a variety of social services, police protection, and economic development efforts.

BIA education programs furnish bureau-funded schools (182 in 1992–1993) with curriculum materials and technical assistance to develop and implement alcohol and substance abuse programs; the programs focus on identification, assessment, prevention, and crisis intervention through the use of referrals and additional counselors at the schools. Boarding schools also depend on a number of BIA personnel—typically social workers, educational psychologists, and special educators—to screen for, intervene with, and monitor students who experience social and mental health problems. Much of this effort takes place within the context of the local Intensive Residential Guidance program. In 1994, the BIA reported that 19.2 percent of all Indian children were in BIA-funded schools (personal communication, C. Gabow).

The BIA also funds programs under the Indian Child Welfare Act that provide a wide range of human services. Managed by tribes, these services often address the social and mental health problems both of Indian adults seeking to retain or reassume parental responsibility for their children and of Indian children subject to the stresses inherent in foster care and adoption. Although the ultimate disposition of the cases is not well documented, Indian Child Welfare workers also play a role in identifying abused adolescents in need of mental health services, and in assuring that these needs are met. However, a lack of treatment resources for children and their families was among the barriers identified in a 1989 BIA/IHS Forum on Child Abuse (U.S. Department of the Interior 1989).

The BIA also plays a major role in the law enforcement and criminal justice systems in many reservation communities. These systems frequently encounter mental health-related issues, such as the detention and diversion of Indian adolescents involved with alcohol and substance abuse, and those who experience serious emotional disturbance; this involvement is likely to increase, as outlined in the joint BIA-IHS Organizational Management Action Plan (U.S. Department of the Interior 1988).

DEPARTMENT OF VETERANS AFFAIRS

The Department of Veterans Affairs (DVA) plays a major role in providing behavioral health services to many American Indian veterans. Under the recent restructuring of the DVA, 2 separate health care programs will continue to provide services to American Indian veterans (Kizer 1995). The Patient Care

Services program provides primary, acute, long-term, and rehabilitative care for American Indian veterans with physical and mental health problems. These services are offered through urban medical centers (e.g., Phoenix, Albuquerque, Denver) and more distant, outpatient satellite programs (e.g., Prescott, AZ; Gallup, NM; Ft. Mead, SD). The DVA has specifically identified post-traumatic stress disorder, substance abuse, and serious mental illness as health problems of special programmatic concern. In addition, Readjustment Counseling Services are offered through over 200 field-based Veteran's Centers. This branch of the DVA provides a range of services, including initial assessment, supportive counseling and self-help groups, referral for more intensive out-patient and in-patient care, and relapse prevention.

TRIBAL HEALTH PROGRAMS

As a consequence of Public Law 93-638 (the Indian Self-Determination and Education Assistance Act) many tribes have assumed administrative control of local health programs, either partially or in their entirety. Administration of programs is negotiated on a tribal basis, leading to considerable variation in program activities and services. An analysis by the IHS Office of Health Program Development (OHPD) provides one of the few, albeit limited, overviews of this system of care (U.S. Department of Health and Human Services 1987). OHPD identified 174 tribal health programs that received substantial IHS funding under Public Law 93-638 in fiscal year 1985 programs; eighty-five percent of the existing programs completed and returned the profiles. Approximately 42 percent of the tribal health programs reported providing mental health services; yet only 3 percent of tribal health staff worked in mental health services, indicating limited provision of such services. Ten percent of the tribal health programs reported that mental health services were not available at all. Programs were not asked about mental health services targeted specifically for adolescents, but the paucity of mental health staff suggests that adolescents are not provided adequate mental health care.

URBAN INDIAN HEALTH PROGRAMS

In 1976, the IHS began to fund urban health programs—many of which differ from IHS reservation-based clinics in their emphasis on increasing access to existing services rather than providing or paying for services directly. There are currently 34 urban Indian health programs that encompass 40 urban areas in 20 states. A study by the American Indian Health Care Association (AIHCA) (1988) provided insight into the nature and scope of these programs. Until recently, urban Indian health programs were not eligible for behavioral health funding through IHS, creating service accessibility problems for the estimated 50 percent of American Indians who live in cities (U.S. Department of Health and Human Services 1989; Bureau of Census 1991). Within this context, many smaller urban Indian health programs offer behavioral health services as part of primary medical care; behavioral health problems that cannot be managed by the primary care provider are referred to outside resources. Other urban programs receive categorical funding for substance abuse or child welfare problems, and address mental health problems within the context of these services. Larger urban programs are able to provide a range of on-site behavioral health services with funds received through such sources as mental health block grants, substance abuse treatment/prevention block grants, and community mental health center funds. On average, expenditures for mental health services represent about 3.8 percent ($600,000 per year) of all ambulatory health care provided by urban Indian health programs. Between 1985 and 1987, the total number of on-site mental health providers ranged from 15 to 20 for all urban programs, representing less than 4 percent of the entire staff. During this period, the average number of users per full-time provider more than doubled, and the number of visits per provider also increased. Several of the respondents in the AIHCA study reported that available services were of poor quality and that waiting periods for appointments were excessively long. A replication of this survey was completed in 1993, and initial results suggested little change (personal communication, F. Miller, AIHCA, 1993).

STATE AND LOCAL SERVICE AGENCIES

Very little information exists about the extent to which local agencies, such as community mental health centers and state psychiatric facilities, serve Indian communities. It seems fair to assume, though, that numerous Indian people obtain care from these settings, especially in urban communities. However, the diverse points of entry into this system—State hospitals, day treatment centers, Social Security Administration, the criminal justice system, detoxification facilities, and vocational rehabilitation centers—yield a confusing and often unmanageable set of service utilization data. For example, in Oregon alone, over 30 service agencies are available to emotionally disturbed Indians. A survey by Denver Indian Health and Family Services, Inc. (an urban Indian health program), revealed that 71 municipal, county, state, and private agencies offered behavioral health services within the immediate metropolitan area (U.S. Department of Health and Human Services 1989). Less than 40 percent of these agencies' patient information systems track ethnicity, although virtually all of them (91 percent) answered affirmatively when asked if they could recall having had an Indian patient in care during the month prior to the survey. This is not, of course, an indication of the extent of care available to Indians from non-IHS agencies.

TRADITIONAL HEALING RESOURCES

The use of traditional healers is thought to be common in many American Indian communities (Powers 1971, 1986). However, little has been published about their role in treating diagnosable behavioral health problems. Ethnographic studies indicate that traditional healers do indeed address problems such depression, substance-related disorders, post-traumatic stress disorder, and seizure disorders (Arbogast 1995; Levy et al, 1987; Kunitz and Levy 1981). Moreover, traditional healing approaches frequently operate side-by-side with Western psychotherapeutic interventions in many tribal mental health programs (Csordas 1999, Guilmet and Whited 1989). Mental health and substance abuse practitioners at some IHS clinics also encourage the use of traditional healers, particularly when individuals describe culturally specific explanations for their distress (J. Almony, personal communication, 1991). Similarly, regional adolescent substance abuse treatment centers all report active involvement of traditional healers in their programs (personal communication, E. Smith, A/SAPB, IHS, 1996)—a finding entirely consistent with IHS policy that respects participation of traditional healers in patient care. These findings about the parallel use of Western and traditional services are consistent with our own work (Gurley et al, in press).

As evident, then, the system of services for treating behavioral health problems among American Indians is a complex, and often fractured, web of federal, state, local, tribal, and community-based services. Despite the wide range of services described here, the availability of these programs varies considerably across communities. Moreover, there can be no doubt that the system is inadequate for the overall needs of American Indians, as underscored by a series of recently emerging studies. Questions about service utilization and outcomes assume critical importance within this complicated service ecology.

CURRENT KNOWLEDGE OF NEED, SERVICE UTILIZATION, AND OUTCOMES

From 1980 to 1995, over 2,000 journal articles and book chapters were published on the behavioral health of American Indians. Slightly more than one third (N=703) of these publications addressed some aspect of service-related care. The most frequent service-related topics were: (1) need for culturally sensitive assessment and care (76 percent); (2) importance of family and community to the treatment process (59 percent); (3) limitations of the delivery system and lack of local input into planning (47 percent); and (4) the role of traditional healing (32 percent). Few service-related publications were empirically based; for example, 69 percent of the relevant publications report no data, either survey-oriented or case example. The relatively few empirically-based publications available employed poorly designed studies in program settings or unreliable IHS service utilization data.

AMERICAN INDIAN CHILDREN AND ADOLESCENTS

The current estimated size of the AI/AN population is just under 1 percent (0.8%) of the total U.S. population, or about 2.3 million people (U.S. Bureau of the Census, Population Projections Program 2000). Their birthrate is currently the highest of any major cultural group in the United States. Consequently, American Indians are considerably younger than the U.S. population as a whole, with a median age of 24.4 compared to 34.4 years (Indian Health Service 1996). Yet, infant mortality is greater among American Indians than among the general population (Indian Health Service 1996). Nationally, the unemployment rates for American Indian males and females are 16.2 percent and 13.5 percent, respectively, significantly higher than the 6.4 percent and 6.2 percent rates for their U.S. All Races counterparts. The median household income for AI/AN is $19,865, compared to $30,056 for the general population; 31.7 percent of American Indian families live below the poverty level, compared to a national rate of 13.1 percent (Indian Health Service 1994). Employment opportunities are especially scarce in most reservation communities (Dehyde 1992). Of the 10 counties in the nation with the highest unemployment rates in 1990, three include Northern Plains Indian reservations. Thirty-seven percent and 28 percent of American Indian and Alaska Native children, respectively, live in single parent families. These rates, which are among the highest in the country, further compound the scarcity of resources available to them. The high rates of adoption and foster care placement, involving Indian children, are unparalleled in any other segment of the population; many of the children go to non-Indian homes. Mortality data indicate that suicide and homicide are the second and third leading causes of death, respectively, for American Indian youth 15 to 24 years of age, exceeded only by accidents (Indian Health Service 1996; Blum et al, 1992); these rates are two to three times the national average. Alcohol-related causes of death rank among 6 of the 10 leading causes of death in this special population.

American Indian children growing up under these stressful circumstances would appear to be at high risk for behavioral and emotional problems. While data on the prevalence of alcohol, drug, and mental (ADM) disorders among American Indian youth are scarce, some evidence suggests that American Indian youth experience more behavioral health problems than their peers in the general population (Blum et al, 1992, Office of Technology Assessment 1990). Although population-based data on adolescent suicide, alcohol, and drug use rates for American Indians are available, little data exist for these and other mental disorders defined according to current diagnostic systems for either adults or adolescents (Office of Technology Assessment 1990).

Suicide rates among American Indians vary greatly among tribes and over time. In Native populations, suicide is primarily a phenomenon of the young, and especially of males (May 1990). Citing Indian Health Service (IHS) data,

May (1990) observed age-specific suicide rates for ages 10–24 to be 2.3 to 2.8 times higher than general U.S. rates; certain communities have experienced much higher rates and clusters of suicides. Furthermore, in a survey of over 13,000 American Indian adolescents, 22 percent of females and 12 percent of males reported having attempted suicide at some time. Over 67 percent of those who reported attempts had made those attempts within the past year. Fourteen percent of the females and 8 percent of the males reported significant feelings of sadness and hopelessness (Blum 1992).

Beals, et al (1997) reported on a follow-up of a school-based psychiatric epidemiological study involving Northern Plains youth, 13-17 years of age. Of the 109 adolescents, 29.4 percent (n=32) received a diagnosis of one or more psychiatric disorders. Altogether, 16.5 percent of the students qualified for a single diagnosis; 12.9 percent met criteria for multiple diagnoses. In terms of the broad diagnostic categories, 5.5 percent of the sample met criteria for an Anxiety Disorder; 4.6 percent for a Mood Disorder (either Major Depressive Disorder or Dysthymia); 13.8 percent for one or more of the Disruptive Behavior Disorders; and 18.3 percent for Substance Abuse Disorders. Only 1 percent was diagnosed with an Eating Disorder. The 5 most common specific disorders were Alcohol Dependence/Abuse (11.0 percent), Attention Deficit/Hyperactivity Disorder (ADHD) (10.6 percent), Marijuana Dependence/Abuse (8.6 percent), Major Depressive Disorder (4.7 percent), and Other Substance Dependence/Abuse (3.9 percent). Beals et al observed considerable co-morbidity among disorders. Specifically, more than half (8 of 15 or 53.3 percent) of those with a Disruptive Behavior Disorder also qualified for a Substance Use Disorder. Similarly, more than half (3 of 5 or 60 percent) of those youth diagnosed with Any Depressive Disorder had a Substance Use Disorder as well.

Beals and her colleagues compared these rates to those reported by Shaffer, et al (1996) and Lewinsohn, et al (1993) for non-minority children drawn from the population at large. American Indian adolescents were diagnosed with fewer anxiety disorders than the Shaffer, et al (1996) sample. However, American Indian adolescents were much more likely to be diagnosed with ADHD and Substance Abuse/Dependence Disorders. The rates of Conduct Disorder and Oppositional Defiant Disorder were also elevated in the American Indian sample. Rates of depressive disorders were essentially equivalent. Similarly, when compared to the Lewinsohn et al (1993) sample, American Indian adolescents demonstrated statistically significantly higher 6-month prevalence rates than did the non-minority children for lifetime prevalence of ADHD (p<0.01) and Alcohol Abuse/Dependence (p<0.01). In addition, American Indian youth had higher 6-month rates of Simple Phobias, Social Phobias, Overanxious Disorder, and Oppositional Defiant and Conduct Disorders than the non-minority children's lifetime rates for those disorders.

Many children and adolescents who suffer from alcohol, drug, and mental disorders (ADM) receive no form of behavioral health services (Burns et al 1993). Several studies indicate that only 16.1 percent to 29.0 percent of youth meeting criteria for a current ADM disorder receive care for that disorder (Anderson et al, 1987; Costello et al, 1988; Bird et al, 1988; Fergusson et al, 1993; Offord et al, 1987). These findings are consistent with other reports on lifetime rates of service utilization (McGee et al, 1990) and parental and teacher ratings of serious emotional and behavioral problems (Zahner et al, 1992). The discrepancy between the need for behavioral health services and their use can be due to cost, lack of transportation, limited availability of child-care for siblings, or geographic distance (Cohen and Hesselbart 1993). Gender, ethnicity/race, and socioeconomic status also have been implicated as possible barriers to service utilization. And, while the question remains open as to whether or not the amount of services consumed varies by ethnicity, minority children and adolescents do receive help from different types of providers and for different problems than their mainstream counterparts (Hoberman1992). Some investigators suggest that these differential service utilization patterns reflect funding emphases, programmatic biases, and organizational barriers; others argue that cultural differences in beliefs about behavioral health servic-es are more salient determinants of help-seeking behavior (Alegria et al, 1991; Rogler and Cortes 1993; Wallen 1992). The latter encompass issues of stigma (Lefley 1989, 1992), problem recognition (Staghezza et al, in press), and assumptions about cultural competence (Cross et al 1989). Clearly, both rea-sons for poor service utilization are true.

Few published studies speak directly to the question of behavioral health service utilization among American Indian youth. The Great Smoky Mountains Study (Costello et al, 1997) examined the prevalence of psychiatric disorders and service utilization among Cherokee and non-Indian youth in western North Carolina. Those researchers found that one in seven Cherokee children with a diagnosable DSM–III–R psychiatric disorder received profes-sional mental health treatment—a rate similar to that for the non-Indian sam-ple. However, Cherokee children were more likely to receive this treatment through the juvenile justice system and in-patient facilities than were the non-Indian children, despite the fact that free mental health services were available to the Cherokee children through the IHS. This study reveals that the behav-ioral health utilization patterns for Indian youth are different than those for non-Indian youth. It also suggests the assertion that the behavioral health needs of Indian children are met by the Public Health Service—thus freeing local authorities from their responsibility for contributing to such care—is sim-ply wrong. Although IHS services may be free, few are oriented toward child behavioral health. As an Office of Technology Assessment (1990) report indi-cated, at that time there were 17 child-prepared mental health professionals within the entire IHS system. This yielded an average of 0.43 providers per 10,000 children, which is less than10 percent of the number recommended by the OTA for the general population. Moreover, in 4 of the 12 IHS Areas there were no child- or adolescent-trained mental health-providers. Eight years later, the circumstances are little different.

Novins, et al (in press) analyzed the relationship between psychiatric diagnosis and the use of alcohol, drug, and mental disorders (ADM) treatment services among the same American Indian adolescents who were the focus of an earlier report by Beals, et al (1997). Sixty-one percent of those youth who met criteria for a psychiatric disorder never used ADM services during their lifetime. The majority who received services were seen through their school (68 percent) and just one adolescent received service from a mental health professional. Of the diagnostic categories examined, only the presence of a substance-related disorder was associated with lifetime service use. Among those youth with a psychiatric disorder who did not receive services, 57.1 percent were recognized as having an ADM problem by a parent, teacher, or employer.

Anticipating the Great Smoky Mountain Study's finding that Indian youth in detention are especially at risk for psychopathology, Duclos, et al (1998) assessed the 6-month prevalence of DSM–III–R psychiatric disorders among a sample of American Indian adolescents held in a juvenile detention facility on a Northern Plains reservation. Forty-nine percent of the detained youth were diagnosed with at least one alcohol, drug, or mental disorder, 12.7 percent with 2 disorders and 8.7 percent with 3 disorders. The most common disorders were Substance Abuse/Dependence (38 percent), Conduct Disorder (16.7 percent), and Major Depression (10 percent). When compared to their counterparts living at large in another Northern Plains community (Beals et al, 1997), the detained youth exhibited a higher prevalence of Substance Use and Conduct disorders. Female detainees were significantly more likely than males to be diagnosed with Major Depression and/or Anxiety Disorders, and were more likely to have 3 or more disorders. Novins et al (1999) again analyzed the relationship between diagnostic status and use of ADM treatment services in this sample. Forty percent of the youth who met criteria for a substance-related disorder and 34.1 percent of those diagnosed with an anxiety, mood, or disruptive behavior disorder reported having received ADM treatment at some point in their lives. Though overall service use was greater among these detained youth than those in the community, the unmet need remained significant (60 percent). While services for substance-related problems were most commonly provided in residential settings, services for emotional problems were commonly provided through out-patient settings. Traditional healers and pastoral counselors provided more than a quarter of these services.

AMERICAN INDIAN ADULTS

From a public health perspective, depressive disorders are of particular interest for intervention: they are common and have serious consequences, such as loss of social contacts, decreased work productivity, and the risk of suicide. In addition, highly effective treatments are available. Earlier studies provide some limited insight into depression among adult American Indians. In a study of a Northwest Coast Indian village (N=100), Shore, et al (1973), found the overall prevalence of psychiatric impairment to be 69 percent—compared with rates of 23 percent, 40 percent, 45 percent, and 57 percent from studies using similar methods in South Africa, two sites in Nigeria, and Nova Scotia. Sampath (1974) found a rate of (DSM–II) neuroses of 116 in 1000 in Eskimos (depression being the most common) compared to rates of 2 in 1000 to 52 in 1000 in other North American populations. However, Murphy and Hughes (1965), in a different Eskimo community, found rates of psychopathology consistent with those of the general Canadian population.

Suicide as a complication of depression is of particular concern. As noted earlier, in some Indian communities, suicide rates are extremely high, as are mortality rates from accidental injury that may represent disguised suicide. The latter often are referred to as "parasuicide" or as quasi-suicidal behavior. The majority of suicides in Indian communities involve alcohol consumption, in which the disinhibiting effects of alcohol combine with severe depressive symptomatology to dramatically increase risk of suicide.

Foulks and Katz (1973) reported the treated prevalence of anxiety neurosis in 5 Alaska Native culture groups to be nearly as high as the prevalence of depression, and for some groups much higher, consistent with the work of Kinzie, et al (1992) in their more recent findings in a Northwest Coast village. These investigators found a wide range of (DSM–II) psychoses, neuroses, and personality disorders. Kinzie, et al (1992) found that the prevalence of alcohol use in general and of affective disorders, in particular among women in a Northwest Indian community, were significantly higher than in the national Environmental Catchment Area (ECA) study.

Although large-scale epidemiological studies of American Indians are lacking, Manson (1992) found that 32 percent of American Indian elders visiting one urban Indian Health Service outpatient facility reported depressive symptoms, a rate dramatically different from those published in regard to elderly Whites. In another investigation, 19 percent of primary care patients had symptoms suggesting significant psychiatric morbidity (Goldwasser and Badger 1989), with more elevated rates among older adults. Lastly, in a survey of older urban Natives, depression and sadness or grieving were reported by 11 percent and 22 percent, respectively (Kramer 1991). Taken together, these limited data suggest that the prevalence of psychiatric illness is likely to be significant among Indian elders, especially in primary care and urban settings.

The American Indian Vietnam Veterans Project (AIVVP) is the only community-based, diagnostically oriented psychiatric epidemiological study to be conducted among American Indian adults within the last 25 years (Manson et al, 1996). It was part of a Congressionally mandated, DVA-funded effort to replicate the National Vietnam Veterans Readjustment Study (Kulka et al,

1990). Results from the latter study fueled significant new programming for White, African American, and Hispanic veterans, but not for other minority veterans, such as American Indians, who were thought to be at equal or greater risk of combat-related mental health problems. Consequently, the AIVVP was designed to: (1) ascertain the prevalence of psychiatric disorders, readjustment problems, and risk as well as protective factors, with special emphasis on Post-traumatic Stress Disorder (PTSD); and (2) describe the nature and extent of related-service use among Indian Vietnam combat veterans. Between 1992 and 1995, a two-stage, cross-sectional survey was conducted of random samples of Vietnam combat veterans drawn from three Northern Plains reservations (N=305) and one Southwest reservation (N=316). The first stage lay-administered interview included the Composite International Diagnostic Interview (CIDI) and a detailed inventory of use of biomedical services (VA, IHS, private) as well as traditional healing options (tribal ceremonials, Native American Church). The second stage entailed clinician administration of the Structured Clinical Interview for Diagnosis (SCID) to a 30 percent sub-sample of these veterans stratified in terms of reported PTSD symptomatology. Current and lifetime CIDI–rates of PTSD among the Northern Plains and Southwestern Vietnam veterans were 31.0 percent and 26.8 percent (current rates); 57.2 percent and 45.3 percent (lifetime rates), respectively. These rates are significantly in excess of their White, Black, and Japanese American counterparts. Likewise, current and lifetime prevalence of alcohol abuse and dependence among the Indian veterans was >70 percent current and > 80 percent lifetime, which was far greater than that observed for the others (which ranged from 11–32 percent current; 33–50 percent lifetime) (Beals, under review, 2000).

Many social groups (e.g., the elderly, males, Catholics, the poor, ethnic minorities) report lower rates of mental health service utilization than do other segments of society (Bromet and Schulberg 1989; Broman 1987; Hu et all, 1991; Shapiro et al, 1984; Tempkin-Greener and Clark 1988; Snowden and Cheung 1990; Sue 1977). These rates cannot be explained solely on the basis of clinical factors. For example, the ECA results indicate that lower use for some groups persists even after controlling for symptomatology. A variety of hypotheses have been generated to explain these differences. For example, attitudinal differences attributable to culture (such as incongruent values and beliefs) are likely to be important (Rodriguez 1987, Cheung 1990, Gary 1987, Kleinman and Good 1985). Acculturation has also been shown to be related to the likelihood of certain types of services utilization (Wells et al, 1987). Similarly, people with serious symptoms may not seek treatment because they, and those in their social network, do not label such symptoms as a "mental problem"; thus, they do not perceive a mental health professional as an appropriate source of help (Link and Cullen 1990). Moreover, people with severe symptoms may not seek treatment because they are unaware or unconvinced that effective treatment is available. People also may avoid seeking treatment because they fear others will see them as a "mental patient" and, consequently, treat them differently (Link 1987; Link et al, 1987; Link et al, 1989). Also, the expression of symptoms (e.g., as somatic or emotional) may differ across cultures (Katon et al, 1982; Angel and Guarnaccia 1989) and thus have a significant effect on the type of service utilized. Attitudinal differences may also arise from racial discrimination perceived or experienced in health settings (Vega and Rumbaud 1991). Barriers intrinsic to behavioral health service systems can deter people from seeking (or continuing) treatment. In addition to financial and logistical concerns, other barriers include anticipated difficulties in navigating the service and insurance systems, language and cultural differences between providers and potential clients, and anticipated (or actual) rebuffs by mental health professionals. Finally, there is clearly an interaction of socioeconomic status and ethnicity in relation to the utilization of services by adults.

Little is known about service utilization for psychopathology specifically among Indian adults. To date almost all of the literature has focused on substance-related disorders (Shore 1974; Kunitz and Levy 1994; Westermeyer and Peake 1983; Westermeyer 1985; Walker et al, 1992–1993,1994). In terms of non-substance related disorder, we know that American Indians appear to use community mental health facilities far less frequently than other segments of the American population (Sue 1977; Willie et al, 1973). In a 3-year survey of 17 community mental health centers in Seattle, Sue (1977) reported that 55 percent of the Indian patients seen did not return after the initial contact—a significantly higher non-return rate than was observed for Black, Asian, Hispanic, or White patients.

The American Indian Vietnam Veterans Project carefully examined the nature and extent of the services used by this segment of the population to address physical as well as mental health problems (Gurley et al, in press). Northern Plains (NP) and Southwestern (SW) veterans differed substantially in their respective use of VA facilities (NP: 26.5 percent, SW: 13.6 percent) and traditional healing options (NP: 4.7 percent, SW: 17.1 percent) for the care of physical health problems. They did not differ in their use of the IHS (NP: 32.8 percent, SW: 29.4 percent) or private biomedical care (NP: 8.6 percent, SW: 8.1 percent) to treat such problems. A similar pattern emerged in terms of their utilization of the care available though these same service mechanisms for treating alcohol, drug, and mental health (ADM) problems. Specifically, Northern Plains (NP) and Southwestern (SW) veterans differed substantially in their respective use of VA facilities (NP: 17 percent, SW: 5.7 percent) and traditional healing options (NP: 5.0 percent; SW: 18.5 percent) for the care of ADM problems. They did not differ in their use of the IHS (NP: 3.9 percent, SW: 3.8 percent) or private biomedical care (NP: 0.9 percent, SW: 1.6 percent) for treating these same problems. Extent of overall service use (combining biomedical and traditional healing options) was similar across these two groups—regardless if for physical or ADM problems—which manifested similar levels of need. However, the kinds of services used varied by availability. For example, VA services were significantly more available to Northern Plains than Southwestern veterans, and, thus, likely used more by the former. IHS and private sources of biomedical care, equally available to both, were used to a similar degree. Traditional healing options, more readily available to Southwestern veterans, were used to a greater extent by them than by their Northern Plains counterparts. Especially noteworthy is the finding that veterans were more likely to use the VA rather than IHS for the care of ADM problems, despite the latter's proximity. This pattern is likely attributable to the stigma attached to seeking behavioral health care within the local community as well as to the belief that fellow veterans are more empathic and understanding of combat-related trauma.

This small, but growing knowledge base represents a promising start for understanding the behavioral health service needs, patterns of use, and barriers to care among American Indian children and adults. There seems little doubt that their needs are great, and that services generally are lacking. But, what contributes to this gap? Is it related to the system of care itself, in terms of funding emphases, programmatic biases, and organizational barriers? Or is it stigma, distrust, and other elements of acceptability? Work is underway with respect to the latter, more consumer-oriented possibilities. However, the former—the structure and financing of care—remains largely unexamined, with the consequences unknown, but easily guessed.

PRESSING ISSUES, FORCES FOR CHANGE

A 1987 study by the Agency for Health Care Policy and Research (Cunningham and Schur 1991) revealed that American Indians are much less likely to have private insurance coverage than any other segment of the U.S. population. For example, only 28.2 percent of the sample, drawn from Indian and Native households on or near reservation lands, reported such coverage. This compared to 74.5 percent coverage for U.S. All Races (80.8 percent Whites, 52.9 percent Blacks, 50.1 percent Hispanics). Even excluding IHS coverage, Indian households in this study had significantly higher rates of public coverage than the total U.S. population (16.9 percent versus 10 percent). Both findings relate directly, albeit in inverse ways, to employment and job opportunities. However, the data also indicate that Indian people who work and have the option to purchase health coverage are less likely to choose private coverage than their non-Native counterparts (e.g., 36.2 percent versus 75.4 percent). In the final analysis, 54.9 percent of American Indian families are either uninsured or entirely reliant on the IHS for health care. And, as noted above, mental health care in particular varies in availability across the IHS system.

The IHS system is undergoing dramatic change as a consequence of tribal options to self-administer federal functions through the contracting or compacting provisions of P.L. 93-638 (Henry J. Kaiser Family Foundation 1996). In fiscal year 1995 the IHS reported that fully 35 percent of its budget flowed through these mechanisms, with significant implications for subsequent resource allocation. Direct contracting of various tribes' proportionate "shares" of the overall IHS system resources has led to a concomitant reduction in Area and Headquarters functions, which have included technical assistance, consultation, quality control, patient information management, and long-term planning. These functions are critical to the IHS', and now tribes' ability to position themselves to recover Medicaid, Medicare, and private reimbursement, as provided for under the 1976 Indian Health Care Improvement Act. But this is a relatively new development, and efforts have been slow to capture the available monies. Concurrently, the move to downsize the federal government has led to fewer resources available, just as tribes are assuming authority, and responsibility, for delivering the related care.

In other areas, such as federal block grant monies for substance abuse and mental health services, Indian communities always have been included among the populations that states enumerate as the basis for their respective allocations from the federal government. However, it is widely acknowledged that these same communities have not shared proportionately in the services supported by these funds. Recognition of this inequity several years ago led to a change in the authorizing language that now enables tribes to apply directly to the Substance Abuse and Mental Health Services Administration (SAMHSA) for block grant funds to support substance abuse prevention and treatment services, independent of the states in which they reside. No such provision is available with respect to mental health block grants, but this option is the subject of increasing discussion.

Several exciting initiatives are underway, supported by SAMHSA, in regard to the strategic planning and implementation of better-coordinated services for AI/AN children who suffer from serious emotional disturbance. One, the "Circles of Care Initiative," supports 9 AI/AN grantee communities in their efforts to redesign local systems of care in a manner more consonant with these rapidly changing circumstances and with local priorities, as rooted in their cultural values. Whether such change at this level—involving the sectors described at the outset of this paper—is possible awaits the conclusion of these initiatives. But the even more important question is: will change in the organization of behavioral health services make a difference in the effectiveness of the care delivered, as measured by the status and functioning of the recipient children and families? The answer has been equivocal elsewhere: hopefully not here.

ACKNOWLEDGMENTS

The preparation of this chapter was supported in part by the National Institute of Mental Health (P01 MH42473; R01 MH48174), the National Institute on Aging (P30 AG15292), the Center for Mental Health Services, SAMHSA, the Robert Wood Johnson Foundation RWJF (032815), and the

Administration on Aging (90-AM-0757).

REFERENCES

Alaska Native Health Board. *Evaluation of Alcoholism Treatment Services in the State of Alaska*. Rockville, MD: Indian Health Service: 1973.

Alaska Native Health Board. *Adolescent Alcoholism: A Relationship to other Mental Problems*. Rockville, MD: Indian Health Service; 1976.

Alegria M, Robles R, Freeman D. Patterns of Mental Health Service Utilization among Puerto Rican Poor. *American Journal of Public Health*, 81(875-879). 1991.

American Indian Health Care Association. *Mental Health Services Delivery: Urban Health Programs*. St. Paul, MN: American Indian Health Care Association; 1988.

Anderson JC, et al. DSM-III Disorders in Preadolescent Children. *Archives of General Psychiatry*. 1987; 44:69-76.

Angel R, Guarnaccia PJ. *Mind, Body, and Culture: Somaticization among Hispanics*. Social Science and Medicine. 1989; 28(12): 1229-1238.

Arbogast D. *Wounded Warriors: A Time for Healing*. Omaha, NB: Little Turtle Publications; 1995.

Beals J, et al. Psychiatric Disorder among American Indian Adolescents: Prevalence in Northern Plains Youth. *Journal of the American Academy of Child and Adolescent Psychiatry*. 1997; 36(9):1252-1259.

Beals J, et al. Posttraumatic Stress Disorder among Vietnam Theater Veterans: A Comparison across Five Racially and Ethnically Distinct Samples. *American Journal of Psychiatry*. Under review.

Bird HR, et al. Estimates of the Prevalence of Childhood Maladjustment in a Community Survey in Puerto Rico. *Archives of General Psychiatry*. 1998; 45: 1120-1126.

Blum RW, et al. American Indian—Alaska Native Youth Health. *Journal of the American Medical Association*. 1992; 267: 1637-1644.

Broman CL. Race Differences in Professional Help Seeking. *American Journal of Community Psychology*. 1987; 32:473-489.

Bromet E, Schulberg H. Special Problem Populations: The Chronically Mentally Ill, Elderly, Children, Minorities, and Substance Abusers. In: Rochefort D, ed. *Handbook on Mental Health Policy in the United States*. New York, Greenwood Press; 1989.

Bureau of Census, U.S. Department of Commerce. *A 1990 Census Profile of American Indian, Eskimo, or Aleut Population*. Washington, DC: Bureau of Census; 1991.

Burns BJ, Thompson JW, Goldman HH. Initial Treatment Decisions by Level of Care for Children in the CAMPUS Tidewater Demonstration. *Administration and Policy in Mental Health*. 1993; 20:231–246.

Charleston GM, Meyers JG, Charleston K. *Indian Alcoholism Program Evaluation, Fiscal Year 1984*, National Report. Rockville, MD: Indian Health Service; 1984.

Cheung YW. Overview: Sharpening the Focus on Ethnicity. *The International Journal of the Addictions*. 1990; 25(5A):573–579.

Cohen P, Hesselbart CS. Demographic Factors in the Use of Children's Mental Health Services. *American Journal of Public Health*. 1993; 83:49–52.

Costello EJ, et al. Psychiatric Disorders in Pediatric Primary Care. *Archives of General Psychiatry*. 1988; 45:1107–1116.

Costello EJ, et al. Psychiatric Disorders among American Indian and White Youth in Appalachia: The Great Smoky Mountains Study. *American Journal of Public Health*. 1997; 87:827–832.

Cross T, Bazron B, Dennis K, Issacs K. *Towards a Culturally Competent System of Care: A Monograph on Effective Services for Minority Children who are Severely Emotionally Disturbed*. Washington, DC: Georgetown University Child Development Center; 1989.

Csordas TJ. Ritual Healing and the Politics of Identity in Contemporary Navajo Society. *American Ethnologist*. 1999; 26(1):3–23.

Cunningham P, Schur C. Health Care Coverage: Findings from the Survey of American Indians and Alaska Natives, *in National Medical Expenditure Survey Research Findings*. Rockville, MD: Agency for Health Care Policy and Research; 1991.

Dehyde D. Constructing Failure and Maintaining Cultural Identity: Navajo and Ute School Leavers. *Journal of American Indian Education*. 1992; 31(2):24–47. 1992.

Duclos CW, et al. Prevalence of Common Psychiatric Disorders among American Indian Adolescent Detainees. *Journal of the American Academy of Child & Adolescent Psychiatry*. 1988; 37(8):866–73.

Fergusson DM, Horwood LJ, Lynskey MT. Prevalence and Comorbidity of DSM-III-R Diagnoses in a Birth Cohort of 15 Year Olds. *Journal of the American Academy of Child and Adolescent Psychiatry*. 1993;32:1127–1134.

Foulks EF, Katz S. The Mental Health of Alaskan Natives. *Acta Psychiatrica Scandinavia*. 1973; 49:91–96.

Gary LE. Attitudes of Black Adults toward Community Mental Health Centers. *Hospital Community Psychiatry*. 1987; 38:1100–1105.

Goldwasser HD, Badger LW. Utility of a Psychiatric Screen among the Navajo of Chinle: A Fourth-year Clerkship Experience. *American Indian and Alaska Native Mental Health Research*. 1989; 3(1):6–15.

Guilmet GM, Whited DL. *The People Who Give More: Health and Mental Health among the Contemporary Puyallup Indian Tribal Community*. Denver CO: University Press of Colorado. 1989.

Gurley D, et al. *Comparative* Use of Biomedical Services and Traditional Healing Options by American Indian Veterans. *Psychiatric Services*. In press.

Henry J. Kaiser Family Foundation. A *Forum on the Implications of Changes in the Health Care Environment for Native American Health Care*. Washington, D.C.: Henry J. Kaiser Family Foundation; 1996.

Hoberman HM. Ethnic Minority Status and Adolescent Mental Health Services Utilization. *Journal of Mental Health Administration*. 1992; 19:246–267.

Hu TW, et al. Ethnic Populations in Public Mental Health: Services Choice and Level of Use. *American Journal of Public Health*. 1991; 81:1429–1434.

Indian Health Service, U.S. Department of Health and Human Services. *IHS Alcoholism/Substance Abuse Prevention Initiative*. Rockville, MD: Indian Health

Service; 1985.

Indian Health Service, U.S. Department of Health and Human Services. *A Progress Report on Indian Alcoholism Activities: 1988.* Rockville, MD: Indian Health Service; 1988.

Indian Health Service, U.S. Department of Health and Human Services. *Trends in Indian Health.* Washington, DC: Indian Health Service; 1994.

Indian Health Service, U.S. Department of Health and Human Services. *Trends in Indian Health.* Washington, DC: Indian Health Service; 1996.

Katon W, Kleinman AG Rosen G. Depression and Somaticization: A Review, Part I. *American Journal of Medicine.* 1982; 72:127–135.

Kinzie JD, et al. Psychiatry Epidemiology of an Indian Village: A 19-year Replication Study. *Journal of Nervous and Mental Disease.* 1992; 180:33–39.

Kizer KW. *Vision for Change: A Plan to Restructure the Veterans Health Administration.* Washington, DC: Department of Veterans Affairs; 1995.

Kleinman A, Good B. *Culture and Depression: Studies in the Anthropology and Cross-cultural Psychiatry of Affect and Disorder.* Berkeley, CA: University of California Press; 1985.

Kramer BJ. Urban American Indian Aging. *Journal of Cross Cultural Gerontology.* 1991; 6(2):205–217. 1991.

Kulka RA, et al. *Trauma and the Vietnam War Generation: Report of Findings from the National Vietnam Veterans Readjustment Study.* New York: Bruner/Mazel; 1990.

Kunitz SJ, Levy JE, eds. Navajos. *Ethnicity and Medical Care.* A. Harwood, ed. Harvard University Press: Cambridge, MA; 1981.

Kunitz SJ, Levy JE. *Drinking Careers: A Twenty-five-year Study of Three Navajo Populations.* New Haven, CT: Yale University Press; 1994.

Lefley HP. Family Burden and Family Stigma in Major Mental Illness. *American Psychologist.* 1989; 44:556–560. 1989.

Lefley HP. The Stigmatized Family. In: Fink P and Tasman A. ed. *Stigma and Mental Illness.* Washington, DC: American Psychiatric Press; 1992.

Levy JE, Neutra R, Parker D. Hand Trembling, Frenzy, Witchcraft, and Moth Madness: *A Study of Navajo Seizure Disorders*. Tucson, AZ: University of Arizona Press; 1987.

Lewinsohn PM, et al. Adolescent Psychopathology: I. Prevalence and Incidence of Depression and other DSM-IIIR Disorders in High School Students. *Journal of Abnormal Psychology*. 1992; 102:133–144.

Link B. Understanding Labeling Effects in the Area of Mental Disorders: An Assessment of the Effects of Expectations of Rejection. *American Sociological Review*. 1987; 52:96-112.

Link B, et al. The Social Rejection of Former Mental Patients: Understanding Why Labels Matter. *American Journal of Sociology*. 1987; 92:1461–1500.

Link B, et al. A Modified Labeling Theory Approach to Mental Disorders: An Empirical Assessment. *American Sociological Review*. 1989; 54: 400–423.

Link B, Cullen FT. The Labeling Theory of Mental Disorder: A Review of the Evidence. In: Greenley J, ed. *Mental Illness in the United States*. Greenwich, CT: JAI Press; 1990.

Manson SM. Long-term Care of Older American Indians: Challenges in the Development of Institutional Services. In: Barresi C, Stull DE, Ed. *Ethnicity and Long-term Care*. New York, NY: Springer Publishing Co; 1992.

Manson S, et al. Wounded Spirits, Ailing Hearts: PTSD and Related Disorders among American Indians. In Marsella AJ, et al, ed. *Ethnocultural Aspects of Posttraumatic Stress Disorder: Issues, Research, and Clinical Applications*. Washington, DC: American Psychological Association; 1996.

May, Philip A. A bibliography on suicide and suicide attempts among American Indians and Alaska Natives. *Omega—Journal of Death & Dying*. 1990; 21(3):199–214.

McGee R, et al. DSM–III–R Disorders in a Large Sample of Adolescents. *Journal of the American Academy of Child and Adolescent Psychiatry*. 1990; 29:611–619.

Murphy JM, Hughes CC. The Use of Psychophysiological Symptoms as Indicators of Disorder among Eskimos. In: Murphy JM, Leighton AH, eds, *Approaches to Cross-cultural Psychiatry*. Ithaca, NY: Cornell University Press;

1965.

Novins DK, et al. Utilization of Alcohol, Drug, and Mental Health Treatment Services among American Indian Adolescent Detainees. *Journal of the American Academy of Child and Adolescent Psychiatry.* 1999; 38(9):1102–1108.

Novins DK, et al. Use of Mental Health and Substance Use Services among Northern Plains American Indian Adolescents. *Psychiatric Services.* In press.

Office of Technology Assessment, U.S. Congress. *Special Report: Clinical Staffing in the Indian Health Service.* Washington, DC: Office of Technology Assessment; 1987.

Office of Technology Assessment, U.S. Congress. *Indian Adolescent Mental Health.* Washington, DC: Office of Technology Assessment; 1990.

Offord DR, Boyle HH, Racine YA. Ontario Child Health Study II: Six Month Prevalence of Disorder and Rates of Service Utilization. *Archives of General Psychiatry* 1987; 44:832–836.

Peake-Raymond MP. and Raymond EV. *Identification and assessment of model Indian Health Service alcoholism projects.* Report to the Office of Program Planning and Evaluation, Washington, DC: Indian Health Service; 1984.

Powers WK. Yuwipi Music In Cultural Context. Wesleyan University; 1971.

Powers WK. *Sacred Language: The Nature of Supernatural Discourse in Lakota.* Norman, OK: University of Oklahoma Press; 1986.

Rodriguez O. Hispanics and Human Services: Help-seeking in an Inner City. Hispanic Research Center Monograph Series. Bronx, NY: Fordham University; 1987.

Rogler LH, Cortes DE. Help-seeking Pathways: A Unifying Concept in Mental Health Care. *American Journal of Psychiatry.* 1993; 150(4):554–561. 1993.

Sampath BM. Prevalence of Psychiatric Disorders in a Southern Baffin Island Eskimo Settlement. *Canadian Psychiatric Association Journal.* 1974; 19:303–367.

Shaffer D, et al. The NIMH Diagnostic Interview Schedule for Children Version 2.3 (DISC-2.3): Description, Acceptability, Prevalence Rates, and Performance in the MECA Study. *Journal of American Academy of Child and*

Adolescent Psychiatry. 1996; 35(7):865-877.

Shapiro S, Skinner E, Kessler L. Utilization of Health and Mental Health Services: Three Epidemiologic Catchment Area Sites. *Archives of General Psychiatry.* 1984; 41:971–988.

Shore JH, et al. Psychiatric Epidemiology of an Indian Village. *Psychiatry.* 1973; 36(1):70–81.

Shore JH. Psychiatric Epidemiology among American Indians. *Psychiatric Annals.* 1974; 4(11): 56-66.

Snowden LR, Cheung FK. Use of Inpatient Mental Health Services by Members of Ethnic Minority Groups. *American Psychologist.* 1990; 45(3):347–355.

Staghezza B, et al. Mental Health Service Utilization among Puerto Rican Children Ages 4 through 16. *Journal of Child and Family Studies.* In press.

Sue S. Community Mental Health Services to Minority Groups: Some Optimism, some Pessimism. *American Psychologist.* 1977; 32(8):616–624.

Tempkin-Greener H, Clark KT. Ethnicity, Gender, and Utilization of Mental Health Services in a Medicaid Population. *Social Science and Medicine.* 1988; 26:989–996.

U.S. Department of Health and Human Services, Indian Health Service, Mental Health and Social Services Branch. *A national plan for Native American mental health services.* Washington, DC: U.S. Department of Health and Human Services; 1989.

U.S. Department of Health and Human Services, Indian Health Service, Office of Program Planning and Evaluation. *Final report: Descriptive analysis of tribal health systems.* Washington, DC: U.S. Department of Health and Human Services; 1987.

U.S. Department of the Interior, Bureau of Indian Affairs. *Organizational Management Action Plan Responsibilities.* Washington, DC: U.S. Department of the Interior; 1988.

Vega, WA and Rumbaud RG. Ethnic minorities and health. *Annual Review of Sociology,* 1991; 17:351–383.

Walker RD, Howard MO, Anderson B, Lambert MD. Substance Dependent American Indian Veterans: A National Evaluation. *Public Health Reports.* 1994; 109(2):235–42.

Walker RD, Lambert MD, Walker PS, Kivlahan DR. Treatment Implications of Comorbid Psychopathology in American Indians and Alaska Natives. Culture, *Medicine & Psychiatry.* 1992–1993; 16(4):555–72.

Wallen, J. Providing culturally appropriate mental health services research for minorities. *Journal of Mental Health Administration.* 1992; 19:288–295.

Wells, K.,Hough RL., Golding J.M., Burnam M.A., and Karno M., Factors affecting the probability of use of general and medical health and social/community services for Mexican-Americans and non-Hispanic whites. *American Journal of Psychiatry.* 1987; 144:918–922. 1987.

Westermeyer, J., Psychiatric diagnosis across cultural boundaries. *American Journal of Psychiatry.* 1985; 142(7): 798–807.

Westermeyer J, Peake E. A Ten-year Follow-up of Alcoholic Native Americans in Minnesota. *American Journal of Psychiatry.* 1983; 140(2):189-94.

Willie CV, Kramers BM, and Brown BS. *Racism and mental health: Essays.* Pittsburgh, PA: University of Pittsburgh Press; 1973.

Zahner GEP, et al. Children's Mental Health Service Needs and Utilization Patterns in an Urban Community: An Epidemiological Assessment. *Journal of the American Academy of Child and Adolescent Psychiatry.* 1992; 31:951–960. 1992.

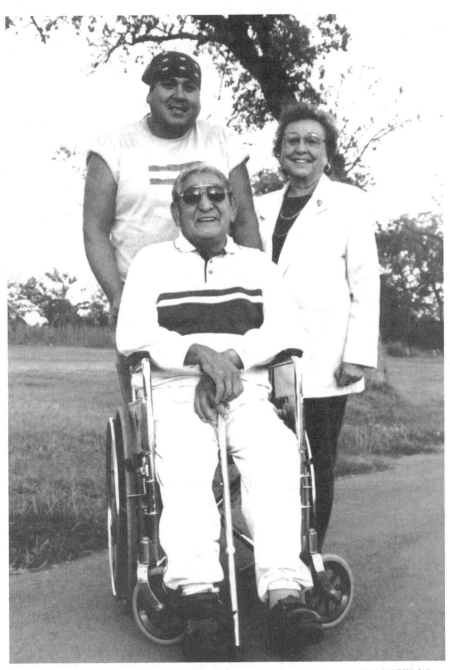

DIABETES IN AMERICAN INDIANS

Yvette Roubideaux and Kelly Acton

iabetes is a serious problem for American Indians and Alaska Natives (AI/AN), who suffer from some of the highest rates of Type 2 diabetes in the world. While the Indian health system has been trying to address this growing problem, rates of diabetes have continued to rise in the AI/AN population, with an alarming trend toward the development of diabetes at increasingly younger ages. Fortunately, there has been increased interest and efforts in the treatment and prevention of diabetes in AI/AN communities due to some significant recent changes in policies and resources for diabetes. Diabetes is a relatively new problem for AI/AN; the Indian Health Service (IHS), tribes, and urban Indian programs are working steadily towards the goal of a diabetes-free future for American Indian communities.

THE GROWING PROBLEM OF DIABETES IN AI/AN COMMUNITIES

While diabetes is now a serious and growing problem for AI/AN communities, reports of diabetes were rare in the AI/AN population prior to World War II. Unfortunately, rates of diabetes have risen to the point where certain Indian communities and tribes have some of the highest rates of diabetes in the world. In studies of the Pima Indians, the prevalence of diabetes has been reported to be at least 50 percent of the adult population over age 35 (Gohdes 1995). Overall, diabetes is four to eight times more common in American

Indians than in the general population (Lee et al, 1995). In a 1996 review of the Indian Health Service national outpatient database, the overall prevalence of diabetes was two to three times higher in AI/AN compared to non-Hispanic whites in all age groups studied (*Morbidity and Mortality Weekly Report* 1999).

Estimates of the prevalence of diabetes for AI/AN as a group tend to obscure the fact that the prevalence of diabetes varies greatly among tribes and regions of the country. In the Strong Heart Study, a longitudinal study of cardiovascular disease in American Indians ages 45–74, age-adjusted rates of diabetes have been found as high as 72 percent in women and 62 percent in men in the Arizona cohort. While the prevalence of diabetes was somewhat lower in the Dakota and Oklahoma cohorts (33–42 percent), the prevalence of diabetes in all three of these groups was still much higher than the U.S. general population (Lee et al 1995). In the Navajo Health and Nutrition Survey, the age-standardized prevalence of diabetes was 22.9 percent for persons age 20 years and older, and greater than 40 percent among Navajo individuals age 45 and older (Will et al 1997).

The most alarming trend in relation to diabetes in AI/AN is the rising prevalence of Type 2 diabetes in children and adolescents, a disease previously considered rare in individuals in these age groups. Type 2 diabetes is thought to be a disease of adults, usually occurring in people aged 30-40 years old, but data from the Pima studies gathered over time have shown significant increases in the number of cases of diabetes in children as young as three and five years old (Dabelea et al 1998). The IHS Diabetes Program recently completed a study of changes in diabetes prevalence over a 7-year period by age group and found a 6 percent increase in the under 15-year-old group, a 28 percent increase in the 15–19 year old group, a 36 percent increase in the 20–24 year old group, and a 32 percent increase in the 25–34 year old group. The rise in cases of Type 2 diabetes in AI/AN children and adolescents is thought to be due at least in part to the increased prevalence of obesity and increased exposure to diabetes in utero due to the high rates of diabetes in the female adult population of child-bearing age.

COMPLICATIONS OF DIABETES

The problem of diabetes has grown to become the fourth leading cause of death for AI/AN (Indian Health Service 1996). Recent analyses by the IHS have shown that mortality rates for American Indians with diabetes are 3.8 to 5.6 times higher compared to non-Hispanic whites (Gilliland et al, 1997). AI/AN also suffer from higher rates of the complications of diabetes compared to the general U.S. population, with 6.8 times more end stage renal disease (Muneta et al, 1993), 3 times greater rates of lower extremity amputations (Valway et al, 1993), and double the amount of cardiovascular disease (Howard et al, 1999).

The impact of diabetes on AI/AN communities and families is not adequately reflected in the statistics and research results. With such high rates of diabetes and its complications, recent amputations, problems related to blindness, access to transportation to dialysis, and coping with the problems related to chronic disabilities are unfortunately common topics of discussion in the daily lives of AI/AN families and community members. Health care providers have difficulties addressing all of the health problems and needs of AI/AN patients due to the long list of diagnoses, medications, and acute conditions that are present and needing attention during a 15-minute clinic visit. Wheelchairs, crutches, canes, and dark glasses are so common they are rarely noticed as unusual.

RISK FACTORS FOR DIABETES

The risk factors for developing diabetes in the AI/AN population have been determined in two recent studies. In the Strong Heart Study, age, parental diabetes, obesity, and a higher degree of American Indian ancestry were associated with the diagnosis of diabetes (Lee et al, 1995). In the Pima studies conducted by the National Institutes of Health, parental diabetes, obesity, degree of Indian heritage, and high calorie–high fat diets were associated with the development of diabetes (Knowler et al, 1993). While there is some evidence for an increased genetic susceptibility for diabetes in AI/AN, it is clear that environmental factors have played a significant role in the elevated rates of diabetes. The lifestyles of AI/AN have changed dramatically over the past century with the transition from a hunter-gatherer society to restriction to the reservation and a more "modernized" lifestyle, including decreases in physical activity, increases in high calorie–high fat diets, participation in the fast food economy, and rising rates of obesity.

TREATMENT AND PREVENTION OF DIABETES

Even though diabetes has grown to be a serious health problem for AI/AN communities, recent studies in the medical literature demonstrate the benefits of treating diabetes and its complications. Some studies are beginning to suggest that Type 2 diabetes may be preventable. In the Diabetes Control and Complications Trial (DCCT Research Group 1993) and the United Kingdom Prospective Diabetes Study (UKPDS Group 1998 a,b), aggressive control of blood glucose in individuals with Type 1 and Type 2 diabetes, respectively, was associated with significant reductions in complications of diabetes. Aggressive control of blood glucose in these studies included not only intensive therapy with medications for diabetes, but also aggressive diet changes, physical activity, structured diabetes education, and a team approach to care. These studies were the first to definitively show that intensive treatment of diabetes can result in better outcomes.

A number of primary prevention trials are currently underway to determine if diabetes can be prevented before it occurs in individuals at risk. The Diabetes Prevention Program is an NIH-funded, prospective multi-center, randomized trial of metformin (a medication normally used to reduce blood glucose levels in patients with Type 2 diabetes) vs. intensive lifestyle change as the interventions intended to prevent progression to frank diabetes in individuals with impaired glucose tolerance (IGT).   Results of this study are highly anticipated, and should be available in the year 2002 (DPP Research Group 1999). Some smaller studies have provided promising results, including the DaQing study in China that found a significant reduction in the risk of developing diabetes in individuals with IGT who implemented the exercise and/or diet interventions compared to control subjects who did not participate in these interventions (Pan X-R et al, 1997).

These studies provide evidence that there is hope for the treatment and prevention of diabetes and its complications. Unfortunately, many AI/AN people with diabetes are unaware of the results of these studies, and believe there is little they can do to control their diabetes. As the rates of diabetes rise in Indian communities and more individuals are seen going to dialysis centers, getting amputations, and suffering from the complications of diabetes, the potential for individuals to develop a sense of fatalism about their diabetes is very high. More efforts and resources are needed to increase awareness and to provide education on diabetes in AI/AN communities and how to best treat it and prevent complications.

STANDARDS OF CARE

The American Diabetes Association (ADA) has developed recommendations for a number of routine examinations and tests that an individual with diabetes should receive on a regular basis, in addition to intensive control of blood glucose. These recommendations are part of the ADA's *Standards of Medical Care for Patients with Diabetes Mellitus*, first published in 1988. A number of routine tests and examinations are recommended to help monitor and prevent the complications of diabetes, including annual foot examinations, eye examinations, and routine laboratory tests such as the HbA1C test (which measures the level of blood glucose control over the past three months) (ADA/Diabetes Care 1999).

Unfortunately, while these routine examinations and tests are associated with improved outcomes, rates of adherence to these recommendations vary greatly, and many studies show low rates of adherence in patients with diabetes (Jacques et al, 1991; Kenny et al, 1993; Worrall et al, 1997; Marshall et al, 1996; Martin et al, 1995; Peters et al, 1996; Zoorab et al, 1996; Brechner et al, 1993; Streja et al, 1999).

ADDRESSING THE PROBLEM OF DIABETES IN THE INDIAN HEALTH SYSTEM

THE IHS NATIONAL DIABETES PROGRAM

The Indian Health Service recognized the growing problem of diabetes in AI/AN communities in the 1970s, and subsequently implemented programs and policies to provide comprehensive services for individuals with diabetes within its system of health programs and facilities. In the Indian Health Care Improvement Act of 1976 (P.L. 94-437), specific language was included to create expanded health care services for diabetes. The Indian Health Service Diabetes Program was established by Congress in 1979 to address the growing problem of diabetes in the American Indian population (Mayfield et al, 1994). This program has grown over the years to become a comprehensive network of diabetes-related resources in the Indian health system, including a National Program office located in Albuquerque, New Mexico and Area Diabetes Consultants in each IHS Area who coordinate the diabetes surveillance data and activities of local diabetes programs in many of the Indian health hospitals and clinics located on or near Indian reservations. The IHS National Diabetes Program's activities include: setting *Standards of Care* for patients with diabetes, published biannually since 1986; developing and maintaining a data surveillance system for diabetes and its complications; providing resources, education, and technical assistance; developing patient education materials; implementing Staged Diabetes Management™ to encourage community involvement in diabetes care; and evaluating the quality and measuring outcomes of diabetes care through the annual IHS Diabetes Care and Outcomes Audit, which is an annual, systematic medical record review of a sample of patients with diabetes seen in participating Indian health facilities.

The Indian Health Care Improvement Act (IHCIA) of 1979 included language to establish "Model Diabetes Programs" in the Indian health system for the purpose of creating programs that would model the translation of diabetes research findings into practice in the unique settings of AI/AN communities. Subsequent reauthorizations and amendments to the IHCIA have led to the establishment of 19 Model Diabetes Programs across the country; the most recent Model Diabetes Program was established in 1995.

The IHS Diabetes Program is actually the most comprehensive rural system of care for diabetes in the country, combining both clinical and public health approaches to the problem of diabetes. Surveillance and evaluation of program activities over time have shown many successes in the care and treatment of diabetes in American Indian communities. For example, the IHS Diabetes Audit is the most comprehensive ongoing national review of diabetes care in the country, and serves as a model for other health care systems. However, despite improvements in the care of diabetes over time, significant disparities in quality of care still exist, primarily due to lack of resources. The rates of diabetes continue their alarming rise in the AI/AN population.

THE SPECIAL DIABETES GRANTS FOR INDIANS PROGRAM

As the Indian Health Service continued to reorganize and downsize in the mid-1990s, many providers in the Indian health care system expressed concern about the future of the IHS Diabetes Program. Clearly, the program and its services were needed, but resources were declining and positions were being eliminated. The Balanced Budget Act of 1997 provided a much-needed injection of funding for new programs for the treatment and prevention of diabetes in Indian country. The specific language of the legislation provided the IHS $30 million each year for the next 5 years ($150 million total) to establish grants for new prevention and treatment services in IHS, tribal, and urban health programs. An additional $3 million was added to the IHS budget through the Department of the Interior Appropriation for diabetes grants. This was the first time that a significant new appropriation of funds for diabetes was added to the IHS budget since 1979, and there was much celebration in the Indian health system for this significant addition of resources. However, once the euphoria subsided, it became clear that $30 million was only a "drop in the bucket" in terms of the real amount of resources needed to address the problem of diabetes in the Indian health system, which includes 556 federally-recognized tribes, over 300 Indian health facilities, and 34 urban Indian programs eligible to apply for funding under this new appropriation.

The IHS is a health care agency with expertise in providing primary health care to patients; it is not an agency that is experienced in developing and managing grant programs. With the announcement of the availability of these new funds, the IHS needed to devise a strategy to distribute these funds as grants to eligible programs, and to provide an opportunity for tribal consultation on this issue. The Director of the IHS convened the "Indian Health Diabetes Workgroup" in 1997 and charged the group with determining a formula for distribution of these new funds for diabetes treatment and prevention services. The workgroup membership consisted of one elected tribal leader from each IHS Area, diabetes scientists, and representatives from national Indian organizations, such as the National Indian Health Board, the National Council of Urban Indian Programs, and the Association of American Indian Physicians.

After intense negotiations and discussion, the workgroup developed a method for distribution of the diabetes-services funds in a non-competitive grant program for eligible IHS, tribes, and urban programs. They devised a formula to determine the exact amount of funding available for each tribe that included calculations of disease burden (diabetes prevalence and diabetes mortality), user population, and an adjustment for tribal size to ensure that small tribes got at least a base level of funding for their programs. A portion of the funding was set aside for the improvement of data collection in each Area to address the problem that some Areas did not have accurate disease-burden data, and as such may not have received their fair share of funding.

The distribution formula was used to calculate the total amount of funding that would be allocated to each IHS Area. A consultation process within each Area determined further distribution to tribes and Indian health programs. The entire process for determining the allocation of this new diabetes funding serves as an excellent example of how federal agencies can implement a tribal consultation process and comply with the spirit of the President's Executive Order for true partnering with tribes.

The Special Diabetes Program Grants for Indians is currently in its third year of operation at the time of this book's publication, and the grants have been successfully administered by the IHS National Diabetes Program. In the beginning, the program faced many challenges in providing the needed training and technical assistance for new programs as administrators developed their grant applications. Delays in the transfer of funds to the Areas and the local programs, and delays in the ability of some programs to comply with adminis-trative requirements and deadlines posed considerable problems. The grant program was subsequently modified to meet the needs of the tribes and pro-grams involved, and a 3-cycle application and renewal process was implement-ed.

The Balanced Budget Act of 1997 included specific language that required the IHS to report on the progress of The Special Diabetes Program Grants for Indians with an interim report in year 2000 and a final report to Congress in year 2002 at the completion of the grant program. The IHS Diabetes Program convened a panel of experts in qualitative research in the fall of 1998 to pro-vide advice and guidance on the development of a methodology for a formal evaluation of the new and expanded diabetes programs. With further techni-cal assistance from experts in program evaluation and the assistance of an eval-uation contractor, the IHS National Diabetes Program developed an assessment tool that was distributed to all 333 diabetes grant recipients in September 1999; The assessment tool also serves as the yearly progress report from recip-ient programs that requested that their progress reports include less narrative and more multiple choice answers. Overall, 99 percent of the programs responded and provided information on the emphasis of their grant program; target groups served, methods for screening, education, physical activity, and nutrition; improvements in services and program infrastructure due to the increased funding; barriers to program implementation; and programmatic and staffing needs (IHS 2000). A comprehensive summary of the results and the history of the grant program were included in the *IHS National Diabetes Program Special Diabetes Program for Indians Interim Report to Congress*, sub-mitted in January 2000.

The *Interim Report to Congress* contained over 20 pages of results that char-acterized the wide variety of prevention and treatment programs implemented under this grant program. In terms of program emphasis, 67 percent of sites emphasized primary and secondary prevention of diabetes and its complications, 32 percent emphasized tertiary prevention of complications, and 41 percent emphasized program planning. The target audiences for these programs include all community members, family members, individuals at high risk for diabetes, and individuals with diabetes in pregnancy. The majority of grant programs indicated substantially increased services available specifically for children, adolescents, and elders. Grant program emphases included activities such as diabetes screening, treatment and prevention activities, diabetes education, physical activity programs, and nutrition programs.

Most grant programs also included activities to improve their diabetes-related services, such as establishing or improving diabetes teams and registries, using flow sheets to track diabetes care and, thus, enhance data collection and monitoring. The grant programs also identified barriers to program implementation, including space and problems with hiring new staff, and they identified significant needs for technical assistance (IHS 2000).

In December 2000, Congress passed the Consolidated Appropriations Act 2001, which included $240 million in additional funding for the Special Diabetes Program Grants for Indians. This Act provided for an additional $70 million in fiscal year 2001, an additional $70 million in fiscal year 2002, and a total of $100 million in fiscal year 2003, thus extending the program an additional year. Congress also changed the requirement for a final report to Congress to year 2003. Congressional direction included recommendations to use this new funding to build on the successes of the original Special Diabetes Program Grants, including the development of special initiatives and model programs. A tribal consultation process was developed to determine how to distribute these new diabetes funds to IHS, tribal, and urban programs.

The IHS National Diabetes Program will continue to administer, monitor and evaluate the grant program, in partnership with the Tribal Leaders Diabetes Committee, in preparation for the final report to Congress in the year 2003. Clearly, this program has been successful in providing much needed new and expanded prevention and treatment services to AI/AN communities. However, since the appropriation was originally designated for 5 years, with one additional year provided in the Consolidated Appropriations Act of 2001, significant advocacy efforts are needed to convince Congress of the need to continue funding for these programs in the future. Language has been included in the reauthorization draft of the Indian Health Care Improvement Act (IHCIA) to continue funding for diabetes programs until the year 2012 when the next reauthorization occurs. Failure to continue funding for these programs beyond year 6 would be devastating for tribes and Indian programs that are working so hard to address the problem of diabetes in their communities.

THE TRIBAL LEADERS DIABETES COMMITTEE

In preparation for Year 2 of The Special Diabetes Program Grants for Indians, the Director of the Indian Health Service reconvened the Indian

Health Diabetes Workgroup, but limited the membership of the workgroup to elected tribal officials from each IHS Area; the original purpose of this meeting was to determine the formula for distribution of grant funds in Year 2. The tribal leaders decided to continue the current formula, and also discussed the importance of having a mechanism for tribal leaders to provide input and consultation on diabetes-related activities in the IHS and other government agencies, with special notice taken of the number of new initiatives related to diabetes in American Indians. They then established themselves as the "Tribal Leaders Diabetes Committee," and drafted a letter asking to be formally recognized by the Director of the IHS and to request administrative support. The request was approved in October 1998, and the Tribal Leaders Diabetes Committee (TLDC) became part of the official consultation process in the IHS. The mission and vision statements of the TLDC are as follows:

> *Mission*: Make recommendations to the Director, Indian Health Service, on issues related to diabetes and its complications in American Indian and Alaska Native people.

> *Vision*: Empowering AI/AN people to live free of diabetes through healthy lifestyles while preserving cultural traditions and values through tribal leadership, direction, communication and education.[1]

The establishment of the TLDC is significant. It is the first time a group of elected tribal officials voluntarily agreed to form a committee with a special interest in a chronic health condition. It is also significant in its demonstration of a true spirit of ongoing partnership between this group and the IHS. Previous workgroups and committees involving tribal leadership often were focused on budget and administrative issues. Perhaps the most important element of the TLDC is the enthusiasm and commitment of these elected tribal officials to help in the fight against diabetes in Indian country. The TLDC is clearly a model mechanism for how to provide tribal consultation and input on federal programs that address a specific condition or disease.

DIABETES EDUCATION SERVICES

The Balanced Budget Act of 1997 also provided authorization for Medicare reimbursement of diabetes education services. In February 1999, the Health Care Financing Administration (HCFA) published proposed rules for *Expanded Coverage for Outpatient Diabetes Self-Management Training Services for Medicare*, which would allow for reimbursement of diabetes education services, but with specific rules and criteria that limit reimbursement to those programs that have obtained proper certification for their diabetes education programs. Currently the only form of certification available is the American Diabetes Association (ADA) Diabetes Education Recognition Program.

---

[1] Mission and Vision Statements as stated in a letter from the TLDC to the Director of the IHS, October 1998.

Experience with this program in the past has revealed problems with cost and a lack of culturally competent criteria in the program that would make it more relevant for Indian health programs (IHS 2000).

The IHS National Diabetes Program is currently working to establish an Indian Health Diabetes Education Accreditation Program that would provide a culturally competent mechanism for Indian health diabetes programs to receive certification for Medicare reimbursement for diabetes education services. The IHS has formed a workgroup that is developing the process for this certification, which would use an updated version of the IHS Diabetes Education Program Criteria based on the National Standards for Diabetes Education, which have also been revised on a national level. This certification process is being developed with input and participation of the TLDC.

SPECIAL INITIATIVES FOR DIABETES IN AMERICAN INDIANS

A number of special initiatives outside of the IHS have also been developed over the past few years to address the problem of diabetes in American Indian/Alaska Native communities.

NATIONAL DIABETES PREVENTION CENTER

The Balanced Budget Act of 1997 also authorized the Centers for Disease Control and Prevention (CDC) to establish a National Diabetes Prevention Center (NDPC) in Gallup, New Mexico. The purpose of the NDPC is to provide guidance and technical assistance related to diabetes prevention research and programs in AI/AN communities, with an initial focus on the Navajo and Zuni tribes, and subsequent national expansion to serve all tribes. The CDC received a yearly appropriation of $2 million directly from Congress, and another $1 million from the Special Diabetes Program Grants for Indians at the request of the TLDC, to establish the new center.

AMERICAN DIABETES ASSOCIATION

The American Diabetes Association (ADA) established a Native American Design Team in 1997 to help assist in the development of a special ADA program for American Indians and Alaska Natives. The members of this team include representatives from all regions of the country, including Indian health professionals, diabetes program personnel, and representatives from the IHS National Diabetes Program. The ADA formally launched the "Awakening the Spirit" Campaign, developed with the assistance of the Native American Design Team, in October 1998 at the "Diabetes in American Indian Communities" National Conference in Albuquerque, New Mexico. The Awakening the Spirit Program consists of a number of activities related to diabetes education, including special educational materials, partnerships with other organizations and efforts, and the adoption of the "Strong in Body and Spirit" curriculum (developed by the Native American Diabetes Project at the

University of New Mexico to be a culturally competent diabetes education program that trains community members to provide education about diabetes). The Awakening the Spirit Campaign is an example of how a national organization such as the ADA can effectively develop culturally competent educational programs with the participation of members of the communities involved.

NATIONAL DIABETES EDUCATION PROGRAM

The National Diabetes Education Program (NDEP) is a national effort to teach individuals with diabetes that they can control their diabetes and prevent complications. The NDEP is a collaborative activity supported by the Centers for Disease Control and Prevention, the National Institutes of Health/National Institute of Diabetes, Digestive and Kidney Diseases (NIDDK), and over 200 public and private sector partners. The goal of the NDEP is to reduce the morbidity and mortality related to diabetes and its complications. Educational messages in all of the NDEP activities focus on the importance of controlling blood glucose and better self-care for diabetes. The five major components of the NDEP include public awareness campaigns, community interventions, health systems interventions, special population activities, and a partnership network.

The NDEP is committed to developing public service messages that are culturally appropriate for communities and populations that are disproportionately affected by diabetes. The NDEP formed four "Special Population Workgroups" (Hispanic, African American, Asian Pacific Islanders, and American Indian) in 1997 to serve as advisors on the development of educational materials for these "special populations." The initial plans for these campaigns were to develop culturally appropriate television, radio, and print ads with educational messages about diabetes.

The NDEP American Indian Workgroup, formed in January 1998, was charged with assisting in the development of culturally-appropriate advertisements for AI/AN communities. The workgroup members include representatives from the Association of American Indian Physicians, the Indian Health Service, the National Indian Health Board, and other health care providers and community members with a special interest and experience in the area of diabetes.

The initial activities of the workgroup involved educating the NIH, CDC, and NDEP contractors on the demographics and characteristics of the American Indian and Alaska Native population. This process included a review of relevant literature and previous efforts to develop diabetes education materials for American Indian and Alaska Natives. The Association of American Indian Physicians also sponsored a series of focus groups to gather information from tribal leaders, Indian health professionals, and American Indian community members on their experiences with current diabetes education materials and their recommendations for how these materials could be improved. (Roubideaux et al, 2000)

The next step in the process included development of draft concepts and messages for pre-testing with members of the target audience. In the initial campaign, the target audience was chosen to be AI/AN with diabetes, and the message was to be focused on the importance of controlling the disease. The overall NDEP public awareness campaign message is "Control your Diabetes for Life" and is based on recent research results that have shown that controlling blood glucose can prevent the complications of diabetes (DCCT Research Group 1993, UKPDS Group 1998).

Draft messages and concepts were pre-tested in a series of focus groups held around the country that included AI/AN with diabetes from a number of tribes. As a result of these focus groups, the overall campaign message was developed. Repeatedly during the focus groups, AI/AN with diabetes asked for advertising that carried a message of hope, that were specific to AI/AN, and that focused on the importance of families, children, and preserving the future and Indian culture. They also wanted the materials to contain pictures of AI/AN representing a number of different tribes, both in modern and traditional dress, to represent the diversity of American Indian people. Participants didn't want materials that presented stereotypes of Indians or that focused only on one region, such as the Southwest. The final NDEP American Indian Campaign message was "Control your Diabetes for Future Generations." With this message as the focus of the American Indian campaign, a 30-second TV public service announcement (PSA), several radio scripts, and a number of print ads were developed.

The Association of American Indian Physicians (AAIP) was selected by CDC to help assist in the dissemination of the NDEP American Indian Campaign materials. The AAIP Diabetes Program's activities include: dissemination of materials at conferences and community events; development of diabetes education packets with newly-developed educational materials; development of a web page for the AAIP Diabetes Program and a toll-free telephone number for information and access to the materials; and formation of a diabetes partnership network of over 200 individuals and organizations. Materials have been mailed to a number of individuals and organizations, including all 333 Special Grants for Diabetes Programs in the Indian health system. The AAIP is encouraging Indian health professionals, programs, and tribes to use these materials in their programs, health facilities and communities to help teach American Indians and Alaska Natives the importance of controlling their diabetes "for future generations."

The NDEP American Indian Workgroup recently developed a strategic plan for the next few years, which includes continued dissemination of current campaign materials, developing new partnerships with other organizations and groups, and the development of a new campaign focus on youth. The workgroup members recognize that the rates of diabetes are increasing, and that it is important to educate children and adolescents about diabetes and how they can reduce their risk factors for this condition. Focus groups will be conducted with American Indian youth to assist in the development of concepts and activities for this new aspect of the campaign. This process of community involvement in the development and dissemination of educational materials for the NDEP is clearly a model program for other government agencies and organizations to follow to ensure the cultural competence and effectiveness of their materials.[2]

FUTURE EFFORTS

While there are currently a number of exciting programs and activities addressing the problem of diabetes in American Indians, more efforts are clearly needed. Diabetes is a chronic disease that individuals can live with for many years. It is a prevalent disease that is present in almost every extended family in some communities. But diabetes is not just a disease of an individual; it is also a disease of a family, and a disease of a community. The risk factors for diabetes are present in individuals, families, and communities. Many AI/AN community events involve large quantities of high calorie-high fat food consumed in large portions that are considered normal and appropriate. Many AI/AN individuals believe that an overweight or obese body image is "normal" or "healthy" for American Indian people, and make comments to friends and relatives about their displeasure with someone who has lost weight, or a baby who is "too thin." And in many communities, the only people engaging in regular physical activity are young children. This community-wide mindset is contributing to the problem of diabetes by inadvertently increasing the risk of every community member for diabetes.

More efforts are needed to provide education to AI/AN about what they can do to reduce their risks for developing diabetes, how they can best care for themselves if they are diagnosed with diabetes, and how to prevent subsequent complications. Educational efforts are needed at all levels to ensure that AI/AN receive the highest quality of diabetes care and treatment.

AI/AN can work to restore health and wellness to themselves, their families and their communities by working together to promote healthy behaviors such as physical activity, providing healthier food choices at community events, and being supportive of those community members who are trying to improve their health. In order to achieve healthier communities, and therefore hopefully reduce risk factors for diabetes, community involvement is needed at all levels, but particularly at the level of tribal leadership. The Special Diabetes Program Grants for Indians has created a mechanism for communities to work together in the fight against diabetes, as 94 percent of the grant programs funded under this initiative are primarily administered by tribes. Clearly, tribes and community members have the opportunity to work to recreate healthy communities that will help reduce their risks for diabetes.

---

[2] This description of the NDEP American Indian campaign was adapted from a manuscript in press for the *IHS Provider* 25(6): 97-100. June 2000.

Tribal leaders and community members have repeatedly requested more prevention efforts to try to stop the rising rates of diabetes. The results of the Diabetes Prevention Program and other primary prevention studies are anxiously being watched for any encouragement and information on how to prevent diabetes from occurring in Indian communities. However, if the DPP shows that medication does help prevent the development of diabetes, significant resources will be needed to develop strategies for screening and identification of appropriate individuals for treatment, and for the increased pharmaceutical cost burden this strategy may bring. Advocacy efforts must start now to find the resources to ensure that AI/AN will not have to settle for a lower standard of care in the prevention and care of diabetes.

Finally, it is important to remember that diabetes was not a significant problem for AI/AN communities prior to World War II. There were no words in traditional languages for diabetes; pictures from the 1800s of AI/AN show healthy, thin, and fit individuals; and the messages of traditional Indian medicine include messages that encourage keeping active, eating healthy foods in moderation, and being mindful of the health of the community as well. While AI/AN may not be able to go back to how they lived centuries ago, they can restore principles of wellness to their communities.

REFERENCES

American Diabetes Association. Standards of Medical Care for Patients with Diabetes Mellitus. *Diabetes Care.* 1999; 22(Suppl. 1): S32–S41.

Brechner RJ, Cowie CC, Howie LJ, et al. Ophthalmic Examination among Adults with Diagnosed Diabetes Mellitus. *Journal of the American Medical Association.* 1993; 270:1714–1718.

Dabelea D, Hanson RL, Bennett PH, et al. Increasing Prevalence of Type II Diabetes in American Indian Children. *Diabetologia.* 1998; 41:904–910.

The Diabetes Control and Complications Trial Research Group. The Effect of Intensive Treatment of Diabetes on the Development and Progression of Long-Term Complications in Insulin-Dependent Diabetes Mellitus. *New England Journal of Medicine.* 1993; 329:977–86.

Diabetes Prevention Program Research Group. The Diabetes Prevention Program. Design and Methods for a Clinical Trial in the Prevention of Type 2 Diabetes. *Diabetes Care.* 1999; 22:623–634.

Gilliland FD, Owen C, Gilliland SS, Carter JS. Temporal Trends in Diabetes Mortality among American Indians and Hispanics in New Mexico: Birth Cohort and Period Effects. *American Journal of Epidemiolgy.* 1997; 145:422-31.

Gohdes D. Diabetes in North American Indians and Alaska Natives. *Diabetes in America*. 2nd Ed. National Institutes of Health/NIDDK; Bethesda, MD; 1995.

Howard BV, Lee TL, Cowan LD, et al. Rising Tide of Cardiovascular Disease in American Indians: The Strong Heart Study. *Circulation*. 1999; 99:2389–2395.

Indian Health Service, US Department of Health and Human Services. *Trends in Indian Health*. Indian Health Service, Washington DC; 1996.

Indian Health Service. *IHS National Diabetes Program Special Diabetes Program for Indians Interim Report to Congress*. (Draft Pending Approval by OMB). IHS National Diabetes Program, Albuquerque, NM 2000.

Jacques CHM, Jones RL, Houts P, et al. Reported Practice Behaviors for Medical Care of Patients with Diabetes Mellitus by Primary-Care Physicians in Pennsylvania. *Diabetes Care*. 1991; 14:712–17.

Kenny SJ, Smith PJ, Goldschmid MG, et al. Survey of Physician Practice Behaviors Related to Diabetes Mellitus in the U.S. *Diabetes Care*. 1993; 16:1507–1509.

Knowler WC, Saad MF, Pettitt DJ, et al. Determinants of Diabetes Mellitus in the Pima Indians. *Diabetes Care*. 1993; 16(Suppl 1): 216–227.

Lee ET, Howard BV, Savage PJ, et al. Diabetes and Impaired Glucose Tolerance in Three American Indian Populations Aged 45-74 Years. The Strong Heart Study. *Diabetes Care*. 1995; 18:599–610.

Martin TL, Selby JV, Zhang D. Physician and Patient Prevention Practices in NIDDM in a Large Urban Managed-Care Organization. *Diabetes Care*. 1995; 18:1124–1132.

Marshall CL, Bluestein M, Chapin C, et al. Outpatient Management of Diabetes Mellitus in Five Arizona Medicare Managed Care Plans. *American Journal of Medical Quality*. 1996; 11:87-93.

Mayfield JA, Rith-Najarian SJ, Acton KJ, et al. Assessment of Diabetes Care by Medical Record Review. The Indian Health Service Model. *Diabetes Care*. 1994; 17:918–923.

Muneta B, Newman J, Stevenson J, Eggers P. Diabetic End-Stage Renal Disease

Among Native Americans. *Diabetes Care*. 1993; 16(Suppl 1): 346–348. 1993.

Pan X-R et al. Effects of Diet and Exercise in Preventing NIDDM in People with Impaired Glucose Tolerance. The Da-Qing IGT and Diabetes Study. *Diabetes Care* 1997; 20:537–44.

Prevalence of Diagnosed Diabetes Among American Indians/Alaskan Natives – United States, 1996. *MMWR*. 1997; 47(42): 901–904.

Peters AL, Legorreta AP, Ossorio RC, Davidson MB. Quality of Outpatient Care Provided to Diabetic Patients: A Health Maintenance Organization Experience. *Diabetes Care*. 1996; 19:601–606.

Roubideaux Y, Moore K, Avery C, et al. Diabetes Education Materials: Recommendations of Tribal Leaders, Indian Health Professional, and American Indian Community Members. *The Diabetes Educator*. 2000; 26(2): 290–294.

Streja DA, Rabkin SW. Factors Associated with Implementation of Preventative Care Measures in Patients with Diabetes Mellitus. *Archives of Internal Medicine*. 1999; 159:294–302.

UK Prospective Diabetes Study (UKPDS) Group. Intensive Blood-glucose Control with Sulphonylureas or Insulin Compared with Conventional Treatment and Risk of Complications in Patients with Type 2 Diabetes (UKPDS 33). *Lancet*. 1998a; 352:837–53.

UK Prospective Diabetes Study (UKPDS) Group. Effect of Intensive Blood-Glucose Control with Metformin on Complications in Overweight Patients with Type 2 Diabetes (UKPDS 34). *Lancet*. 1998b; 352:854–65.

Valway SE, Linkins RW, Gohdes DM. Epidemiology of Lower-Extremity Amputations in the Indian Health Service, 1982–1987. *Diabetes Care*. 1993; 16 (Suppl 1): 349–352.

Will JC, Strauss KF, Mendlein JM, et al. Diabetes Mellitus and Navajo Indians: Findings from the Navajo Health and Nutrition Survey. *Journal of Nutrition*. 1997; 127:2106S–2113S.

Worrall G, Freake D, Kelland J, et al. Care of Patients with Type II Diabetes: A Study of Family Physicians' Compliance with Clinical Practice Guidelines. *Journal of Family Practice*. 1997; 44:374–381.

Zoorob RJ, Mainous AG. Practice Patterns of Rural Family Physicians based on the American Diabetes Association Standards of Care. *Journal of Community Health*. 1996; 21:175–182.

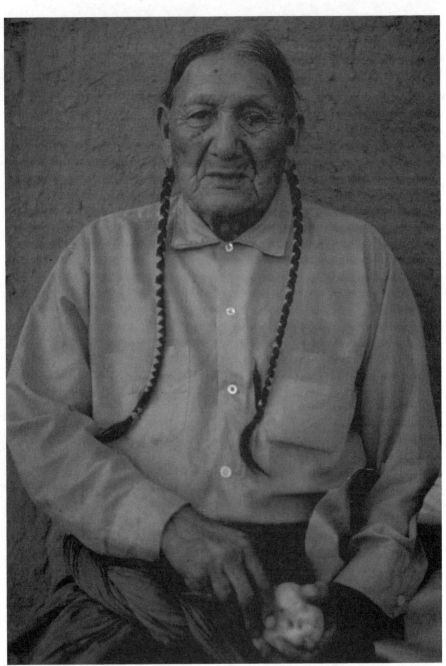

CARDIOVASCULAR DISEASE

Yvette Roubideaux

Cardiovascular disease (CVD), which refers to diseases involving the heart or blood vessels, is the leading cause of death for American Indians and Alaska Natives (AI/AN), and rates are increasing. However, the problem of CVD and its treatment and/or prevention receives little attention in discussions on Indian health. It is usually regarded as merely a complication of diabetes, not as a health problem responsible for more deaths among AI/AN than any other cause. This is unfortunate, since many of the risk factors for cardiovascular disease are modifiable and the disease itself may be prevented. Fortunately, we know much about CVD in American Indians primarily due to the Strong Heart Study, but more efforts are needed to evaluate the treatment and prevention of CVD in AI/AN. Public health efforts will need to play an important role in these efforts, and policy changes are clearly needed to help adequately address this increasing health problem in Indian communities.

THE GROWING PROBLEM OF CARDIOVASCULAR DISEASE IN AMERICAN INDIAN/ALASKA NATIVE COMMUNITIES

For many years, cardiovascular disease was believed to be rare in AI/AN. Rates of CVD were very low in the first half of the 20th century, and small studies found few or no cases of CVD in AI/AN (Gilbert 1955, Fulmer and Roberts 1963). Even though diabetes is a major risk factor for cardiovascular disease, rates of CVD in the Pima Indians for many years were surprisingly lower than the general population (Howard et al, 1999). However, while rates of CVD are declining in the general population (McGovern et al, 1996), AI/AN deaths from CVD have increased to be equal, and in some areas, higher than the general population (IHS 1997, Lee et al 1998, Howard 1999). CVD is the number one cause of death for AI/AN age 65 and older, as in the general population, but it is also the number one cause of death for AI/AN as young as age 45 (IHS 1997).

While some of the measured increase in CVD may be due to better data and correction of racial misclassification, this increase in cardiovascular disease in AI/AN is a real and significant phenomenon, and providers in the Indian health system are noticing the rise in cases of CVD in their daily practices. The Strong Heart Study, the first large epidemiologic study of CVD in AI/AN, deserves much of the credit for providing evidence of the rise in CVD rates reported in AI/AN communities. The Strong Heart Study was initiated in 1988 to study the rates of cardiovascular disease and its risk factors in 12 tribes in three distinct regions of the country: Arizona, Oklahoma, and North/South Dakota. Over 4500 individuals ages 45–74 have participated in this study which involved a baseline examination in Phase I (1989–1991) and a repeat examination in Phase II (1993–1995) of those same individuals who were still alive (Howard et al, 1992, 1999). This research design (longitudinal cohort) allowed for measuring rates of CVD risk factors, prevalence and mortality at baseline, and changes in the rates of CVD and its risk factors over time. The Strong Heart Study has been conducted in a culturally sensitive manner, with active participation of local community members in all phases of the study, and is well-accepted in the participating communities.

The major risk factors for cardiovascular disease in the general population are diabetes, hypertension, high cholesterol, obesity, and smoking. Rates of CVD in the general population are declining due to the success of public health efforts and policies that have provided education and awareness of CVD and its risk factors, improvements in rapid diagnosis and treatment, and prevention efforts that have promoted healthy lifestyles and led to a significant decline in the risk factors for heart disease. However, the lifestyles of AI/AN have also dramatically changed over the past decade, and have resulted in higher fat diets, lower rates of exercise, increased rates of smoking, and obesity. In addition, rates of diabetes, which is a major risk factor for cardiovascular disease, have increased in epidemic proportions in AI/AN (Lee et al, 1995).

The Strong Heart Study has better defined the risk factors for CVD in American Indians. These risk factors include diabetes, hypertension, obesity (percent body fat), smoking, high plasma insulin levels, low HDL cholesterol, high LDL cholesterol, high triglyceride levels, and albuminuria (Welty et al, 1995; Howard et al, 1995, 1996a, 1996b, 1999, 2000). Diabetes is the greatest risk factor for CVD in AI/AN; CVD rates are two to four times higher in

AI/AN men and women with diabetes than those without diabetes (Howard et al 1996b). There were also regional differences in the rates of cardiovascular disease risk factors in the Strong Heart Study, including higher rates of diabetes and obesity in Arizona, lower rates of hypercholesterolemia in Arizona, higher rates of hypertension in Arizona and Oklahoma, and higher rates of smoking in North/South Dakota (Welty 1995). The Navajo Health and Nutrition Survey also found high rates of cardiovascular disease risk factors, including obesity, diabetes, hypertension, smoking, high triglycerides, low HDL cholesterol and low physical activity levels (Mendlein et al, 1997). Rising rates of the risk factors for CVD have clearly contributed to the rising rates of CVD in AI/AN communities.

TREATMENT AND PREVENTION OF CARDIOVASCULAR DISEASE IN AMERICAN INDIAN/ALASKA NATIVE COMMUNITIES

The treatment of cardiovascular disease involves recognition of the symptoms, rapid evaluation and treatment, utilization of new and aggressive therapies, and proper rehabiliative care to improve function and prevent further complications. Primary prevention of CVD involves reducing risk factors through healthy lifestyles and identification and treatment of conditions that are risk factors for CVD, such as diabetes, hypertension, and high cholesterol levels. The most significant disparities in care for AI/AN in the Indian health system are in the emergent treatment of cardiac symptoms such as acute chest pain and shortness of breath. Morbidity and mortality from CVD remain high likely due to disparities in the quality of acute cardiac care.

Treatment of CVD in the general population has improved markedly, with improved emergency medical systems, rapid identification and treatment of chest pain and heart attacks, new emergency treatments that help dissolve clots that may block the coronary arteries, and new emergency procedures that help restore blood flow to the heart during heart attacks and heart failure. These improvements in the quality of care for CVD patients have clearly contributed to the declining death rates for heart disease in the general population.

For example, the most effective treatments to save lives during heart attacks must be started within the first hour or two of the onset of symptoms, and delays in care can mean greater damage to the heart and even death. Many cities in the U.S. set as a goal for their emergency medical systems a time frame of 30 minutes from onset of symptoms to diagnosis and treatment. This problem of access to high quality cardiac care is a serious issue in the Indian health system, and may help explain why death rates from CVD remain high in the AI/AN population.

There are many challenges in the treatment of cardiovascular disease in AI/AN communities. The Indian Health Service is a primary care system, with few sub-specialists available within the system. Therefore, AI/AN with heart disease, including those patients suffering heart attacks and heart failure, must be referred for both emergency and non-emergency cardiac care to tertiary-care hospitals (public/university and private hospitals) for evaluation by cardiologists and for diagnostic procedures and interventions. Treatment may be delayed by transportation, distance, and cost factors, and unfortunately, delays in care for heart attacks and strokes may result in increased complications and deaths. Indian health facilities often do not have access to updated equipment, the latest medicines, or treatments for CVD and are subsequently often unable to handle complex cases. Also, since many of the providers in the Indian health system are primary care providers, they may not be up-to-date on the latest treatments for heart disease. Furthermore, treatment is often delayed due to difficulty in getting initial medical care if the patient lives far from the Indian health facility, and if paramedics are unavailable during transport to the hospital. It is not unusual for AI/AN to have to travel for an hour or more to the local IHS facility, and then have to be transported another hour or more to the nearest tertiary-care facility, thus potentially delaying treatment by several hours.

Education and awareness of the symptoms and treatment of CVD in AI/AN communities are also problems, especially since many providers still believe that cardiovascular disease rates are lower in AI/AN compared to the general population. While AI/AN are very familiar with diabetes and its symptoms, there is little education available for community members on the symptoms of heart disease and the need for prompt treatment. In addition, AI/AN often present with atypical symptoms due to the presence of diabetes, which is often associated with "silent" ischemia and atypical symptoms of heart disease. Also, AI/AN may have difficulty describing their symptoms due to cultural or language factors.

Prevention of CVD in American Indian/Alaska Native communities is difficult due to the high prevalence of risk factors and recent lifestyle changes. Obesity, diets high in fat, and low rates of physical activity are common on Indian reservations, and as with the near epidemic of diabetes, changing community habits is difficult, since some risk factors and unhealthy behaviors are considered normal in some communities. The poor access to quality medical care present in the Indian health system also contributes to poor control of conditions that are risk factors for cardiovascular disease, such as diabetes, hypertension, and high cholesterol. Without understanding that these conditions are risk factors for CVD, AI/AN may not request screening for these conditions, and may not understand that they need to aggressively control these diseases to prevent CVD. Contract health funding may not be available for routine screening tests for CVD, and diagnoses may be unnecessarily delayed.

SPECIAL INITIATIVES FOR CARDIOVASCULAR DISEASE

The Indian Health Service has attempted to make arrangements for specialty services and referrals for the treatment of CVD on a local or regional basis, and from time to time, cardiologists have been on staff in larger Indian health facilities. For example, the Native American Cardiology Program at the University of Arizona is staffed by IHS and university cardiologists who provide tertiary care for referrals and who travel to conduct cardiology clinics in Indian health facilities on reservations in the Southwest. Similar referral systems have been implemented in other regions of the country, including the Plains and Alaska. A special clinic designed to provide pharmacy-based treatment of high cholesterol levels has been established at the Sante Fe Service Unit. However, most AI/AN patients do not have access to these limited services and must be referred to non-Indian health facilities for cardiac care, often using Contract Health Services, Medicare, Medicaid, or private insurance. Once patients are referred outside the Indian health system, they may encounter providers who are not culturally competent in the care of AI/AN, and may not understand the unique challenges in caring for AI/AN patients with cardiovascular disease.

Clearly, more efforts are needed to improve the treatment and prevention of CVD in AI/AN communities. There have been no studies that evaluate the effectiveness of specific interventions for cardiovascular disease in AI/AN, and there are no published studies on the prevention of CVD in AI/AN. However, there are a number of initiatives that are being developed for the prevention and treatment of CVD in AI/AN.

The National Heart, Lung and Blood Institute (NHLBI) in the National Institutes of Health has initiated a project entitled "Building Healthy Hearts for American Indian and Alaska Natives." This project is designed to promote healthy lifestyles and reduce the prevalence of heart disease and its risk factors through prevention strategies designed specifically for AI/AN tribes (Lising 1998). The Alaska Native Women's Wellness Project (WISEWOMAN) has recently been funded by NIH to develop a community-based program to reduce CVD risk factors among Alaska Native women, through health education, screening, and both primary and secondary interventions involving lifestyle interventions to reduce risk factors (personal communication, Stillwater 1999). The Pathways project, funded by NIH, is a multi-site school-based intervention for children in grades 3-5 to reduce the prevalence of obesity through classroom education, physical activity, and family involvement. American Indian schools are included in this intervention study, and participation of local community members is a vital part of the program (Lising 1998). The Checkerboard Cardiovascular Curriculum is an example of a culturally appropriate school curriculum to teach 5th grade AI/AN children about cardiovascular health. This program was implemented in rural New Mexico in Indian communities, and has shown positive results in terms of increasing the knowledge and physical activity of participating children (Harris et al, 1988). Another curriculum, the "Southwestern Cardiovascular Curriculum", has been used in rural northwestern New Mexico with teachers and students, to teach about healthy habits and lifetime skills (Lising 1998).

There are a number of new community-based prevention programs being implemented under the Special Grants for Diabetes in Indians Program administered by the IHS National Diabetes Program that promote healthy behaviors and address some of the risk factors for diabetes and cardiovascular disease (See chapter 8 for more on diabetes). Many programs promote primary and secondary prevention of diabetes, physical activity, nutritional education such as cooking classes, community activities such as health fairs and school activities, and some focus on high-risk individuals with hypertension, obesity, and smoking cessation (IHS 2000).

Over half of the Special Diabetes Grants for Indians Programs are providing education on the healthy use of commodity foods. For many years, the USDA Food Distribution Program on Indian Reservations has provided commodity foods to low-income AI/AN given the problems experienced in rural areas with access to food stores. Unfortunately, many of these foods were high fat, processed foods that were different from the traditionally low-fat meats and vegetables that AI/AN ate as a part of their diet in the past. For example, large packages of cheeses and lard were routinely distributed; since access to other healthier foods was limited by distance and poverty, AI/AN incorporated these high fat foods in their diet. . Fry bread is an example of a modern adaptation to available food sources. It is actually not a traditional Indian food, but was easily made with the flour and lard received through the USDA commodity program – the manner in which it is made is inconsistent with the lifestyle and habits of many tribal traditions. It is likely that the commodity foods program inadvertently contributed to unhealthy eating habits in Indian communities and the increased rates of obesity, diabetes, and cardiovascular disease. However in recent years, the USDA has been working to lower the levels of fats and sugars in commodity foods and to distribute healthier foods, including more high-quality fruits and vegetables (Lising 1998).

The Diabetes Prevention Program, a large, multi-center intervention trial designed to determine if the development of diabetes can be prevented in individuals with Impaired Glucose Tolerance has both a medical and lifestyle intervention. The lifestyle intervention consists of a healthier diet and physical activity, and promotes the same healthy behaviors that can reduce the risk of CVD. A positive result for the lifestyle intervention in preventing diabetes will provide more evidence to support adoption of these healthy behaviors, because not only will they help reduce the occurrence of diabetes, they will likely reduce the rates of CVD as well by reducing common risk factors.

FUTURE EFFORTS

Given the rising rates of cardiovascular disease in American Indian/Alaska Native communities, efforts are clearly needed to help improve the treatment and prevention of CVD and its risk factors. Even though many of the community-based activities addressing diabetes also indirectly help improve healthy behaviors that may reduce CVD rates as well, specific interventions are needed for CVD.

Education on the symptoms of CVD, appropriate treatment, and the need for rapid evaluation if symptoms develop are needed for all community members, and specific educational activities are needed. More information needs to be developed to distribute to tribe members at community events and health fairs, and public service announcements and posters need to be developed to send these messages. Any educational messages developed for AI/AN should be culturally competent, easy to understand, relevant to the habits of the target audience, and must involve community members in the development and dissemination process (Roubideaux et al, 2000a). The National Diabetes Education Program's American Indian Campaign is an example of using the principles of social marketing and a very participatory process to develop educational messages and products; it can serve as a model for a similar campaign on reducing risks for heart disease (Roubideaux 2000b).

Education of health providers in the Indian health system is needed to ensure that AI/AN patients receive the highest quality care when they present with symptoms of CVD, and receive timely, emergent treatment for CVD conditions. In a preliminary study utilizing Strong Heart Study medication data, participants had significantly lower rates of medication usage, such as aspirin, beta blockers, and nitrates, for a variety of cardiovascular conditions (e.g., past heart attack or heart failure), that would be considered a standard of care in the general population (personal communication, Henderson J, 2000). Unfortunately, while there are very good systems in place to measure the quality of diabetes care as in the IHS Diabetes Audit, there are no systems in place to measure the quality of care for cardiovascular disease. More data is needed to determine whether Indian health providers are meeting standards of care for CVD.

Indian health systems also need to review the services available for CVD, and to determine if they are meeting appropriate standards of care. Pre-hospital personnel, such as paramedics and EMTs, need to be up-to-date in Advanced Cardiac Life Support (ACLS) and carry adequate equipment to transfer potentially unstable patients over long distances, responding to emergencies if needed. Emergency rooms also need to carry the most up-to-date equipment, keep it in working order, and have available the most recent cardiac medications for emergency treatment of myocardial infarction, heart failure, and stroke. Emergency room personnel, including nurses and physicians, need to be trained in the most updated techniques and medications for cardiac care. Drug dosages and delivery schedules of emergency medications such as thrombolytics (medications to dissolve blood clots blocking the arteries to the heart) must be posted in easily accessible places. Health systems also need to review their referral policies and practices to make sure that patients are getting timely referrals to cardiologists who are culturally competent and familiar with the Indian health system.

Indian communities and tribes need to consider what they can do in terms of public health strategies to educate their members on the symptoms of cardiovascular disease, the need for quick treatment, and how to reduce risk factors. Tribal leaders and community members need to take an active role in the education and prevention of CVD, and act as role models of healthy behavior themselves. Tribes and Indian health facilities need to collaborate more on education and prevention activities to address the growing problem of CVD.

Tribal leaders also need to advocate for more funding, education, and treatment of CVD and its risk factors. While advocacy for diabetes funding has never been a more popular cause, it is rare to hear about tribal leaders going to Washington to advocate for funding for CVD awareness. However, because the rates of CVD are rising, and it is the number one cause of death in AI/AN as young as 45, tribal leaders need to help advocate for more funding and programs for prevention and treatment. In particular, given the DHHS policy on tribal consultation, tribal leaders should especially focus their efforts on increased funding for research and interventions from the National Institutes of Health/National Heart, Lung, and Blood Institute.

With more public health and prevention efforts, and with tribes taking the lead in advocacy and assurance of quality, timely care, the rising rates of cardiovascular disease can be stopped, and the risk to Indian communities can be reduced. The falling rates of CVD mortality in the general U.S. population are evidence that the problem of heart disease can be addressed through education, better treatment strategies, and community-based education on healthy lifestyles and the reduction of risk factors. It is time for tribal leaders and Indian communities to take the lead in building stronger and healthier hearts in AI/AN communities.

REFERENCES

Gilbert J. Absence of coronary thrombosis in Navajo Indians. *California Medicine*. 1955; 82:114–115.

Fulmer HS, Roberts RW. Coronary heart disease among the Navajo Indians. *Annuals of Internal Medicine*. 1963; 59:740.

Harris MD, Davis SM, Ford VL, Tso H. The Checkerboard cardiovascular curriculum: a culturally oriented program. *Journal of School Health*. 1988; 58:104–107.

Howard BV, Welty TK, Fabsitz RR, et al. Risk Factors for Coronary Heart Disease in Diabetic and Non-diabetic Native Americans. The Strong Heart Study. *Diabetes*. 1992; 41(Suppl. 2):4–11.

Howard BV, Lee ET, Cowan LD, et al. Coronary Heart Disease Prevalence and its Relation to Risk Factors in American Indians. The Strong Heart Study. *American Journal of Epidemiology*. 1995; 142:254–68.

Howard BV, Lee ET, Yeh JL, et al. Hypertension in adult American Indians. The Strong Heart Study. *Hypertension*. 1996; 28:256–64. 1996.

Howard BV, Lee ET, Fabsitz RR, et al. Diabetes and Coronary Heart Disease in American Indians. The Strong Heart Study. *Diabetes*. 1996; 45 (suppl.3): S6–S13.

Howard BV, Lee TL, Cowan LD, et al. Rising Tide of Cardiovascular Disease in American Indians: The Strong Heart Study. *Circulation*. 1999; 99:2389–2395.

Howard BV, Robbins DC, Sievers ML, et al. LDL Cholesterol as a Strong Predictor of Coronary Heart Disease in Diabetic Individuals with Insulin Resistance and Low LDL: The Strong Heart Study. *Arterioscler Thrombosis Vascular Biology*. 2000; 20:830–835.

Indian Health Service. *Trends in Indian Health*. Rockville MD: Department of Health and Human Services; 1997.

Indian Health Service. *IHS National Diabetes Program Special Diabetes Program for Indians Interim Report to Congress*. (Draft Pending Approval by OMB). Albuquerque, NM: IHS National Diabetes Program, 2000.

Lee ET, Howard BV, Savage PR, et al. Diabetes and Impaired Glucose Tolerance in Three American Indian populations aged 45–74. *Diabetes Care*. 1995; 18:599–610.

Lee ET, Cowan LD, Welty TK, et al. All-Cause Mortality and Cardiovascular Disease Mortality in Three American Indian Populations, Aged 45–74 Years, 1984-1988. The Strong Heart Study. *American Journal of Epidemiology*. 1998; 147:995–1008. 1998.

Lising M. *Building Healthy Hearts for American Indians and Alaska Natives. A Background Report*. Bethesda, MD: NIH/NIDDK, 1998.

McGovern P, Pankow J, Shahar E, et al. Recent trends in acute coronary heart disease, mortality and morbidity, medical care and risk factors. *New England Journal of Medicine*. 1996; 334:884–890.

Mendlein JM, Freedman DS, Peter DG, et al. Risk Factors for Coronary Heart

Disease among Navajo Indians: Findings from the Navajo Health and Nutrition Survey. *Journal of Nutrition.* 1997; 127:2099S–2105S.

Roubideaux Y, Moore K, Avery C, et al.   Diabetes Education Materials: Recommendations of tribal leaders, Indian health professional, and American Indian community members. *The Diabetes Educator* 26(2): 290–294. March-April 2000. (2000a)

Roubideaux Y. The National Diabetes Education Program American Indian Campaign. *The IHS Provider.* 2000; 25(6): 97–100.

Welty TK, Lee ET, Yeh J, et al. Cardiovascular Disease Risk Factors among American Indians. The Strong Heart Study. *American Journal of Epidemiology.* 1995; 142:269–87.

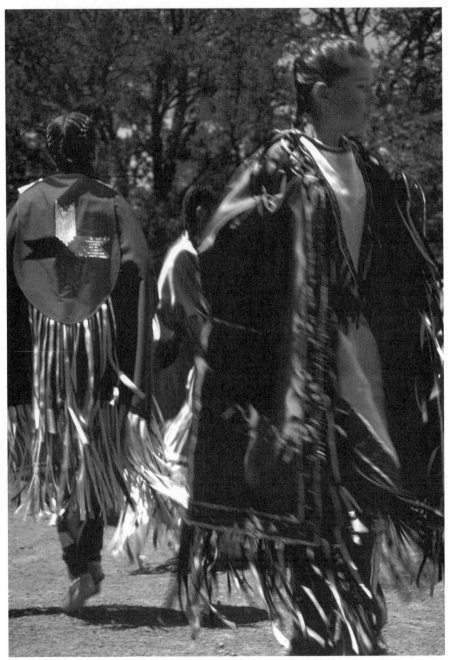

PHOTO BY ALEJANDRO LOPEZ AND ARIE PILZ
COURTESY OF THE NATIONAL INDIAN YOUTH LEADERSHIP PROJECT

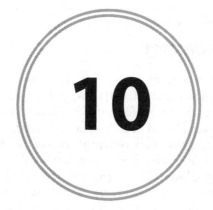

CANCER: A GROWING PROBLEM AMONG AMERICAN INDIANS AND ALASKA NATIVES

Linda Burhansstipanov

This chapter provides an overview of the growing problem of cancer among American Indian and Alaska Native (AI/AN) communities. It includes a brief overview of the culturally-specific historical cancer information with brief explanations of how cancer rates have risen– noting that at the same time, most communities are unaware of the presence and impact of cancer in their communities. Geographic and cultural distributions of cancer, including tribal variability of selected forms of cancer, are summarized based on Indian Health Service data, which illustrate why cancer data cannot be generalized from one geographic region or tribe to another. Cancer risk factors and the relationship between risk factors and carcinogens are explained; this includes selected risks, such as genetic/familial risk, behavioral risk factors, tobacco, high fat or high calorie food consumption, other dietary factors and cancer prevention and control, alcohol, sedentary lifestyle, and poverty. Prevention and early detection programs implemented in Indian Country are briefly described. Clarification is included regarding cancer screening examinations, cancer diagnosis, screening examination versus diagnostic tests, and access issues related to early detection and treatment. Lack of access to culturally acceptable cancer services, IHS Contracted Health Services, and urban Indian health system issues are described to help understand long intervals between time of diagnosis and implementation of cancer treatment.

Descriptions of AI/AN cancer patients, traditional Indian medicine and cancer care, and related cancer care issues are briefly explained. Finally, cultural issues related to early detection and treatment and barriers to participation in cancer prevention and control programs are summarized.

HISTORICAL PERSPECTIVE

At the turn of this century, cancer was considered a rare disease among American Indian people (Levin 1910). The disease was so rare that some authors suggested that American Indians never had cancer. (Hrdlicka, 1905) However, skeletal remains found in archaeological investigations of Indian burial grounds in Alaska and New York verify that cancer did indeed exist, but suggested that cancer was not a common disease among these people (Ritchie, et al 1932). However, since World War II, and even more strikingly within the past twenty years, nearly every American Indian and Alaska Native community has experienced suffering and death from this dread disease among their family members. (Lanier, et al 1993; Burhansstipanov, et al, 1999a; Burhansstipanov, 2001)

Both AI/AN and non-natives alike are less aware of the growing cancer dilemma than they are of alcohol, violence, diabetes, and other well-publicized and common conditions within one's community. In the last half of the twentieth century, cancer has become the leading cause of death for Alaska Native women, and is the second leading cause of death among Alaska Native men (Cobb, et al 1997; Valway, et al 1992; DHHS 1998). Cancer is currently the third leading cause of death for American Indians and Alaska Natives of all ages (DHHS/OPEL/IHS/IHS 1997; Cobb, et al 1997), and is the second leading cause of death among American Indians (both sexes) over age 45 (Cobb, et al 1997). Cancer is the third most frequent reason for hospital stays among Indian Health Service beneficiaries served by the Alaska Area Native Indian Health Service (DHHS, 1998). Cancer rates which were previously reported to be lower in American Indian and Alaska Natives have been shown to be increasing in the past 20 years (DHHS/OPEL/IHS 1998; Cobb, et al 1998). Incidence rates among Alaska Natives have exceeded "U.S. All Races" rates for most types of cancer. Cancer rates are similarly increasing for Canadian bands (Lanier, et al 1989). (Burhansstipanov 2001)

LACK OF AWARENESS OF THE GROWING CANCER PROBLEM

The general lack of awareness is partially due to racial misclassification in statistical data collection that has subsequently resulted in under-counting the number of cancer incidence and mortality cases in AI/AN. As a result, providers are misinformed about the significance of cancer within specific Native communities (e.g., Northern Plains) and may be less aggressive in their efforts to identify and refer cancer symptoms. Until recently, federal agencies, such as the

National Cancer Institute (NCI) were more likely to discount cancer as a problem because the primary sources for their data summaries were from Arizona and New Mexico, where Native American cancer incidence and mortality rates are lower than for Indian communities from other parts of the United States.

Unfortunately only one-third of the 50 State Health Departments directly support or sponsor cancer prevention and control services for American Indians and Alaska Natives (Michalek, et al 1994) which reinforces this misconception of cancer as not being a significant health problem among this population. Health problems such as alcoholism, substance abuse, diabetes, and domestic violence are very visible within AI/AN communities and educational efforts targeting these problems are widely dispersed among Native communities (e.g., almost all AI/AN communities provide alcohol and diabetes programs and many more are addressing domestic violence issues within their communities). Many AI/AN cultural beliefs discourage open discussion of cancer (discussed later), which contributes to cancer being prioritized as a lesser problem.

Although cancer is a growing problem for AI/AN, in comparison with other racial groups, the disease has overall lower incidence and mortality rates among tribes located in Arizona and New Mexico, and in other selected geographic areas (Creagan 1972; Black 1980; Mahoney, et al 1989; Horner 1990; Horm 1992, 1996; Gaudette 1993; Hampton 1984, 1989, 1992; Sorem 1985; Mao 1986; Miller 1992, 1996; Valway 1992; Nutting 1993; Eidson 1994; Burhansstipanov 1995, 1997, 1999b, 2000a). While mortality rates are lower among this population, survival from most types of cancer is the poorest of any racial group.

These issues and many others which affect cancer prevention and control efforts within AI/AN communities are discussed and prioritized in the 1992 *National Strategic Plan for Cancer Prevention and Control to Benefit the Overall Health of American Indians and Alaska Natives*. This plan was developed by the "Network for Cancer Control Research among American Indian and Alaska Native Populations" and was published in a special National Cancer Institute Monograph (Burhansstipanov and Dresser 1994). The plan informed both federal agencies and tribal leaders that cancer is now a major public health problem for AI/AN, and that steps should be taken to inform them of this change in cancer epidemiology.

Based on IHS, National Cancer Institute SEER data, and the National Center for Health Statistics of the Centers for Disease Control and Prevention, types of cancer identified to be of most concern among American Indians and Alaska Natives include: lung, colorectal, breast, prostate, uterine cervix, stomach, pancreas, and gallbladder (Burhansstipanov, et al 1994). American Indians living in New Mexico and Arizona have incidence rates for stomach, uterine cervix, primary liver, and gallbladder cancers that are higher than rates for the "U.S. All Races" population. American Indians have the highest gallbladder cancer incidence rate (10.9) of any racial group. (DHHS, NIH 1992).

Lanier's work in Alaska among the Eskimo, Athapaskan Indians, and Aleuts also identifies elevated cancer incidence and mortality rates (Lanier et al, 1989). Lanier is recognized by both Natives and non-Natives as an investigator whose data and findings is consistently of high quality and typically has few racial misclassification or ICD coding errors. Data from the Alaska Native Tumor Registry indicate that Alaska Natives have excessive cancer incidence of the cervix uteri, colorectum, gallbladder, kidney, oral cavity and pharynx.

GEOGRAPHIC AND CULTURAL DISTRIBUTION OF CANCER

CANNOT GENERALIZE CANCER DATA FROM ONE GEOGRAPHIC REGION TO ANOTHER

UNAVAILABILITY OF ACCURATE REGIONAL CANCER SURVEILLANCE DATA FOR AI/AN. Cancer surveillance data for AI/AN populations from one geographic region may not accurately reflect the incidence of cancer experienced by AI/AN populations in other regions. There are only two regions of the country that have accurate AI/AN data: New Mexico and Alaska. Although some federal agencies question the accuracy of IHS databases, both IHS and National Cancer Institute (NCI) Surveillance, Epidemiology, and End Results (SEER) data for New Mexico and Alaska are included in the tables in this section to illustrate the similarity of data. Table 10.1 displays the most common cancer mortality sites (e.g., lung, breast, colon, prostate), as well as cancer sites that are disproportionately high in AI/AN (e.g., kidney, stomach, and gallbladder) in comparison with other racial groups. Table 10.1 clearly illustrates why geographically specific data, even though derived from excellent cancer tumor registries cannot be used to generalize to other AI/AN communities.

Comparison of data on indigenous peoples from these two regions with cultural differences and lifestyle differences demonstrates that data on one AI/AN population cannot be extrapolated to all descendants of the indigenous people of North America (Cobb, et al 1998, 1997; Burhansstipanov, et al 1998d, 1994, 1999a, Hampton 1989, 1998, 1992). There are no accurate regional cancer surveillance data for the rest of the AI/AN population.

URBAN AMERICAN INDIAN / ALASKA NATIVE DATA. Over 60% of the American Indian/Alaska Native population reside in urban centers (Dept. of Commerce 1992). Urban AI/AN diagnosed with cancer rarely are documented as American Indians or Alaska Natives by hospital-based cancer registries; although racial misclassification is a problem in all regions, the prevalence of racial misclassification appears to be greater among urban dwelling AI/AN. People living in urban areas may sometimes be of mixed descent—tribal and non-tribal. For example, the American Indian populations of Los Angeles County and Orange County represent over 250 different tribes, predominant-

Cancer Site	New Mexico AI Females (&) and Males (%)				Alaska AN Females (&) and Males (%)			
	IHS ABQ Female[a]	SEER NM Female[b]	IHS ABQ Male[a]	SEER NM Male[b]	IHS AK Female[a]	SEER AK Female[b]	IHS AK Male[a]	SEER AK Male[b]
All Sites	100	99	134.4	123	187	179	218.6	225]
Breast	10.3	[8.7]	#	#	21.4	[16]	#	#
Cervix	4	[8]	--	--	5.2	*	--	--
Ovarian	9.6	[7.3]	--	--	6.5	*	--	--
Prostate	--	--	21	16.2	--	--	7.4	*
Colon & Rectum	5.5	*	15.8	[8.5]	24.3	24.0	27.0	27.2
Kidney & Renal Pelvis	7.9	*	9.1	*	11.9	[7.4]	14.1	[13.4]
Lung & Bronchus	11.5	*	9.2	[10.4]	46.5	45.3	70.3	69.4
Stomach	6.7	*	8.9	[11.4]	5.2	*	18.9	[18.9]
Gallbladder	4.8	[8.9]	12	#	3.2	*	2.1	#

a   Cobb N and Paisano RE 1997

b   Miller et al, 1996.

*   rate not calculated when fewer than 25 deaths

[Italic]   rates based on fewer than 25 deaths are included only for the top five most common types of cancer death for ethnic groups. These rates may be subject to greater variability than other rates that are based on larger numbers.

data not available

TABLE 10.1 AGE ADJUSTED CANCER MORTALITY DATA
BURHANSSTIPANOV ET AL, 2000A

	Both Sexes		Males		Females	
	Cancer Site	Rate	Cancer Site	Rate	Cancer Site	Rate
US All Races	Lung	49.6	Lung	74.4	Lung	31.4
	Colon/Rectum	18.7	Prostate	26.0	Breast	27.1
	Breast	15.2	Colon/Rectum	23.1	Colon/Rectum	15.6
	Ill Defined/Unk	11.9	Ill Defined/Unk	14.9	Ill Defined/Unk	9.7
	Prostate	9.9	Pancreas	10.0	Ovary	7.8
All IHS	Lung	30.5	Lung	41.9	Lung	21.7
	Ill Defined/Unk	12.5	Prostate	17.3	Breast	14.3
	Colon/Rectum	12.1	Ill Defined/Unk	13.5	Ill Defined/Unk	11.7
	Breast	7.8	Colon/Rectum	13.2	Colon/Rectum	11.2
	Prostate	7.3	Stomach	8.3	Pancreas	6.5

	Both Sexes			Both Sexes	
	Cancer Site	Rate		Cancer Site	Rate
Aberdeen	Lung	69.2	Nashville	Lung	38.1
	Colon/Rectum	24.2		Colon/Rectum	14.2
	Ill Defined/Unk	18.1		Breast	11.1
	Breast	14.5		Ill Defined/Unk	9.7
	Pancreas	9.6		Prostate	9.1
	Prostate	9.6			
	Stomach	9.6	Navajo	Ill Defined/Unk	15.0
Alaska	Lung	57.2		Stomach	9.0
	Colon/Rectum	25.8		Prostate	8.7
	Ill Defined/Unk	17.9		Liver/Intrahep	7.1
	Kidney	13.0		Gallbladder	6.9
	Stomach	11.7			
			Oklahoma	Lung	27.6
Albuquerque	Ill Defined/Unk	13.4		Colon/Rectum	9.9
	Lung	10.4		Ill Defined/Unk	7.7
	Colon/Rectum	10.1		Breast	7.4
	Prostate	9.2		Prostate	5.8
	Kidney/Renal	8.4			
			Phoenix	Lung	16.8
Bemidji	Lung	70.4		Ill Defined/Unk	14.0
	Colon/Rectum	23.3		Liver/Intrahep.	7.0
	Ill Defined/Unk	22.3		Breast	6.2
	Liver/Intrahep.	10.3		Prostate	6.0
	Pancreas	10.2			
			Portland	Lung	42.9
Billings	Lung	55.4		Colon/Rectum	15.2
	Ill Defined/Unk	22.0		Ill Defined/Unk	11.8
	Colon/Rectum	21.6		Breast	10.3
	Prostate	15.4		Prostate	9.5
	Pancreas	14.9			
			Tucson	Ill Defined/Unk	20.5
California	Lung	16.7		Pancreas	11.7
	Colon/Rectum	10.0		Liver/Intrahep.	10.4
	Ill Defined/Unk	7.1		Stomach	9.1
	Breast	5.0		Kidney/Renal	9.0
	Stomach	4.2			

* All rates per 100,000 per year, adjusted to the 1970 US standard population

TABLE 10.2. FIVE LEADING CAUSES OF CANCER MORTALITY *by Average Annual Age-Adjusted Rates*, 1969-1993, by IHS Area. IHS Areas Compared to US All Races*
Source: Paisano and Cobb, 1997

ly Sioux, Navajo, Chickasaw, Choctaw, Apache, and Cherokee, as well as tribes indigenous to California. Urban misclassification occurs because health care forms may lack the option of identification (i.e., no AI/AN racial category) or hospitals may have a policy of not asking for race information due to legal constraints. One commonality is that the urban Indians, like their reservation relatives, are likely to lack access to cancer treatment services (Burhansstipanov 2000b).

RISK FACTORS

Traditional lifestyles practiced by AI/AN ancestors helped prevent the development of cancer. These lifestyles included vigorous daily exercising (e.g., hunting, gathering, obtaining food for family and community), reserving tobacco for ceremonial use only, and consuming low fat (e.g., game meats) and high fiber (e.g., beans, squash, corn) foods.

AI/AN traditional lifestyles have gradually been replaced with contemporary lifestyles, incorporating many habits known to have a direct relationship to specific types of cancer: sedentary lifestyles, habitual tobacco use, and high-fat/low-fiber diets. These lifestyle changes are directly related to the types of cancer (e.g., lung, colon) that are increasing in both incidence and mortality in AI/AN communities; clearly there is substantial reason for AIAN to incorporate many of the practices of the ancestors. (Burhansstipanov, et al 1999a).

RISK FACTORS AND CARCINOGENS

"Cancer risk factors" include agents (e.g., high consumption of dietary fat) which, based upon scientific evidence, increase the likelihood of developing one or more types of cancer. In comparison, "carcinogens" include certain man-made and natural chemicals that cause cancer (Doll and Peto 1981). For example, smoking and smokeless tobacco are carcinogens that cause changes that turn a normal cell into a cancer cell (NIH Pub No. 87-2059). When exposed to a carcinogen, given enough frequency, duration and/or exposure to that factor, a specific type of cancer will eventually develop in most people. For example, chronic tobacco use causes nearly 90 percent of lung cancer. There are substantial data to support that chronic tobacco use has a causal relationship to cancer rather than only a "risk" for developing cancer.

Risk factors may be regional and depend on lifestyles in that area. Welty has shown that the high rate of smoking (56% for men and 48% for women) among the Sioux Nation living in North and South Dakota is closely related to their high lung cancer mortality rates. Intensive smoking cessation and prevention programs are likely to have the greatest impact on reducing preventable cancer deaths, e.g., lung cancer, within their community (Welty, et al 1993). Similar programs in New Mexico where the incidence and risk factors are less (e.g., AI in Arizona rarely are chronic/habitual tobacco users), may not result in as significant of a decrease in incidence and risk factors.

Risk Factors	Breast	Cervix	Colo-rectal	Lung	Prostate	Gall-bladder	Stomach	Pancreas
Habitual tobacco use		●[1]	●[2]	●			●	●
High fat/calories	●		●		●[1]	●		
Low fiber/fruits and/or vegetables		●	●	●	●[1]		●	
Food preservation							●[3]	
Alcohol misuse	●		●	●	●[1]			
Multiple sexual partners		●	●[2]		●[1]			
Menarche age 12 or younger	●							
Early Age at First Coitus		●						
Late age (30+) at first Birth		●		●				
Diseases/disorders	●[4]	●[5]	●[6]		●[7]	●[8]	●[9]	●[10]
Air pollution				●				
Chemical exposure (e.g., occupational)			●[11]	●[12]	●[13]		●[14]	
Ionizing radiation	●		●	●[15]			●	
Socioeconomic	High	Low	Low	Low	●[1]		Low	
Genetics/family history	●[16]	●[1]	●		●[1]	●	●[17]	
Increasing after age ___	30	50	50		65			30
Hormone(s)		●	●	●		●		
Other					●[18]			

[1]Possible risk factor
[2]Risk for anal cancer
[3]Pickled, salted, smoked foods
[4]Previous breast disease
[5]Human Papilloma Virus (HPV), Herpes Simplex Type 2
[6]Human Papilloma Virus (HPV) may be related to anal cancer; inflammatory bowel disease; polyps, clostridia, syphilis
[7]Urinary tract infection
[8]Biliary disease; gallstones, cholescystitis, ulcerative colitis
[9]Pernicious anemia; atrophic gastritis
[10]Diabetes
[11]Asbestos
[12]Asbestos, arsenic, mustard gas manufacture, copper smelter workers, nickel
[13]Cadmium exposure; rubber industry
[14]Nitrosamines/nitrites
[15]Uranium mining; atom bomb survivors
[16]Mother or sister
[17]Blood Type A
[18]Geographic Distribution (higher rates in the North); may be screening phenomenon

TABLE 10.3. SUMMARY CHART — RISK FACTORS FOR SPECIFIC CANCER SITES
Source: Burhansstipanov and Dresser, 1994

A summary of cancer risk factors for the eight most common cancer sites among American Indians and Alaska Natives is shown in Table 10.3 (Burhansstipanov, et al 1994).

GENETIC/FAMILIAL RISK

Advances in genetic research related to cancer have escalated in recent years. As chromosomes are mapped as part of the Human Genome Project, greater insight has been gained about the complexity of the human gene. Through such research, over 100 specific oncogenes have been identified, such as p53, *ras*, HER-2/neu, p16, *myc*, BRCA1 and BRCA2. Some oncogenes are found in many tumors, such as p53. Others, such as BRCA1 and BRCA2 are specific for particular types of cancer: breast and ovarian cancer. This does not mean cancers are inherited (e.g., passed from parent to child), but all cancer is genetic. Thus the genetic changes observed in cancer tumors rarely result from .inheriting those genes directly from the parents. The tumors result from accumulated damage to the cells throughout life. This means that there will be more and more genetic tests available to assist with the diagnosis and eventually with the treatment of cancer in the future. Cancer diagnosis and treatment research are changing continually as scientists learn more about these oncogenes.

CANCER BEHAVIORAL RISK FACTORS

Most cancers have external causes and to a great extent are preventable by living a healthy lifestyle (e.g., not smoking tobacco, daily exercise). Likewise, other factors and behaviors are strongly associated with increased risk for developing cancer, such as high-fat/calorie and low-fiber diet, habitual tobacco use, poverty, and so on. Unfortunately, the factors and behaviors that are associated with increased cancer risk have escalated among AI/AN since World War II.

TOBACCO

Habitual tobacco use is estimated to be responsible for about 30 percent of cancer in people of all races and tobacco use is responsible for causing 90 percent of all lung cancer (DHHS 1991). The chronic use of tobacco is estimated to be responsible for over 400,000 deaths annually; tobacco use is responsible for more than one of every six deaths in the United States and is the most important single preventable cause of death and disease in our society (DHHS 1991). Based upon Behavioral Risk Factor Surveillance System data from 1985–1989, Native communities in the northern states and urban areas are more likely to be habitual tobacco users than are people of other races (e.g., 50–80 percent of individuals from selected American Indian communities in Montana are habitual tobacco users) (Goldberg, et al 1991; Sugarman, et al 1992).

CEREMONIAL VERSUS CHRONIC TOBACCO USE The hazards of chronic smoking and smokeless tobacco use are well documented in numerous publications;

however, there is a difference between ceremonial and chronic tobacco use. Not all tribes include tobacco in ceremonies, but many tribal groups who do use tobacco spiritually do not feel it should be associated with chronic use/abuse of tobacco. Ceremonial tobacco use varies greatly among tribes and specific ceremonies involving tobacco are not described since Native Americans reserve the right to privacy regarding the ceremonial use of tobacco. Native respondents to survey questionnaires and other inquiries are likely to refuse to answer or provide an inaccurate response to these types of questions.

Tobacco is a carcinogen and habitual tobacco use or exposure is responsible for causing nearly 90 percent of all lung cancer. Tobacco also causes cancers of the following sites: larynx, oral cavity, esophagus, bladder, kidney, pancreas, and stomach. In addition, women who smoke may be at higher risk for developing cervical cancer than are non-smoking women.

The risk for developing lung cancer is proportional to the amount smoked daily and the duration of time smoked (DHHS 1991). Lung cancer mortality increases with increasing doses, as determined by number of cigarettes smoked daily, smoking history, and inhalation patterns. Those who smoke two or more packs a day have death rates 15 to 25 times greater than non-smokers.

Lung cancer is rare in individuals who have never smoked. Cessation of cigarette smoking results in a gradual decrease in lung cancer risk. After 10 to 20 years of cessation, lung cancer rates for former smokers approach the rates of lifelong non-smokers (DHHS 1991).

An exception to smoking as a cause of lung cancer is uranium exposure in mine workers, primarily Navajo, and their families. (Their families are exposed through the contaminated work clothes that the miners wear home.) A large proportion of lung cancer experienced by Navajos is due to working in uranium mines.

Lung cancer is exceptionally difficult to treat. The primary reason is that it is almost always diagnosed in late stages when it has already spread throughout the body. Health care providers understand that the best technique for addressing lung cancer is to prevent it from occurring (e.g., to not habitually smoke tobacco products). Nearly 90 percent of lung cancer patients die within five years of diagnosis; survival improves modestly when lung cancer is detected at an early, localized stage (DHHS 1991).

American Indians and Alaska Natives do not have protection from developing lung or other types of tobacco-related cancers. Dr. Thomas Welty, retired Medical Epidemiologist for the Aberdeen Indian Health Service, South Dakota, stresses, "If Indians smoke, they get cancer just as other populations do" (Welty 1992).

SMOKELESS TOBACCO USE. Smokeless tobacco products are primarily used by youth rather than elders; the products include moist or dry snuff and chewing tobacco. All smokeless tobacco products contain substantial amounts of nicotine. Smokeless tobacco use increases one's risk of developing leukoplakia, gingival recession, nicotine addiction, and mouth and lip cancer, Both of these cancers are very aggressive.

HIGH-FAT OR HIGH-CALORIE FOOD CONSUMPTION

Individuals need to reduce their daily fat intake to 30 percent or less of total calories. Diets high in fat, saturated fat, and cholesterol are linked to increased risk of chronic health problems, which are disproportionately high in Native Americans in comparison with other racial groups: coronary heart disease, obesity, diabetes, and certain forms of cancer. Those cancers include, but are not limited to breast, colon and rectum, endometrium, ovary, and gallbladder. High-fat and high-calorie food consumption may also be associated with prostate cancer.

Dresser (1994) of the National Cancer Institute emphasizes that a variety of foods eaten in moderation will not cause cancer; however, she cites that a 1987 review of the literature conducted by Albanes on caloric intake, body weight, and cancer indicated that a large number of epidemiological investigators found an association of high relative body weight and high caloric intake with an increased risk of cancer of the breast, colon, rectum, prostate, endometrium, kidney, cervix, ovary, thyroid, and gallbladder (Albanes 1987). Although the relationships among caloric intake, dietary macro-nutrients, (e.g., fat), and body weight are complex and require further investigation, Albanes' review suggests that reducing caloric intake and relative body weight may lead to a considerable decrease in cancer risk in humans. In laboratory studies on mice with multiple tumors, Albanes also indicated that total caloric intake was an important determinant of tumorigenesis, and that body weight may be a more sensitive indicator for this effect than is caloric intake alone. These findings, among others, implicate obesity as a potential risk factor for the development of cancer (Albanes 1987, Burhansstipanov and Dresser 1994). Almost half of AI/AN over age 45 are overweight or obese. Programs that assist in decreasing obesity contribute to a reduction in risk for multiple types of cancer (e.g., breast, colon) as well as other serious health conditions experienced by AI/AN communities (i.e., diabetes, cardiovascular disease).

DIET AND FOOD SELECTION

Traditional American Indian diets did not include "fry bread" or any other contemporary foods that are made with lard or cow products, such as beef, milk, or butter. The types of foods consumed in the past (i.e., prior to contact with Europeans) were based on availability and included foods that were primarily low in fat, such as fish and game (e.g., deer, antelope, buffalo), corn, squash, beans, rice, roots. High-fat foods included seeds, nuts, and occasionally high-fat protein foods like bear or whale (for Alaska Natives).

Over the last thirty years, the traditional foods consumed by the ancestors of American Indians and Alaska Natives have been replaced by processed and commercially prepared foods, the variety and quality of which have been limited. Foods traditionally prepared over slow fires have been replaced with pan or deep-fat frying cooking methods.

LOW FIBER FRUITS AND VEGETABLES. Dietary fiber is primarily found in fruits and vegetables, with a good secondary source in whole grains. There appears to be a protective chemo-preventive effect against certain types of cancer by consuming fruits and vegetables; cruciferous vegetables (e.g., cabbage, broccoli) are particularly beneficial. The current National Cancer Institute Dietary Guidelines stress consuming at least five servings of fruits and vegetables per day (A serving is typically measured as one piece of fruit or one-half cup of cooked vegetables). The traditional American Indian way of measuring a serving was the amount that fit into one's hand (which is usually about one-half cup). Unfortunately, the majority of Native Americans today rarely consume five servings of fruits and vegetables daily. There are several reasons for this:

• These foods are expensive and most elder Native peoples live below the poverty level.

• Elders grew up on foods other than vegetables and may not have acquired a taste for them.

• These foods are unfamiliar to the population and people may not have learned to cook with them (other than in canned form through the USDA food commodities program).

• Elders who subsist on the USDA food commodity program typically receive five servings of vegetables per week and thus these foods are not accessible.

• The markets on many reservations are unable to obtain fresh fruits and vegetables and people are hesitant to purchase wilted, dried out, and costly foods.

Regular consumption of fruits and vegetables appears to help prevent several forms of cancer. Cancers of the cervix, colon, lung, stomach, and possibly the prostate decrease if one's diet includes high consumption of fruits and vegetables (Burhansstipanov and Dresser 1994).

ALCOHOL AND CANCER RISK

Prevention of alcohol abuse is a health priority among AI/AN communities. In studies with other races, alcohol—combined with cigarette—use presents an even greater risk for cancer than if tobacco products were used alone; alcohol is a powerful solvent and may enhance body absorption of carcinogens.

Epidemiologic data indicate that the combination of chronic alcohol consumption and tobacco use substantially increases the risks of cancers of the oral cavity, esophagus and pharynx (DHHS 1986). No alcohol–cigarette use studies have been conducted with AI/AN.

Alcohol abuse is among the top health problems cited by AI/AN nations, communities, and organizations. Alcohol misuse and abuse affects all aspects of one's health, one's family, and one's community. Excessive alcohol intake increases the risk of heart disease, high blood pressure, chronic liver disease, and some forms of cancer. In addition to the well-known problems caused by alcohol abuse (e.g., violence, accidents), alcohol may be a risk factor for prostate cancer. It is a known risk factor for cancer of the lung, breast, colon, and rectum (Burhansstipanov, et al 1994).

SEDENTARY LIFESTYLE

Strongly correlated with obesity among Native Americans is the contemporary trend of leading a sedentary and non-physically active lifestyle, exercise is a major contributor to attaining and maintaining normal body weight. Aerobic exercise on a regular basis helps prevent obesity, coronary heart disease, and diabetes.

POVERTY

Poverty has been well established to be a risk factor for cancer (National Academy of Sciences 1999; Harras, et al 1996). More than one-quarter (28%) of American Indian and Alaska Native people of all ages live in poverty, which is more than twice the national average. Almost two-thirds (61%) of American Indian and Alaska Native elders live in poverty (Dept of Commerce 1992).

These are just a few examples of factors, lifestyles, and behaviors that are related to cancer risks. Obviously, if such behaviors and conditions continue, the cancer incidence and mortality rates will continue to rise among AI/AN.

PREVENTION AND EARLY DETECTION

CANCER SCREENING EXAMINATIONS

Screening tests are performed when the patient has no symptoms. Screening for some cancers is important because it can help the health care provider make an early diagnosis and treat it before it spreads. Examples of screening tests include Pap testss (for early detection of cervical cancer), mammograms (for early detection of breast cancer), sigmoidoscopy (for early detection of colon cancer), and digital rectal examination (for early detection of prostate cancer). Screening guidelines and recommendations are updated regularly and are available from the Cancer Information Service of the NCI or the American Cancer Society. Some screening tests remain controversial. For example, the research that has been conducted on prostate cancer screening and mortality is inconclusive. This type of incomplete information makes it very difficult to develop specific screening guidelines. Clearly, there is much still to be learned about prostate cancer, screening, and its subsequent treatment.

As a generalization, according to the American Cancer Society, a cancer-related check-up should be performed by a physician every three years for persons aged 20–39 and annually for those aged 40 and older. Screening guidelines are specific to each type of cancer. Some persons at particular risk for certain cancers may need more frequent screenings and should discuss this with their doctor. The checkup in elders should always include exams for cancer of the breast, uterus, cervix, colon, rectum, prostate, mouth, skin, testes, thyroid, and lymph nodes, as well as health behavior counseling (i.e., how to quit smoking, etc.).

There are some cancers that are more common in AI/AN and as a result, require screening on a more frequent schedule. For example, AI/AN women have disproportionately high incidences and mortality rates for cervical cancer, and it also occurs in American Indian women at a younger age than it does in most other racial groups. The standard screening guidelines for cervical cancer state that a woman have a Pap test and pelvic examination every year until she has had three or more consecutive, normal examinations and can then have the Pap test performed less frequently at the discretion of the woman and the physician. However, since AI/AN women appear to experience disproportionately high rates of the disease, the Indian Health Service recommends annual Pap test. The schedule may be reduced for elder Indian women, but only at the discretion of the woman and her provider.

CANCER DIAGNOSIS

Cancer is a term that describes over 100 different types of diseases and cancer sites; every cancer site is diagnosed through specific tests. For example, the tests used to diagnose colon cancer differ from those that are used to diagnose liver cancer or mouth cancer. A diagnosis of cancer is not confirmed until a biopsy of the suspected tumor verifies that the cells collected are examined under a microscope and are identified as cancer cells.

Cancer diagnosis techniques are continually changing. All of these tests require expertise to conduct the screening exam and interpret the results, which usually requires some type of certification or qualification by the health provider. Likewise, the equipment and machines have very specific qualifications and they too must be approved by a designated accrediting body. For example, a mammogram performed on an older machine may not be specific enough to find small tumors and does not have the acuity of state-of-the-art machines. There were so many problems with old or inaccurate machines, that in 1992 the Mammography Quality Standards Act was passed. This act mandates that the medical facilities that perform and interpret mammography tests must be certified by the Food and Drug Administration (FDA). Because of Acts such as this one, today's mammograms are about 94 percent accurate in women over age fifty.

It is not unusual for two providers to interpret test results differently and to differ on the type of treatment prescribed. For these and other reasons the patient is always advised to obtain second and third opinions of their diagnosis. This is not an insult to the original provider who diagnosed the cancer, but rather is prudent patient behavior. Unfortunately, the patient who uses IHS contracted health services may have difficulty obtaining a second medical opinion from a facility other than the one contracted facility. But there are other oncologists within the same facility who may be used for a second or third consultation and opinion. Health providers should encourage patients to obtain a second opinion—it is better to have an accurate diagnosis than to erroneously diagnose and treat the wrong condition. Public health policies are needed that guarantee all patients, regardless of poverty level, have access to a second opinion.

SCREENING EXAMINATION VERSUS DIAGNOSTIC TESTS

Cancer diagnoses are not made through basic screening examinations. When a screening test is abnormal, it means that diagnostic tests need to be conducted to find out why the test is abnormal. This difference between screening examination results and a cancer diagnosis needs to be clarified by the provider with the patient. For example, when women are notified that their screening mammogram had an abnormal result, the provider will tell the woman what type of follow-up test is required. The abnormal film means something looks unusual, or suspicious, but it does not mean that the unusual section of the film is a cancerous tumor. Very few of the abnormal films are actually cancer.

Cancer differs from other health problems (e.g., diabetes, cardiovascular disease) in that it comprises over 100 different diseases, of which multiple types of screening and diagnostic tests are required to accurately determine the presence of cancer in the body. Cancer research, specifically genetic cancer research, is likely to provide major changes in the ways cancer is detected and treated in the near future, and improvements are needed for many types of cancer screening and diagnosis. To date the early detection of ovarian, pancreatic, and brain cancer is insufficient to diagnose most of these cancers while in early stages of development (e.g., in situ, stage I). Innovative laboratory research is currently underway that is likely to improve cancer (1) prevention; (2) screening or early detection; (3) diagnosis; (4) treatment; and (5) quality of life following cancer treatment.

ACCESS ISSUES RELATED TO EARLY DETECTION AND TREATMENT

LACK OF ACCESS TO CULTURALLY ACCEPTABLE CANCER SERVICES

The Indian Health Service (IHS) has the primary role in providing services for American Indians and Alaska Natives, and is perceived by many as a culturally acceptable provider of health care to this special population. However, the IHS lacks sufficient budget, personnel, facilities, and resources to provide high-quality, comprehensive cancer screening services to all urban and reservation Indians without collaboration from other agencies such as the CDC and state health departments.

IHS CONTRACTED HEALTH SERVICE. The Indian Health Service (IHS) has no oncologists or similar cancer specialists on staff. Cancer diagnoses and treatment are conducted via the IHS contracted health services when follow-up tests and services are not available from local IHS service units. The official federal policy regarding the IHS Contract Health Services is to place Indian patients on a "priority list" to transport them for follow-up services as monies are available. However, the U.S. Congress determines how much money is allocated to the IHS Contract Health Services budget and IHS policies are restricted by the availability of those monies; this creates an incredibly frustrating situation for both providers and patients. IHS Contract Health Services requires that the provider place the patient on a priority list to receive recommended follow-up diagnosis, treatment, and/or care. As monies are available, the American Indian patients are provided travel and accommodations to the specified health care setting that has a contract with IHS to provide the recommended tests and procedures. The frustration from this system is that many American Indian elders wait on priority lists for months at a time until money is available. It is widely known that early treatment is essential for cancer diagnoses. Both the provider and the patient become victims of delayed access to services, and meanwhile if cancer is present in the patient's body, it continues to grow. This delay in obtaining access to diagnostic and treatment services is among the primary reasons for the poor survival from cancer among American Indians and Alaska Natives.

Medical services are not always available to the AI/AN cancer patients and are perceived by some as a common reason for the low rates of use of these services. For example, breast cancer screening was assessed through the 1989 Survey of American Indians and Alaska Natives (SAIAN), which was a subset of the National Medical Expenditure Survey. The SAIAN found that only 23 percent of the women reported ever having had a mammogram (AHCPR, 1991). Another common reason cited for not using IHS services is the unavailability or inaccessibility of a nearby IHS facility. For example, American Indians living in the rural New York (e.g., Seneca Reservation) area must travel over 500 miles one-way to access IHS hospital services in Cherokee, North Carolina.

American Indians living in Denver must travel 390 miles one-way to Ignacio, Colorado to obtain IHS services (Burhansstipanov and Morris, 1998). Some American Indian people choose convenience over culturally acceptable services and those who have access to private health insurance are also likely to use other services. Clearly the majority of American Indian women are medically underserved and are under-screened for breast cancer.

URBAN INDIAN HEALTH. Although American Indians and Alaska Natives are eligible to receive comprehensive health services free of charge from the Indian Health Service (IHS), only about 10 percent of urban American Indians use IHS. The IHS has made significant improvements in the overall health of Native people, specifically related to infectious diseases and in prenatal, infant, child, and youth care. However, cancer primarily affects elders and the IHS is only financially supported by Congress to meet about a third (34 percent) of the documented health care needs of communities (NIHB 1997). Thus, the health, welfare, and education of AI/AN fall below the national average (DHHS/OPEL/IHS 1997). When given a choice, most Tribal Nations and urban Indian clinics focus their limited, insufficient funds on protecting the next generation. Elder health issues, such as cancer, remain a lower priority among most tribes and urban Indian clinics (Michalek, et al 1996a and 1996b). The major reasons for urban American Indians not accessing IHS is their perceived ineligibility for services provided by the Tribe and/or inaccessibility to an IHS facility. For example, Los Angeles county AI/AN have no IHS-supported health care services other than referrals. In Colorado, although 43 percent of the American Indian population lives in Denver, the closest IHS facility is 390 miles away in the southwest corner of the state, and therefore virtually inaccessible.

HOW DO URBAN AMERICAN INDIANS AND ALASKA NATIVES ACCESS CANCER CARE?

This can become a very challenging experience. Native American Cancer Research is a national program providing cancer support to American Indians and Alaska Natives living on the North American continent. Program staff receive calls from Native cancer survivors who share their experiences with accessing care, support groups, and so on; by far, the most frustrating experiences revolve around delay of treatment for urban dwelling Native women with breast cancer. There are many obstacles facing patients trying to access care and the process for overcoming these obstacles is never the same—even when the same health care facility and when the same cancer site (i.e., breast) exists in two different patients.

Urban-dwelling Natives who have lived off the reservation for 6 months or more are typically ineligible for tribal health services (according to tribal policies, not IHS). Therefore, many of the urban-dwelling AI/AN cancer patients must be served through Medicare or Indigent Care Services. However, when going through the Department of Social Services to apply for Medicare, typically there is at least a three-month delay before getting the patient approved for Medicare. Invariably, sometime during the application process, the patient is told that she is not eligible for services because she is Indian and is supposed to use the IHS. The documentation explaining why she is ineligible to receive IHS services must be submitted and then the Medicare process is initiated all over again.

Eligibility of cancer patients for the Americans with Disabilities Act (ADA) has varied in the last decade resulting in some cancer patients being classified as eligible and others not. ADA support is of particular concern for cancer patients (of all races) who experience long-term fatigue, which is frequently a permanent side-effect of cancer treatment (e.g., chemotherapy).

PAYER OF LAST RESORT. Among the reasons for long intervals between the time of diagnosis (i.e., biopsy) and initiation of treatment is that government agencies must determine who is the payer of last resort. The state/county (indigent programs) and federal (Medicare and IHS) programs all have documents that state they are the last payer.

Some Social Service personnel suggest that urban Indian women return to the reservation for follow-up diagnostic tests or treatment, being totally unaware of (1) the limited availability of cancer screening, diagnosis, and treatment services available for tribal or IHS facilities, (2) tribal nations' requirements of having to currently be a resident (e.g., live on the reservation for at least six months) to be eligible for services, (3) the distances people have to travel to access IHS facilities, and (4) the lack of cancer specialists within the IHS system.

AI/AN CANCER PATIENTS AND TRADITIONAL INDIAN CEREMONIES

On the other end of this continuum, American Indian cancer patients may refuse to initiate treatment until they have participated in traditional Indian ceremonies. This typically requires a return to their reservation and a traditional Indian healer and ceremonies often require many months of preparation. Native American Cancer Research is a non-profit, Indian owned and operated organization that coordinates a National Native American Cancer Survivors' Support Network which functions on the North American continent. To date, when the Native Cancer Support Network has contacted traditional Indian healers and ask for their assistance in getting a woman into western medical care within a few weeks of diagnosis, the healers have been totally supportive. Most feel that cancer is a white man's disease and therefore, the treatment needs to include Western Medicine. In such cases, the healers have performed less rigorous ceremonies requiring only a day or two. The AI/AN cancer patient begins the treatment feeling spiritually stronger and cleaner. Once the adjuvant therapy has been completed and the patient is strong enough to participate in a ceremony, the healers can conduct a complete ceremony (usually requiring three to five days of ceremonial events which may or may not include fasting).

CANCER RISKS FROM RESERVATION TO URBAN

Many tribal nations are concerned that during their years living on the reservation they have been exposed to environmental pollutants that may be responsible for their current increase in cancer prevalence. For example, the Department of Energy stores nuclear wastes on several reservations, and concern has been raised that the storage containers may have leaked radiation. Prepubescent reservation Indian girls may be exposed to high levels of irradiation which could be associated with the development of breast cancer while in their 30s or early 40s. Such hypotheses will require many years of data collection to accept or reject.

LACK OF CANCER TREATMENT MONIES

After gaining access to screening programs and enduring long waiting lists, cancer patients must till face a severe lack of funding for treatment programs. One stellar program, The California Breast Cancer Treatment Fund, provides selected treatment services to Californians without health insurance or health care coverage. This program was initiated in 1996 by Blue Cross of California Public Benefit Program (now known as The California Endowment). The Treatment Fund pays for standard treatments such as lumpectomy, mastectomy, radiation therapy, chemotherapy, and hormonal therapy; it does not pay for social worker services, bone marrow or peripheral stem cell transplants, breast reconstruction, wigs, hospice services, nutrition services, alternative or complementary treatments, home health care, or treatment for recurrent or refractory disease. The Treatment Fund has been an incredibly effective and efficient organization helping American Indian breast cancer patients and other women of all ethnicities.

CULTURAL ISSUES RELATED TO EARLY DETECTION AND TREATMENT

Many tribes regard cancer as a white man's disease because it was a very rare condition prior to the European presence on the North American continent (Hampton 1989). For many Native American cancer patients, the disease is not discussed and is considered a form of punishment, shame, and guilt. A few tribes consider cancer to be a condition for which the patient experiences physical challenges which may enable the rest of the tribal members to have fewer health problems (i.e., they wear the pain so that their community will be spared the pain). Some tribal beliefs regard the person with cancer as being contagious with the cancer spirit and therefore he or she is ostracized by others in their community. Still others prohibit surgery to treat cancer for fear that

1. Cancer is a "White man's" disease.
a. "I tried to act white when I was young and that is why the Creator gave me a white man's disease."
b. "Cancer didn't exist until white men brought the disease with them from Europe."
2. Punishment (from your actions or a family member's actions).
a. "I didn't think I had acted badly, but I must have because now I have cancer."
b. "I got cancer because my son drinks and beats his wife and so that is why I have cancer, as a punishment for his bad behavior."
3. "Wear the pain" to protect other members of one's communities
a. "If I carry my cancer with dignity and do not show the pain, I can protect my community and neighbors from something bad."
b. "My cancer helps to protect my village so that is why I do not get Western medicine to treat it. If I was treated, someone else would have to protect my home from danger."
4. Natural part of one's path and the lessons to learn
a. "Before I was born, my spirit selected cancer for me to learn some lessons ... things that are important for me or my family to learn. Cancer is not a bad thing ... it is just part of my path and my lessons. It is not upsetting. It has helped me greatly."
b. "My cancer diagnosis was a blessing .... not an easy or pleasant blessing, but now, looking back, it was the best thing that happened to me ... I stopped drinking, I live a good life, I am in good health, and I appreciate every day the Creator has given me and my wife. My life is full of living, laughing and loving ... because of cancer."
5. Results from a curse from someone, or a personal violation of tribal mores (stepping on a frog, urinating on a spider)
a. "I got cancer from my cousin ... she put a curse on me."
b. "My cancer was caused because I urinated on a spider. I didn't see him, but it made him angry and he gave me cancer."
6. Contagious "Cancer Spirit"
a. "I got cancer because my daughter played with the daughter of ___ who has the cancer spirit. So it is her fault that I have cancer."
b. "I caught my disease from that machine [ed. Mammography machine]. I didn't have it before that machine touched me. Now I got it."

TABLE 10.4. EXAMPLES OF CULTURAL PERCEPTIONS OF CANCER DIAGNOSIS
Source: Burhansstipanov, et al 1999c

Arctic Slope, AK
Southcentral Foundation, AK
South East Alaska Regional Health Consortium, AK
Cheyenne River Sioux Tribe, SD
Hopi Tribe, AZ
Poarch Band of Creek Indians, AL
Consolidated Tribal Health Project, CA
South Puget Intertribal Planning Agency, WA
Cherokee Nation of Oklahoma, OK
Navajo Nation, AZ/NM
Native American Community Health Center, Inc., AZ
Native American Rehabilitation Association, OR

TABLE 10.5. CDC BREAST AND CERVICAL CANCER TRIBAL PROGRAMS

one's body and spirit are missing a part after the surgery and therefore the individual can never find their ancestors when they move to "the other side" (i.e., death) (Burhansstipanov 1997). Table 10.4 summarizes examples of cultural beliefs related to cancer diagnosis.

BARRIERS TO PARTICIPATION IN CANCER PREVENTION AND CONTROL PROGRAMS

In comparison with other ethnic groups, American Indians and Alaska Natives seldom utilize early cancer detection screening programs (Burhansstipanov 2001). Clinical trials are research studies conducted with people to find better ways to prevent and treat cancer. AI/AN are rarely successfully recruited to participate in clinical trials or "state of the art" treatment programs. When they are recruited, they typically are not "retained" throughout the duration of the study, but withdraw and cannot be evaluated. There are numerous barriers that explain these low utilization and participation rates.

POLICY BARRIERS. Barriers which affect American Indian and Alaska Native participation in cancer early detection and screening programs include poverty, psychosocial, sociocultural, and "policy" barriers. There are numerous "policy" barriers that are specific to Indian Country as well as those policies that affect people of all colors. An example of a policy that is likely to improve screening related to the reproductive organs (e.g., cervix, breast, prostate, testicles) is to mandate that the gender of health providers be the same as for the patient.

CENTERS FOR DISEASE CONTROL AND PREVENTION (CDC) BREAST AND CERVICAL CANCER CONTROL PROGRAM (BCCCP). Another example of a policy barrier lies within the Centers for Disease Control and Prevention (CDC) National Breast and Cervical Cancer Early Detection Program (NBCCEDP). These are the programs currently funded by the CDC to provide breast and cervical cancer screening services to women who are (1) 50 years of age and older; (2) live at 200 percent below the federal poverty level; and (3) are un- or under-insured. This program has been in existence since 1990 and gradually expanded to all 50 states and to twelve tribal programs (See Table 10.5).

In 1999 and 2000 the CDC program modified its cervical cancer screening guidelines based on current scientific evaluation of the efficacy of ongoing cervical cancer screening. As a result, women who have had a normal Pap test three consecutive times within a five-year period of time are no longer required to return to the clinic for annual Pap tests. Several Native programs have expressed concern over this policy change; among the more commonly expressed concerns is that it so difficult to get Native American women to come in annually—most women are tested about every 18 months. How often will women show up for cancer screening once the constant vigilance is lessened? At least two tribal programs are actively reviewing their screening data records to determine the frequency of Native women having a normal Pap and then on the next Pap to have dysplasia or in situ cancer. Results are not yet available.

NIH CLINICAL TRIALS. Another public health policy that needs expansion is Cancer Care Trials (CCT). CCT includes screening, prevention, treatment, and supportive care cancer trials. To date, approximately 80 percent of almost every CCT comprises populations who have at least a college education and likewise are categorized in the middle and upper socioeconomic levels. Since AI/AN in general have less education and live in poverty, it is no wonder that the inclusion of AI/AN, particularly in cancer prevention trials, is proportionately low. Special policies need to be implemented that allow for longer amounts of time to recruit eligible AI/AN into CCT. Most recruitment protocols allow 30 minutes, yet when working with medically underserved populations, such as AI/AN, those protocols need to be expanded to one and one-half hours. The recruitment language also needs to be easier to understand (i.e., using common English rather than medical or research jargon). Likewise, these programs may have policies which are dependent on insurance companies, or that require that patients pay for their own medication. Such a policy inadvertently prohibits any poor or uninsured people from having access to quality treatment provided through the clinical trial. This is one of many reasons why the majority (i.e. 80 percent) of participants of clinical trials are upper middle class and have higher income and education levels.

POLICIES TO SUPPORT NURSING TRAINING FOR THE IMPLEMENTATION OF QUALITY SCREENING SERVICES. Another policy that can improve the quality of care for AI/AN is to promote and support nurses' training to allow them to do clinical breast examinations and Pap smears rather than relying on medical doctors for such screening examinations (Kottke, et al in press; Kottke, et al unpublished observations). The nurses who have undergone an intensive screening training program supported by the Mayo Clinic and implemented by Mary Alice Trapp, RN (in a program called the Native Web) have more accurate screening findings than do a comparison group of physicians.

SCREENING SERVICES AS BUSINESSES. This is an emerging policy that results in under-served populations becoming unserved populations. For example, a screening facility may refuse to schedule mammograms for under-screened populations unless a community-based organization can guarantee enough participants for the facility to make a profit. Screening facilities are businesses and this policy is in accordance with standard business practices. For populations in which the recruiting for screening programs is very time-consuming, organizations may be unable to make such a guarantee, and subsequently, the business policy may result in the population remaining unscreened (Burhansstipanov, 2001).

POVERTY BARRIERS. Poverty has multiple, confounding effects on life priorities other than cancer (e.g., food, rent, clothing); health priorities other than cancer (e.g., alcohol/substance abuse, violence, accidents, suicide, diabetes, obesity, cardiovascular disease); lack of medical insurance or access to an IHS facility; lack of access to telephone communication; the lack of transportation to a medical facility; and the lack of availability for child care during the visit to the medical facility. Obviously, these barriers affect people of all colors who live in poverty and are not racially or ethnically specific.

Volunteerism is a luxury of middle and upper class. Policies are needed which address the need to pay cancer survivors, or others who live in poverty, to perform roles that are typically done by volunteers (e.g., lay health advisors, outreach workers) in other communities.

PSYCHOSOCIAL BARRIERS. Psychosocial factors affect people of all colors and include, but are not limited to, level of education; practices, and beliefs about health and disease; daily customs, lifestyles, and beliefs; language or non-verbal communication styles; and fear of using health services based on cultural practices or unpleasant past medical experiences. Examples of psychosocial barriers among American Indians and Alaska Natives are related to misconceptions about cancer and the lack of cancer education. Some of the identified misconceptions might be a result of cancer education materials being written at a very high literacy level (e.g., most National Cancer Institute materials are written for persons with an average of grade 11 or higher[1]), whereas the average reading comprehension of large segments of the target population (within all ethnic groups) may be as low as grade five. Most psychosocial factors can be addressed through educational interventions.

SOCIOCULTURAL BARRIERS. Sociocultural barriers include culturally irrelevant cancer education and recruitment materials, culturally specific beliefs about cancer (e.g., to discuss the disease is to invite the cancer spirit into one's body), and other misconceptions such as one cannot walk the spirit path of their ancestors if a body part is removed (e.g., mastectomy).

Culturally competent interventions are needed to find acceptable strategies to address these barriers. For example, the Native American Women's Wellness through Awareness (NAWWA) project being implemented in Denver and Los Angeles provides Native Sisters who assist in personalizing the cancer screening process (Burhansstipanov, et al 2000a; Burhansstipanov, et al 1998). For example, one woman requested that she be accompanied to a sweat lodge ceremony on the evening of her mammography screening so that she could participate in a cleansing and spiritual ceremony to help eradicate evil cancer spirits that may have been introduced during screening. The Los Angeles site has also had clients who requested that a female medicine woman be present to smudge and bless the woman both prior to and following early detection breast cancer screening.

Many psychosocial and sociocultural barriers can be addressed on a one-on-one basis using lay health advisors or navigators, such as the Native Sisters. Policies directing hospitals and tribal health care settings to provide salaried employment of such navigators to implement support are necessary.

---

[1] Since 1992, the NCI has made efforts to disseminate easy-to-understand materials.

CONCLUSIONS

Cancer is a growing health problem throughout AI/AN communities. Tribal programs need to incorporate public health policies to improve AI/AN ability to access state of the art cancer screening, diagnosis, and treatment services. These policies need to incorporate cultural beliefs relevant to the local AI/AN communities. Likewise, the policies need to address barriers to participation in cancer interventions, such as poverty, psychosocial, and sociocultural issues. Some policies address issues affecting all medically underserved communities (e.g., those living in poverty, other racial groups) and thus those tribal public health policies could be used as models for other communities. There is a need for the assessment of culturally relevant cancer policy-based interventions that have been designed to address documented barriers within AI/AN communities. Likewise, some research needs to be done to determine how standard cancer protocols need to be modified to be culturally acceptable to Native American cancer patients and their families. Health care policies are also needed to address the access to quality cancer care issues and culturally competent strategies to reduce the interval between diagnosis and initiation of treatment.

ACKNOWLEDGMENTS

Native American Cancer Initiatives Research has been supported by the following organizations and agencies:

Foundations / Trusts / Businesses

The Susan G. Komen Breast Cancer Foundation (Dallas, TX, and the Los Angeles and Denver Affiliates)

AVON Breast Health Leadership Award (New York City, NY)

California Community Foundation (Los Angeles, CO)

The Graham Foundation (Colorado Springs, CO)

Robert Wood Johnson Foundation

The Kettering Family Foundation (Denver, CO)

A.V. Hunter Trust (Denver, CO)

The Breast Cancer Fund (San Francisco, CA)

Paul's Big Screen TV (La Habra, CA)

Federal Agencies

National Institutes of Health, National Cancer Institute (Bethesda, MD)

National Institutes of Health, National Institute of Human Genome Research (Bethesda, MD)

Department of Defense (Ft. Detrick, MD)

Centers for Disease Control and Prevention (Atlanta, GA)

REFERENCES

Agency for Health Care Policy and Research. *National Medical Expenditure Survey, Access to Health Care: Findings from the Survey of American Indians and Alaska Natives.* Pub. No. (DHHS) 91-0028. Washington, D.C.: Government Printing Office; 1991.

Albanes D. Caloric intake, body weight, and cancer: a review. <u>Nutr Cancer</u>. 1987;A:9:199–217

Black WC, Key CR, Epidemiologic pathology of cancer in New Mexico's tri-ethnic population. *Pathology Annuals.* 1980; 15:181- 194.

Burhansstipanov L, Olsen S. Cancer Prevention and Early Detection in American Indian and Alaska Native Populations. *Cancer Prevention in Diverse Populations: Cultural Implications for the Multi-disciplinary Team.* Frank-Stromborg M and Olsen SJ. Oncology Nursing Society. Mosby Publisher: St Louis, MO. 2001.

Burhansstipanov L, Dignan MB, Bad Wound D, Tenney M, Vigil G. Native American Recruitment into Breast Cancer Screening: The NAWWA Project. *Journal of Cancer Education.* 2000a; 15:29–33.

Burhansstipanov L. Urban Native American Health Issues. *Cancer.* 2000b;88: 987–93.

Burhansstipanov L, Hampton JW, Tenney MT. American Indian and Alaska Native Cancer Data Issues. *American Indian Culture and Research Journal.*1999a;23:3:217–241.

Burhansstipanov L. Community-Based Projects: Theory versus Reality. *Cancer Control: Journal of the Moffitt Cancer Center.*1999b; 6:6: 620-626

Burhansstipanov L and Morris S. Breast Cancer Screening among American Indians and Alaska Natives. *Federal Practitioner.* 1998a 15:1: 12–25.

Burhansstipanov L. Editorial of Cancer Mortality among Native Americans. *Cancer.* 1998d 83:11: 2247–2250.

Burhansstipanov L, *Cancer Among Elder Native Americans.* Denver, CO: Native Elder Health Care Resource Center, University of Colorado Health Sciences Center; 1997.

Burhansstipanov L and Dresser CM. *Native American Monograph #1: Documentation of the Cancer Research Needs of American Indians and Alaska Natives.* NIH Pub. No. 94-3603, Bethesda, MD: National Cancer Institute. 1994.

Cobb N and Paisano RE. Patterns of Cancer Mortality among Native Americans. *Cancer:* 1998: 83:11: 2377–2383.

Cobb N, Paisano RE. *Cancer Mortality among American Indians and Alaska Natives in the United States: Regional Differences in Indian Health, 1989-1993* IHS Pub. No. 97-615-23. Rockville, MD: Indian Health Service; 1997.

Creagan E.T., and J.F. Fraumeni. Cancer mortality among American Indians, 1950–67. *Journal of the National Cancer Institute.* 1972:49:956–967.

Department of Commerce, Bureau of the Census. *Selected social and economic characteristics by race and Hispanic origin for the United States. American Indian Population by Tribe for the United States, Regions, Divisions, and States: 1990.* CPH-L-99. Washington, DC: Government Printing Office, 1992.

Department of Health and Human Services. *Healthy People 2010: Objectives for the Nation — Draft for Public Comment.* Washington, DC: Government Printing Office; 1998.

Department of Health and Human Services. *Healthy People 2000: National Health Promotion and Disease Prevention Objectives.* Pub. No. (DHHS) 91-50212. Washington, DC: Government Printing Office; 1991.

Department of Health and Human Services, Public Health Service National Institutes of Health, National Cancer Institute. *Report of the Special Action Committee, 1992: Program initiatives related to Minorities, the Underserved and Persons aged 65 and over.* Appendices A, B, C. Washington, DC: Government Printing Office; 1992.

Department of Health and Human Services, Office of Planning, Evaluation and Legislation. *Regional Differences in Indian Health: 1997.* Rockville, MD: Indian Health Service; 1997.

Department of Health and Human Services, Public Health Service, National Institutes of Health, National Cancer Institute. *Volume III: Cancer: Report of the secretary's task force on Black and minority health.* Pub. No. (DHHS) 1986-621-605:00171. Washington, DC: U.S. Government Printing Office. 1986b.

Doll R. and R. Peto. The causes of cancer: quantitative estimates of avoidable risks of cancer in the United States Today. *Journal of the National Cancer Institute*. 1981:66:1191–1309.

Eidson M, Becker TM, Wiggins CL, Key CR, Samet JM. Breast cancer among Hispanics, American Indians and non- Hispanic whites in New Mexico. *International Journal of Epidemiology* .1994:23(2):231–7.

Gaudette, L.A, Gao RN, S. Freitag S, Wideman M. Cancer incidence by ethnic group in the Northwest Territories, 1969-1988. *Public Health Reports* 5(1):23-32; 1993.

Goldberg HI, Warren CW, Oge LL, Driedman JS, Helgerson SD, Pepion DD, LaMere E. Prevalence of behavioral risk factors in two American populations in Montana. *Preventative Medicine*. 1991:7:3:155–160.

Hampton JW, Conquering cancer among Indians requires education, lifestyle changes. *National Indian Health Board Reporter*. 1984: 3:10–11.

Hampton JW. The heterogeneity of cancer in Native American populations. *Minorities and Cancer*, ed. Jones LA, New York, NY: Springer-Verlag; 1989.

Hampton JW. Cancer prevention and control in American Indians and Alaska Natives. *American Indian Culture and Research Journal*. 1992:16:41–49.

Hampton JW. The Disproportionately Lower Cancer Survival Rate with Increased Incidence and Mortality in Minorities and Underserved Americans. *Cancer*: 1998:83:8:1687–1689.

Harras A, Edwards BK, Blot WJ, Ries LAG. *Cancer Rates and Risks*. Bethesda, MD: National Cancer Institute; NIH Pub. No. 96-691. 1996.

Horm JW, Devesa SS, Burhansstipanov L. Cancer incidence, mortality, and survival among racial and ethnic minority groups in the United States. Schottenfeld D and Fraumeni, Jr. JF. eds. *Cancer Epidemiology and Prevention*. Oxford University Press: New York; 1996.

Horm JW, Burhansstipanov L Cancer incidence, survival, and mortality among American Indians and Alaska Natives. *American Indian Culture and Research Journal*. 1992:16:3:27–28.

Horner RD Cancer mortality in Native Americans in North Carolina. *American Journal of Public Health*. 1990:80:940–944.

Hrdlicka A. Diseases of the Indians, more especially of the Southwest United States and Northern Mexico. *Washington Medical Annals*. 1905:6:3/72 - 3/94.

Kottke T, Trapp, MA. The quality of Pap test specimens collected by nurses in breast and cervical cancer screening clinic. *American Journal of Preventive Medicine*. In Press

Kottke T, Trapp M. Implementing Nurse-Based Systems to Provide American Indian Women with Breast and Cervical Cancer Screening. *Mayo Clinic Proceedings*. 1998; 73(9): 815.

Lanier AP, Kelly J, Smith B, Amadon C, Harpster A, Peters H, Tantilla H, Key, Davidson AM. *Cancer in the Alaska Native Population: Eskimo, Aleut, and Indian Incidence and Trends 1969-1988*. Alaska Area Native Health Service: Anchorage, AK: 1993.

Lanier AP, Bulkow LR, Ireland B. Cancer in Alaska Indians, Eskimos, and Aleuts, 1969-83: Implications of etiology and control. *Public Health Report*. 1989:104:658–664.

Levin I. Cancer among the American Indians and its bearing upon the ethnological distribution of the disease. *Z Krebsforsch*. 1910; 9:423-425. 1910.

Mahoney MC, Michalek AM, Cummings KM, Nasca PS, Emrich LJ. Cancer mortality in a northeastern native population. *Cancer*. 1989:64:187–190.

Mao Y, Morrison H, Semenciw R, Wigle D. Mortality on Canadian Indian reserves 1977–1982. *Canadian Journal of Public Health*. 1986:77:263–268.

Michalek AM, Mahoney MC, Tome D, Tenney M, Burhansstipanov L. Tribal-based Cancer Control Activities: Services and Perceptions. *Cancer Supplement*. 1996a. 78:7.

Michalek AM, Mahoney MC, Burhansstipanov L, Tenney M, Cobb N. Urban-based Native American Cancer Control Activities: Services and Perceptions. *Journal of Cancer Education*. 1996b;11(3).

Michalek AM, Mahoney, MC. Provision of cancer control services to Native Americans by state health departments. *Journal of Cancer Education*. 1994:9:145–147.

Miller BA, Kolonel LN, Bernstein L, Young JL, Swanson GM, West DW, Key

CR, Liff JM, Glover CS, Alexander GA, Coyle L, Hankey BF, Percy C. *Racial/Ethnic Patterns of Cancer in the United States 1988-1992*. Pub. No. (NIH) 96-4104. National Cancer Institute. Bethesda, MD: 1996.

Miller BA, Ries LAG, Hankey BF, Kosary CL, Edwards BK (eds.). *Cancer Statistics Review: 1973-1989*. Pub. No. (NIH) 92-2789, National Cancer Institute. Bethesda, MD: 1992. I.3-I.7.

National Academy of Sciences, Institute of Medicine, *IOM Minority Cancer Study: The Unequal Burden of Cancer*. National Academy Press. Washington, DC. 1999.

National Indian Health Board. *Quarterly Board Report*, NHB. Denver, CO; 1997.

Nutting PA, Freeman WL, Risser DR, Helgerson SD, Paisano R, Hisnanick J, Beaver SK, Peters I, Carney JP, Speers MA. Cancer Incidence among American Indians and Alaska Natives, 1980 through 1987. *American Journal of Public Health*. American Public Health Association, Washington, DC. 1993:83:11:1589.

Ritchie WA, Warren SL. The occurrence of multiple bone lesions suggesting myeloma in the skeleton of a pre-Columbian Indian. *Am J Roentgenol*. 1932:28:622-628.

Sorem KA. Cancer incidence in the Zuni Indians of New Mexico. *Yale Journal of Biological Medicine*: 1985:58:489–496.

Sugarman J.R., C.W. Warren, L.L. Oge, S.D. Helgerson. Using the behavioral risk factor surveillance system to monitor year 2000 objectives among American Indians. *Public Health Reports*. 1992:107:4:451, 454.

Valway S. Kileen M, Paisano R, Ortiz. E. *Cancer Mortality among Native Americans in the United States: Regional Differences in Indian Health, 1984-88 and Trends Over Time*. Rockville, MD: Indian Health Service. 1992.

Welty TK, Zephier N, Schweignam K, Blake B, Leonardson. Cancer risk factors in three Sioux tribes: use of the Indian-specific health risk appraisal for data collection and analysis. *Alaska Medicine*.1993:35:4:265.

Welty, T. Cancer and Cancer Prevention and Control Program in the Aberdeen Area Indian Health Service. *American Indian Culture and Research Journal*. 1992; 16(3): 117–137.

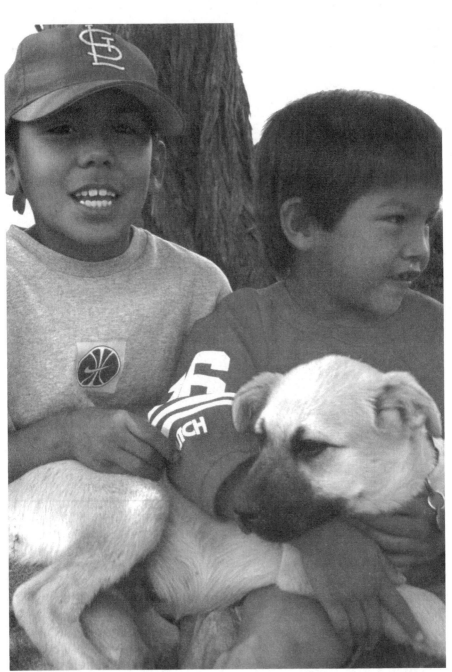

HEALTH SURVEILLANCE, RESEARCH, AND INFORMATION

Yvette Roubideaux and Mim Dixon

In the public health arena, the professions of epidemiology, biomedical research, health systems research, and health education are considered distinct specialties, each with its own types of training, funding streams, and activities. In Indian Country, these types of activities tend to be lumped together due to the following factors: they generally are not a source of direct patient care; they are generally focused at universities and agencies outside of the Indian health system; they require quantitative skills that are not well understood by most people; and the benefits of these activities are not always readily apparent to American Indian/Alaska Native communities.

When funding is not available to meet the most basic health care needs, tribes are reluctant to have Indian Health Service (IHS) dollars diverted from direct patient care to data collection and research. Yet, most tribes understand that measuring health disparities provides powerful information to convince Congress and the American public that funding for Indian health must be increased to bring the health status of American Indians and Alaska Native (AI/AN) people to the level of the rest of the U.S. population.

Tribes also recognize the need to translate research findings into useful information for Indian health providers and AI/AN consumers. Perhaps because so much medical research has been conducted in the past using AI/AN populations without any apparent benefit or results returning to the community, tribes now insist that the research findings benefit the very people who are the subjects of the research.

In this information age, various types of data and information are necessary to provide health services. Policy makers need information on the demography and health status of American Indians and Alaska Natives (AI/AN) so that they can identify unmet needs, monitor health status over time, and take responsibility for funding services at an appropriate level. Health care managers need information to assess the quality of care and health outcomes, so that they can identify opportunities for improvements in their health care systems. They also need information on the costs of delivering services and revenues, in order to maximize the resources available to meet local needs. Health care providers need research to understand the best strategies to prevent and treat diseases in the most effective and culturally competent ways. And consumers need information and education that translates medical research into an accessible format that allows them to make informed choices about their lifestyles and treatment plans.

Good public health policy supports data collection, research, evaluation, and monitoring of health status, quality of care, and new approaches for more effective assessment and treatment. Given the recent changes and trends in the Indian health system, there are a number of special challenges for meeting these information needs in AI/AN health care delivery systems.

HEALTH SURVEILLANCE

Monitoring the health status of the AI/AN population will be critical to help inform public health administrators and policy leaders, and is an essential resource for other public health functions. It is also clear that there are both local and national needs for data to monitor health status, and strategies are needed to ensure that these data are as accurate and as useful as possible.

The IHS Public Health Support Workgroup recently identified the core public health functions and essential public health services that are needed at local, regional, and national levels in the Indian health system, and that are necessary to continue to improve the health status of AI/AN (Public Health Support Workgroup 1999). The 10 core public health functions as defined by the DHHS Public Health Functions Steering Committee are:

1. Monitor health status to identify community health problems;

2. Diagnose and investigate health problems and health hazards in the community;

3. Inform, educate, empower people about health issues;

4. Mobilize community partnerships and coalitions to identify and solve health issues;

5. Develop policies and plans that support individual and community health efforts

6. Enforce laws and regulations that protect health and ensure safety;

7. Link people to needed personal health services and assure the provision of health care;

8. Assure a competent public health and personal health care workforce;

9. Evaluate effectiveness, accessibility, and quality of personal and public health services;

10. Research for new insights and innovative solutions to health problems.

Many of these core public health functions involve acquiring, analyzing, and disseminating information.

Many tribes are so small that there is a problem developing accurate estimates of the incidence and prevalence of diseases, particularly diseases that are not very common. Rates of diseases are usually reported as the number of cases (numerator) per number of people in the community at risk (denominator, usually population number) at one point in time (prevalence) or over a certain period of time (incidence). Unfortunately for small communities, when the numbers used in these calculations are smaller, the calculated results are less accurate, and not comparable to other results calculated with larger numbers. In addition, when the numbers used in the calculations are small, changes in the numbers of cases may or may not represent stable estimates and may overestimate trends or suggest trends that are not real; and, if the numbers in either the number of cases or the number of people at risk in the population are inaccurate, then the calculated rate is inaccurate also. So, for example, a single occurrence of a rare disease in a small population in a single year could generate a rate that appears to reflect an extraordinarily high prevalence of the disease. This can lead to a comparison with disease rates in other populations that results in a skewed picture of the situation. It is possible that health administrators could believe that there was a local epidemic of a certain disease, and choose to invest funding into programs for that disease. However, if the numbers are small, and the data used for this decision are inaccurate, and if the numbers next year show no cases or fewer cases, then the allocation of funds in the previous year may not have been the most cost-effective.

This problem with small numbers has a significant impact on health surveillance in the Indian health system and creates a paradox for health administrators and tribal leaders. There are clear reasons for gathering data on a national level: larger numbers provide more accurate estimates of rates of disease, and overall health status statistics are useful for national program planning, priorities, and funding decisions. In addition, overall health status statistics are useful in advocacy efforts of tribes and national Indian organizations, and overall statistics help track the health of the AI/AN population as a whole over time, which is an important public health function.

However, there are also clear needs for gathering data to monitor health status at the local/community level. There may be regional variations in the incidence and prevalence of certain diseases, and local data are needed to set local priorities that are relevant for the community and responsive to their unique needs. Local data are also needed to help in program planning, decision-making, and local allocation of funds. Also, local data are needed for advocacy efforts relevant to each tribe and their needs. Due to problems with the IHS Resource and Patient Management System (RPMS), tribes with their own resources may want to purchase another more efficient or effective data system for use in their local health care facilities.

NATIONAL DATA

There are a variety of data sources that are used to monitor the health status of AI/AN on a national basis. The Indian Health Service (IHS) has a Program Statistics Branch in its Headquarters Office that receives data from each of the 12 Areas and produces two annual reports. One is a composite picture of the entire Indian health system entitled *Trends in Indian Health*. The other report provides similar information for each of the 12 Areas and it is entitled *Regional Differences in Indian Health*. These two reports have become the standard reference documents for data on AI/AN morbidity, mortality, rates of certain diseases and conditions, and the quantity of various services provided through the Indian Health Service.

Data sources used by the IHS in these annual reports include: the U.S. Census Bureau projections; Vital Statistics reported by states to the National Center for Health Statistics; patient care statistics that are derived from IHS automated data systems[1]; and data that are collected and reported by various branches within IHS[2]. However, there are problems with many of these data sources. For example, state birth and death records do not provide tribal affiliation and the race category is often miscoded to under-represent the number of American Indians; furthermore, the cause of death is frequently reported inaccurately. Data from the IHS automated data systems are subject to recording, inputting, and transmitting errors (Indian Health Service 1997). Also, var-

---

[1] In the IHS, reporting systems that are used include the Monthly Inpatient Services Report, the Ambulatory Patient Care System, Contract Health Care System, the Clinical Laboratory Workload Reporting System, the Pharmacy System, the Urban Projects Reporting System, and the Dental Data System (Indian Health Service 1997).

[2] These include the Chemical Dependency Management Information System, the IHS Nutrition and Dietetics Program Activity Reporting System, the IHS Community Health Activity Reporting System, the IHS Community Health Representative Information System, the Project Data System, the Sanitation Deficiency System, and the IHS Health Education Resource Management System (Indian Health Service 1997).

ious Service Units and Areas do not submit their reports in a complete and timely way. These problems are recognized by the statisticians, who make statistical adjustments for these deficiencies in order to produce more accurate data.

Through these reports, the tribes and the IHS are able to document health service needs and use these data as they advocate for annual appropriations from Congress. Reporting of national indicators and data is required as a part of the DHHS budget process. Each agency must identify, monitor, and report a number of key indicators each year under the Government Performance and Results Act (GPRA). While the purpose of this reporting is to help better inform Congress on performance of each DHHS agency, these numbers must be accurate and participation rates must be high in order to ensure that an accurate picture of the performance of the Indian health system is presented.

The importance of gathering national data is acknowledged by tribal leaders who have consistently agreed that maintenance of a national database for health statistics reporting should remain a national activity that is not divisible among tribes through contracting or compacting. The Indian Health Design Team (IHDT) that was convened by the Director of the IHS in 1995 with representation from Indian leaders and IHS officials issued its final report in 1997 with the following recommendation for IHS Headquarters:

> Focus on core functions of advocacy for Indian health, leadership, empowerment to I/T/Us. Be a voice for Indian people and build partnership with tribes. Document our health needs, support a nation-wide Indian health network, and maintain an Indian health data bank (Indian Health Design Team 1997).

At the current time, tribal leaders regard Headquarters IHS as the appropriate organization to conduct this activity, but they envision a time in the future when an independent national AI/AN organization could assume this responsibility (Baseline Measures Workgroup 1996).

While there is a general recognition of the value of a nationwide database on Indian health, compacting tribes may regard the reporting of their health statistics to the Indian Health Service as optional, or they may choose to use a different system of data collection. However, if a significant number of tribes and facilities do not report to a "national" database, then the information is less accurate and less representative of the health of all AI/AN people. Efforts are needed to bring together IHS and tribal leaders to determine common measures that tribes are willing to report for the purpose of maintaining a national database, but that do not place an unreasonable administrative demand on the local health personnel.

A Baseline Measures Workgroup was formed in 1995 with representation from contracting and compacting tribes and federal representatives. They attempted to identify a core set of data that tribes could use on a voluntary basis. In their final report, the Baseline Measures Workgroup (BMW) states:

> The BMW strongly supports the principle that Self-Governance Tribes have the legal right to negotiate reporting requirements on an individual basis during compact negotiations. However, Self-Governance Tribes must consider provisions that would assure reporting of information to IHS that it needs to provide to the Congress with justification for appropriations. Provision should also be made for data used by IHS/Tribes as a basis for compact resource methodology and the planning/evaluation process. This should not preclude eliminating reporting requirements that Tribes find burdensome and which are not essential to meeting IHS and Tribal information needs. (Baseline Measures Workgroup, 1996)

Thus, the movement toward self-governance acknowledges that each tribe has the sovereign right to collect and report any data it chooses. However, if tribes choose to report different types of information, or information using different parameters of measurement, the national database will become less valid.

LOCAL/COMMUNITY DATA

Data on the health status of the local community can be very useful for local planning, priority setting, and funding allocations. Tribes also often need local data to apply for additional resources and grants; because there are regional and even tribal variations in the rates of many diseases and health conditions, national data is often not relevant to the local situation. For example, while the national prevalence of diabetes according to IHS/CDC data is approximately 10–20 percent, the local prevalence of diabetes on the Pima reservation is over 50 percent in adults age 35 and older. In this case, the local data are more helpful in program planning, priority setting, and advocacy for more diabetes-related funding. In fact, during the allocation of funds under the Special Diabetes Grants for Indians Program (See chapter 8), inaccurate or absent local/tribal data on disease burden (diabetes prevalence and mortality) may have resulted in tribes receiving a smaller grant than actually needed.

Measuring local or tribal data on health status is difficult for a number of reasons. The small numbers of cases for certain diseases may make local estimates unstable, as discussed previously. In addition, tribes or local health programs may not have health professionals (such as epidemiologists or statisticians) with the expertise to measure and interpret health status data accurately; it also may be difficult to define the population to use in the calculations. For example, prevalence is defined as the number of cases of a disease in a population at a certain point in time. Defining the number of people in the population can be difficult. There are three basic choices: (1) the people who use the I/T/U facility at a given time (user population); (2) the people who have ever used the I/T/U services (service population); or (3) the entire population of the tribe. There are benefits and drawbacks to using each of these numbers depending on what is being measured, and the population must be relatively stable to obtain accurate measurements. For example, if a significant number of tribal members travel back and forth to urban areas, numbers measured at one point in time may not be the same when re-checked at a later date.

A number of initiatives are being developed to help tribes and local programs measure accurate local data on health status. One of the purposes of the Baseline Measures Workgroup was to create standardized measures that could be used by Indian health programs and tribes to measure both national and local data; the specifics of how to calculate these data were included in the report. However, since the report of the Baseline Measures Workgroup, there has not been an evaluation of the extent of use of these measures in Indian health and tribal programs.

The Indian Health Service has funded four regional Tribal Epidemiology Centers, and the purpose of these centers is to provide technical assistance and data monitoring for the tribes and Indian health programs in those regions. The quality of data in the regions with Tribal Epidemiology Centers has improved, and these centers provide regional training and technical assistance on data collection and evaluation. They also conduct a number of research and evaluation studies to monitor the health status of the AI/AN population in their region.

The Northwest Tribal Epidemiology Center has developed an innovative *Indian Community Health Profile* that is an instrument to assess the overall health status of AI/AN communities. This instrument consists of 15 recommended indicators that are easy to measure for a community of 1,000–5,000 members. The measures are designed to be used only for local purposes, and cover multiple areas of health including socio-demographic, health status, mental health and functional status, health risk factors and positive health behaviors, and environmental issues. The local community can determine which indicators are relevant and will help them meet their particular needs. The Northwest Tribal Epidemiology Center has been funded by IHS to pilot this process in up to five communities (Northwest Tribal Epidemiology Center 2000). This program is an example of how a regional Tribal Epidemiology Center can help build the capacity of local programs to measure their own data on health status using a very relevant, participatory process.

URBAN DATA

Unfortunately, accurate and comprehensive data do not exist on the health status of urban AI/AN. While the IHS funds 34 urban Indian programs across the country, these programs are under-funded, and each program provides a different level of services. Some programs are only able to provide social services and assistance in referrals to other sources of care, while other programs provide direct clinical services. Because most of these programs cannot provide comprehensive services, urban AI/AN may not use these programs for all of their health needs, and may use multiple other sources of care. As a result, tracking the health status of urban Indians is very difficult, and requires the use of multiple data sources. However, many non-Indian urban health programs and clinics may not record the ethnicity of their clients, so the number of AI/AN using their services is often missing or under-counted.

There is only one published study of the health status of urban Indians in one city (Grossman, et al 1994), but the methodology required to complete the study is likely not feasible in other urban areas without university researchers to assist in the data effort. The lack of accurate data in urban areas significantly impedes the ability of these programs to advocate for more funding, since they cannot provide data to justify increased levels of funding or services. More efforts are clearly needed to develop effective strategies to measure the health status of urban Indians.

MONITORING THE QUALITY OF CARE

It is important for Indian health programs and facilities to measure the quality of care that they provide to AI/AN. Data on the quality of care can help guide decisions that can improve services and health outcomes. Information on the quality of care is also needed for accreditation, reimbursement, participation in managed care plans/networks, program development/implementation, obtaining outside resources or funding, providing feedback to Indian health care providers, and ensuring that consumers are receiving the highest quality of care.

Strategies for evaluating the quality of care have changed over time. Quality assurance was common in the 1980s, but it tended to focus on identifying "bad" providers who did not meet the standards of care and reporting requirements. Quality improvement was common in the 1990s as a method to assess the "processes" of care, and design better strategies for care. Quality improvement strategies often involved teams of providers working to identify less efficient or unnecessary steps in the process of care. In the late 1990s, quality measurement became more important as a strategy to measure the quality of care delivered by health systems or health organizations, with a focus not just on processes of care but also on measuring outcomes. In addition, quality measurement involves recording indicators of quality in a uniform way to facilitate comparisons among health programs. Monitoring the quality of care has become an essential component of the trend towards managed care, where plans try to deliver the highest quality services at the lowest cost compared to their competitors. Recently, there has been a significant backlash from the public as they suspect that the driving force for managed care is lowering costs, not improving quality. As a result of the suspicions of the general public, it is even more important for health care organizations to demonstrate both internally and externally that they deliver the highest quality of care and do not make unnecessary compromises on the basis of cost.

While it is important for Indian health programs to measure quality, it is difficult to measure because quality is actually a concept, and cannot be measured directly. However, quality measurement addresses this problem by attempting to make observations about quality, through the measurement of specific indicators of quality care that can be accessed directly. This requires knowledge of what the standards of care are for the particular indicators being measured.

Health care quality can be observed or measured in three basic domains: patient satisfaction, access to care, and clinical performance. Within each of these domains, indicators of quality can be measured on the structure, process, and outcome of care. For example, measuring clinical performance is the most common way to measure quality; indicators of structure include whether or not the health program has systems in place to hire and support quality health care providers. Indicators of process include whether or not the health program provides the right kinds of care at the right time for certain conditions. Outcome indicators include whether after getting care or services, the patient's health status improves. Accurate measurement of these indicators of quality requires personnel knowledgeable on how to measure these indicators, what data sources are needed, and how to correctly calculate and interpret the findings. In addition, if the programs want to compare their results with other similar programs or with national data, they have to make sure that they measure the data in the same manner so that valid comparisons can be made.

Whether the Indian health system has the capacity to measure the quality of care accurately on a national or a local basis has not been formally evaluated. While many Indian health programs participate in some of the national efforts, (such as the Government Performance Reporting Act (GPRA), the Joint Commission on Accreditation of Healthcare Organizations (JCAHO) or the IHS National Diabetes Audit), not all programs have the capacity to measure quality. In a pilot study for the National Indian Health Board, a sample of Indian health programs was asked if they measured a number of common quality indicators (Roubideaux 1998). Overall, while most programs had the capacity to measure quality, they often did not have accurate or comparable data, and most programs were unable to provide actual data for the survey, even though they stated that they did make the observations. For many of these programs, time and resources were a significant factor. The person responsible for quality improvement was often also responsible for other program functions, especially in small facilities. While the number of facilities interviewed in this survey was small, the results were informative about the capacity of a random selection of Indian health programs to measure quality, and indicative of a need for more training, technical assistance, and resources for quality measurement.

Critics of the trend toward tribal management of Indian health programs have expressed concern about the possibility that the quality of care under tribal management would decrease. As a part of the National Indian Health Board's survey of tribal leaders and health directors (Dixon, et al 1998), participants were asked about their impressions of the quality of care over the past three or four years. Overall, tribal leaders and health directors believed that the quality of care had improved in the Indian health system, and those respondents from tribally managed programs more commonly perceived that the quality of care was "better" compared to respondents from IHS direct service programs. While this study was an observational study to assess the perspectives of tribal leaders and tribal health directors and only provided qualitative data, more studies are needed to assess the changes in the quality of care over time and among different types of health programs in a quantitative, comparable way.

FINANCIAL MANAGEMENT INFORMATION

Health care managers need information about the costs of the services that they deliver in order to set rates at a level that compensates them appropriately; they also need computerized billing systems that track revenues. While these types of information are taken for granted in the private medical sector, comprehensive and workable systems have not been available in most of the Indian health system. As tribes take over the management of Indian health programs, one of the improvements they are most likely to make is the acquisition of computers and billing software (Dixon, et al 1998). In addition, as more I/T/U providers participate in managed care networks, updated financial systems will be needed to comply with the administrative requirements of the managed care plan in order to receive reimbursement for services.

RESEARCH TO HELP IMPROVE THE HEALTH OF AMERICAN INDIAN/ALASKA NATIVE COMMUNITIES

One of the problems in providing the highest quality of care for AI/AN communities is the lack of specific and culturally relevant research and data to help inform Indian health providers and administrators on the most effective treatment and prevention strategies. For many health conditions, there is ample research in the medical literature on the most effective health practices for the general population, but there is no evidence that these strategies will be effective for all AI/AN with the same conditions. Literature searches for research conducted with adequate samples of AI/AN to yield accurate results often reveal few or no publications for most conditions.

This lack of adequate or relevant research on effective approaches to the health problems of AI/AN is due to a number of factors. The agencies that fund clinical research, especially the National Institutes of Health, demand very rigorous methodologies in the projects that they fund, and these include having a sample size that is large enough to ensure that the results are statistically valid. In addition, many research designs for treatment and prevention strategies cannot be adequately conducted with small numbers of participants, which precludes doing the research in some Indian communities.

The advisory structure for most federal research agencies draws upon the leading scientists in the field of the research that the agency funds. There are few AI/AN with postgraduate degrees in the health and behavioral sciences, subsequently AI/AN are not represented at the table when research agencies develop their agendas. However, the Federal Executive Order on tribal consultation provides another avenue for federal agencies to incorporate the needs of AI/AN communities in their planning processes.

The number of researchers interested in conducting research in AI/AN communities is low, due to both a lack of trained personnel, and the low numbers of researchers willing to take the time to conduct culturally relevant research in Indian communities and also meet time-consuming requirements for tribal approvals. Since many successful, well-trained researchers are faculty at universities, they often need to "publish or perish," and research with small communities often doesn't result in publications or large amounts of funding. For many researchers, the costs of conducting research in AI/AN communities are too high, and they choose to work with other populations.

These problems create a self-defeating cycle that fails to promote quality research in Indian health. Since funding agencies are reluctant to fund small community studies, so university researchers are reluctant to spend a lot of time trying to do research with Indian communities. In addition, there are few AI/AN researchers who have the experience and reputation to receive funding, and there are few mentors available with experience working in Indian communities to help them. So AI/AN researchers may get discouraged and abandon their efforts to do research. Therefore funding agencies do not get many quality applications for AI/AN research, and as a result, they do not fund research in Indian communities.

Researchers also get discouraged because, if they try to do research in Indian communities, they often make the mistake of not involving the community and the result is a lack of community cooperation. Research in AI/AN communities must be done with maximal participation of the community in all phases of the research, while establishing real partnerships with tribes and Indian communities.

DEVELOPING TRIBAL PARTNERSHIPS FOR RESEARCH

American Indian and Alaska Native communities are wary of researchers. Too often research has been conducted in Indian Country without people perceiving any potential benefits from their participation in the research. In a health care delivery system that is already so under-funded that even basic health services are lacking, AI/AN people reject the added insult of being treated "like guinea pigs" or being experimented upon. Furthermore, there is a dark history of federally-funded research projects that were conducted without the full consent and understanding of individual participants or their tribes.[3]

AI/AN populations are sometimes attractive to researchers because the higher-than-average incidence of certain types of diseases makes it easier for them to conduct clinical trials to determine whether vaccines, medications or treatments for those diseases are effective. Theoretically, the AI/AN communities should benefit the greatest from the development of effective treatments, because their tribal members are at greatest risk for the disease. However, people also perceive that they are accepting a risk by participating in drug trials in order that an even larger population may benefit. They resent that pharmaceutical companies are becoming wealthy as a result of this type of research, while the Indian communities are remaining impoverished.

Most tribes are not "anti-science," but they are concerned about the ethical conduct of research and the need for culturally appropriate research that acknowledges that traditional cultures embody knowledge that should be valued by scientists of all cultures. The Alaska Federation of Natives (AFN) made this statement in their Board Policy Guidelines for Research:

> Alaska Natives share with the scientific community an interest in learning more about the history and culture of our societies. The best scientific and ethical standards are obtained when Alaska Natives are directly involved in research conducted in our communities and in studies where the findings have a direct impact on Native populations. (Joseph-Fox and Kekahbah 1999)

In addition to the protections of informed consent, the AFN policy calls upon researchers to fund a Native Research Committee appointed by the local community to assess and monitor the research project, to hire and train Native people to assist in the study, to include Native viewpoints in the final study, to give credit to Native resource people, and to report the major findings of the study to the Native Research Committee in a non-technical summary.

Tribal people do not want to be regarded as research subjects, but rather as partners in research; many tribes have developed tribal codes and policies that

---

3 For example, the federal government conducted experiments in the 1950s in which they injected radioactive materials into people, including Alaska Natives, without fully disclosing the risks.

govern research on tribal lands and with tribal members. Some of the larger tribes have their own Institutional Research Boards (IRBs) that perform the human subjects review activities found in universities and government agencies. Several Area Health Boards have hired epidemiologists who apply for grant and contract funding to conduct tribally directed health research.[4]

In 1994, the Alaska Native Science Commission was formed to help broaden the participation of Alaska Native people in the research process. The goals of the Alaska Native Science Commission are:

- Facilitate the inclusion of local and traditional knowledge into research and science.;

- Participate in and influence priorities for research;

- Seek participation of Alaska Natives at all levels of science.;

- Provide a mechanism for community feedback on results and other scientific activities;

- Promote science to Native youth;

- Encourage native people to enter scientific disciplines;

- Ensure that Native people share in economic benefits derived from their intellectual property. (Joseph-Fox and Kekahbah 1999)

American Indian and Alaska Native people want to be part of the process to set the agenda for research in their communities.

RESEARCH NEEDS IN INDIAN COUNTRY

In 1996, the National Indian Health Board surveyed tribal leaders, tribal health directors, and urban Indian clinic directors to identify the priorities for health services research in Indian Country. Based upon the responses from 163 people[5], an advisory committee identified the following as the top ten research priorities (Joseph-Fox and Kekahbah 1999):

1. Addiction Prevention/Treatment/Aftercare with an emphasis on Alcoholism;

2. Diabetes/Dialysis Care and Services;

---

[4] Among the leaders are the Northwest Portland Area Indian Health Board and the Alaska Native Health Board.

[5] This represented 20 percent of the people who were mailed the two-page questionnaire.

3. Alternatives to Long Term Care;

4. Accessibility of State Block Grant Funding to Indian Health Programs;

5. Measuring Unmet Needs/ Research to Establish Need for Continuing IHS Funding;

6. Recruitment and Retention of Health Professionals;

7. Medicaid and Medicare.

This survey formed the basis for a Health Services Research Agenda Building Conference that was held in 1996 to identify specific kinds of research needed in each topic area.[6] Typically, the conference participants were interested in the kinds of pragmatic research that would lead to improvements in the health services for AI/AN communities. They wanted to know how best to solve a particular problem. For example, in the addiction category, conference participants recommended research on the most effective treatment modalities, identifying enforcement policies that reduce domestic violence, and assessing the future impacts of prevention of fetal alcohol syndrome.

HEALTHY PEOPLE 2010

The U.S. Department of Health and Human Services, working with a consortium of over 600 organizations and agencies, has developed national health objectives called *Healthy People 2010*. The intent of this effort is to increase quality and years of healthy life and to eliminate health disparities.

Healthy People 2010 has developed ten leading health indicators:

1. Physical Activity

2. Overweight and Obesity

3. Tobacco Use

4. Substance Abuse

5. Responsible Sexual Behavior

6. Mental Health

7. Injury and Violence

---

[6] Unfortunately, the federal agencies that funded the conference never produced a final report. However, much of the material has been summarized by Joseph-Fox and Kekahbah (1999).

8. Environmental Quality

9. Immunization

10. Access to Health Care (D.H.H.S. 2001)

For the Indian health system to join this effort and benefit from the nationwide focus on these important issues, support must be available to develop data that will measure progress and compare the status of AI/AN with other populations.

TRAINING MORE AMERICAN INDIAN/ALASKA NATIVE RESEARCHERS

There are some current efforts to increase the number of AI/AN researchers who can conduct high-quality research and successfully apply for grant funding from agencies such as the National Institutes of Health. The Native Elder Resource Center in the Division of American Indian and Alaska Native Programs at the University of Colorado Health Sciences Center has a newly developed Native Investigator Program that provides intensive mentoring and training in research methodologies for AI/AN individuals with doctoral level training (MD or PhD).

Recognizing the low numbers of AI/AN researchers, a special American Indian Alaska Native Research Network was recently formed by a group of 13 AI/AN researchers to provide a forum for AI/AN who do research to network, collaborate, and support each other. Within a short time, this new network grew to approximately 150 members. Hopefully these efforts will help increase the number of successful AI/AN researchers who can help conduct the research that is needed to help improve the health of Indian communities.

The National Institutes of Health (NIH) convened a Roundtable Conference on American Indian Research Training Needs in August 1999, and a number of AI/AN researchers participated, discussed current issues, and made recommendations for program development, funding, and training programs at the NIH and other agencies. Major issues discussed included: issues of credibility with the American Indian community; needs of new basic-science investigators; medical doctors and professionals who want to do research; and programs that have worked to encourage and engage students. Specific recommendations were developed in eight areas: outreach to AI/AN researchers and communities; grant application process and approval procedures; working with non-traditional grant recipients; working with tribal colleges; mentoring and training for students, young faculty and MDs; pre-college initiatives; and understanding and respecting American Indian/Alaska Native culture (NIH/IHS 1999).

As a result of this initiative, the IHS and the NIH have recently announced their plans to fund up to five Native American Research Centers for Health (NARCH) to conduct culturally relevant research and to help provide training and mentoring for AI/AN interested in research. Tribes and tribal organizations are eligible to apply, in collaboration with other organizations such as universities and medical centers. Hopefully, other recommendations from the NIH conference will be implemented soon to promote high-quality, culturally competent research in Indian communities.

HEALTH EDUCATION AND HEALTH PROMOTION

Health education often involves the translation of research results into an understandable format for consumers so that they can make informed choices. Many tribes have health promotion and disease prevention programs that provide community health education to reduce unintentional injuries, provide tobacco cessation programs, and encourage healthy lifestyles. However, tribes usually do not have the resources to develop and deliver the types of sophisticated educational materials or social marketing messages that are aimed at the rest of the country through media such as television. Even when mainstream public service messages are delivered through the airwaves to the televisions of AI/AN viewers, the messages may not be effective because of vast cultural and economic differences.

In his summary of the progress of public health in the 20th century, Jonathan E. Fielding stated, "Public health has learned that all interventions to promote health must be culturally relevant." (Fielding 1999) Federal and state agencies sometimes try to develop messages for audiences that are segmented on the basis of race or language. For example, there may be a health education campaign in Spanish to reach Hispanic Americans. However, there is little understanding of the need for tribally-specific health education messages—one approach to meet the needs of AI/AN tribes often does not work for other tribes. In fact, the "generic Indian" is a stereotype that undermines any effort to make a responsible and respectful response to the public health challenges in Indian Country.

Messages and artwork in health education materials must be based on knowledge of the local culture. For example, the owl is often used in the dominant American culture as a symbol of wisdom, but the owl is considered a bad omen in many tribes; while the color red can symbolize "stop" in the dominant American culture, among the Ponca tribe the color red is positive because it represents sunrise; seal oil is a big part of the Eskimo diet and any publications about cholesterol designed for Eskimos should include seal oil as a low cholesterol fat.

While tobacco settlement money is funding smoking prevention programs aimed at youth in many states, substance abuse is a complicated issue for Indian tribes. American Indian spiritual practices may involve the use of tobacco, which is seen as a gift from the Creator. So, tobacco cessation programs for those tribes that use tobacco ceremonially must be respectful of the differences between intermittent spiritual use of tobacco and daily habitual tobacco abuse. Through trials and evaluations, the health education profession has learned that all solutions must be at the community level:

> In the final analysis, the most appropriate center of gravity for health promotion is the community. . . State and national governments can formulate broad policies regulating production and commerce, provide leadership, allocate funding, and generate data for health promotion . . . But the decisions on priorities and strategies for social change affecting the more complicated lifestyle issues can best be made collectively as close to the homes and work places of those affect as possible. This principle assures greater relevance and appropriateness of the programs to the people affected, and it offers greater opportunity for people to be actively engaged in the planning process. (Green 1999)

Nowhere is this more true than in Indian Country, where local conditions affect the choices and behaviors of individuals. For example, most AI/AN communities do not have large chain grocery stores, so their choice of foods is limited to the local store and the U.S. Department of Agriculture (USDA) commodity foods programs that rarely offer low-fat foods, such as low-fat cheese and egg substitutes. It is difficult to promote a diet lower in saturated fat when items are not available locally. Another example of community factors influencing outcomes is that messages to encourage individuals to seek cancer screening tests may be futile if Indian Health Service (IHS) facilities do not offer mammography or sigmoidoscopy. Approaches to behavior change must take place in the context of a coordinated program of community support for that change.

Working at the community level provides the opportunity to develop an understanding and respect for the cultural practices that may put people at risk for disease. For example, the Sundance ceremonies that comprise an important spiritual activity for the Lakota people include piercing the skin and flesh offerings that could lead to the transmission of the human immunodeficiency virus (HIV) through exposure to blood that has been infected with the virus. The Aberdeen Area Office of the Indian Health Service has provided training to spiritual leaders on the use of universal precautions since 1988 (Giroux, et al 1997). They have published guidelines and provided to the spiritual leaders and dancers free medical supplies, such as disposable scalpels and needles, puncture-proof hazardous waste disposal containers, bleach, and latex gloves.

As the National Institutes of Health (NIH) and the Centers for Disease Control and Prevention(CDC) seek to translate scientific findings into health education materials for tribes, it is important they develop materials that are tribally specific. Because AI/AN communities are small and widely dispersed, it is a challenge to find cost-effective ways to do this. Computer technology should allow these federal agencies to design templates for health education materials in which the scientific information is valid and consistent, and then culturally specific information can be adapted for use by individual tribes. These agencies also need to provide more funding for communities to develop their own culturally relevant education materials, as many tribes and health programs lack the funding and personnel for these efforts.

MARKET RESEARCH

Social marketing is an important strategy for health promotion and disease prevention in communities. However, social marketing requires research to identify the knowledge, attitudes, and beliefs of people in AI/AN communities. Market research is needed to develop public health campaigns that are specifically targeted to AI/AN populations. The distinctive languages, cultures, symbols and beliefs of AI/AN render market research with other groups often not applicable to AI/AN communities. It is necessary to find out what motivates AI/AN individuals to make lifestyle changes. Motivating factors are likely to be different from the dominant American culture because AI/AN cultures have less emphasis on individualism, competition, and consumerism. Focus groups with AI/AN communities to develop heart disease prevention education materials found that people were more motivated to make lifestyle changes if they felt that it would help others in their family.

Focus groups are an excellent approach to social marketing research in Indian Country. The cultural patterns of verbal communication and low literacy levels make other forms of research, such as mailed surveys, less successful. While face-to-face interviews also may work well, the focus group allows people to stimulate one another with ideas and to confer on the best way to represent cultural beliefs and symbols.

However, there are many challenges for conducting focus groups with tribes, including obtaining tribal council permission; locating a suitable facility in which to hold the focus groups; creating incentives and reducing barriers for participation; and constructing groups that are representative of the target audience. Selecting a Native American facilitator who is known to the tribe and trusted, developing an interview guide that is relevant and understandable, and maintaining confidentiality without offending other family and tribal members are also significant challenges.

Tribes need training on how to conduct their own focus groups, develop their own community-based programs, and adapt scientific information for their own use. Tribes need forums, such as annual meetings or newsletters, to provide opportunities to share with one another methods and approaches that have been proven successful in health education and prevention in Indian

Country. Models of effective, participatory approaches to the design and dissemination of culturally appropriate education materials need to be replicated and funded (See chapter 9).

SUMMARY

The information and data needs for Indian health programs, tribes, health care administrators, health care providers, and consumers are substantial. Clearly, information is needed on the health status of AI/AN communities, the quality of care delivered to AI/AN, the cost-effectiveness of health services, treatment and prevention strategies, and the most effective educational strategies for AI/AN people so that they can improve their health. However, gathering this information requires knowledge, data systems, personnel, collaboration and cultural sensitivity to the needs of the population. There also needs to be a special effort to define the needs for both national and local data, and strategies to achieve the highest quality data in both areas. Tribal leaders need to advocate for more resources and funding to help the Indian health system meet its own needs for information and data.

Innovative strategies to meet these information needs are long overdue. Current effective strategies must be continued and replicated, such as the development of tribal epidemiology centers, training and technical assistance, and collaborative efforts to define mechanisms for measurement. Indian health leaders need to make sure that these essential public health functions survive despite all the recent changes in the Indian health system. Strategies to meet the information and data needs in Indian health are excellent investments in the future health of Indian people.

ACKNOWLEDGEMENTS

Mim Dixon would like to thank Pamela Iron, Diane Miller, Matilde Alvarado, the Laguna Pueblo, the Ponca Tribe of Oklahoma, and the Bristol Bay Native Corporation for their contributions to the information about cultural differences, derived from focus groups in 1998 and 1999 as part of a project, "Strengthening the Heartbeat of American Indian and Alaska Native Communities," under contract with Native American Management Services with funding from the National Heart, Lung and Blood Institute.

REFERENCES

Baseline Measures Workgroup. *Baseline Measures Workgroup Report. Final Report.* Rockville MD: Indian Health Service; 1996.

Department of Health and Human Services (DHHS). Available at www.health.gov/healthypeople. *Healthy People 2010*. Accessed on January 7, 2001.

Dixon M, Shelton BL, Roubideaux Y, Mather D, Smith CM. *Tribal Perspectives on Indian Self-Determination and Self-Governance in Health Care Management*. Denver CO: National Indian Health Board, 1998.

Fielding J E. Public Health in the Twentieth Century: Advances and Challenges in *Annual Review of Public Health*, Volume 20, 1999, Fielding JE, Lave LB, Starfield B (eds). Palo Alto, CA: Annual Reviews. 1999.

Giroux J, Takehara J, Asetoyer C, Welty T. HIV/AIDS Universal Precaution Practices in Sun Dance Ceremonies. *The IHS Primary Care Provider*. 1997; 22:4.

Green LW. Health Education's Contributions to Public Health in the Twentieth Century: A Glimpse Through Health Promotion's Rear-View Mirror in *Annual Review of Public Health*, Volume 20, 1999, Fielding JE, Lave LB, Starfield B (eds). Palo Alto, CA: Annual Reviews. 1999.

Grossman D, Krieger J, Sugarman J, Forquera R. Health Status of Urban American Indians and Alaska Natives: A Population-Based Study. *Journal of the American Medical Association* .1994; 271(11): 845–850.

Joseph-Fox Y, Kekahbah TM. *Establishing a National Health Services Research Agenda for American Indians and Alaska Natives*. Denver, CO: National Indian Health Board; 1999.

Indian Health Design Team. *Design for a New IHS: Final Recommendations of the Indian Health Design Team, Report Number II*. Rockville, MD: Indian Health Service; 1997.

Indian Health Service. *Trends in Indian Health*. DHHS, Rockville, MD: Indian Health Service; 1997.

National Institutes of Health/Indian Health Service. *Roundtable Conference on American Indian Research Training Needs. Final Report.*; Bethesda MD: National Institutes of Health. 1999.

Northwest Tribal Epidemiology Center. *Indian Community Health Profile*. Northwest Portland Area Indian Health Board; 2000.

Public Health Support Workgroup. *Public Health Support Workgroup Report. Executive Summary*. Rockville MD: Indian Health Service; 1999.

Roubideaux Y. Quality Measurement in Indian Health Facilities. A Pilot Study for the National Indian Health Board. In: Dixon, et al. *Tribal Perspectives on Indian Self-Determination and Self-Governance in Health Care Management*. Denver, CO: National Indian Health Board; 1998.

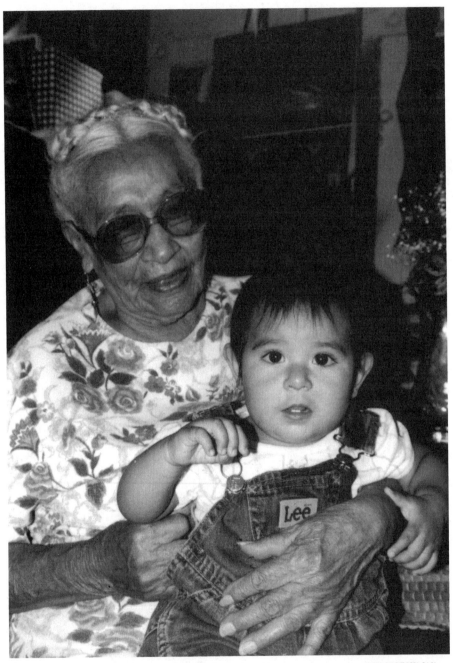

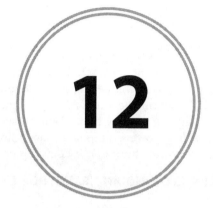

FEDERAL AND STATE POLICY TO STRENGTHEN INDIAN HEALTH

Mim Dixon and Yvette Joseph-Fox

In the last two centuries, the federal government has assumed the primary responsibility for Indian health care. Senator Daniel K. Inouye, Chairman of the Senate Select Committee on Indian Affairs for more than 8 years and former Vice-Chairman for 6 years, is often quoted as saying that American Indians have "the first pre-paid health plan." They paid for their federal health care with more than 400 million acres of land. However, the federal government has not lived up to its obligations. Indian health care is persistently under-funded by Congress.

Many states are only now beginning to recognize tribal sovereignty and accept responsibility for American Indians and Alaska Natives (AI/AN) as state citizens who are entitled to the same state programs that are provided to other citizens of the state. While the federal government is responsible for paying most of the bill for Indian health care, state policies have tremendous impact on the level of funding available to serve tribes and urban Indian people.

Any public health policies that affect tribes should be developed in consultation with tribal governments. The recommendations that are presented in this chapter reflect positions endorsed by national Indian organizations, including the National Indian Health Board (NIHB) and the National Congress of American Indians (NCAI).[1] A broad consensus was developed through tribal consultation and tribal representation in the development of these positions.

---

[1] The National Indian Health Board represents all federally recognized tribes and also serves as the health committee of the National Congress of American Indians.

However, each tribe is a sovereign entity and not every tribe has endorsed every recommendation in this chapter.

The purpose of this closing chapter is to present an agenda for public health policy in the 21st century that reflects the needs of American Indian and Alaska Native people and the official recommendations of national tribal organizations. Following a discussion of guiding principles, this agenda is organized into four sections: (1) funding for the Indian Health Service; (2) funding from other DHHS agencies; (3) strengthening self-determination and self-governance for tribes; and (4) creating healthier AI/AN communities.

It is not possible to anticipate every public policy issue that will be forthcoming in the next decade. However, the legal and historic basis for Indian health care provides guidance for future policy development.

GUIDING PRINCIPLES OF INDIAN HEALTH POLICY DEVELOPMENT

Fundamental to the recommendations in this chapter are some guiding principles, most of which were developed in conjunction with a national effort to recommend protections for AI/AN in Medicaid managed care programs (Dixon 1998). These principles were intended to guide decisions as states develop their Medicaid managed care programs, and as the Health Care Financing Administration (HCFA) exercises its federal trust responsibility with regard to federally-recognized tribes in the approval process for Medicaid state plans and waivers. However, the principles also apply to state and federal policy development related to other health care issues.

BASIC TENANTS OF FEDERAL INDIAN POLICY

There are three basic tenants of federal Indian policy: tribal sovereignty, the government-to-government relationship, and the federal trust responsibility (See chapter 1). Whether policies under consideration relate to health or any other aspect of Indian life, they must be consistent with these cornerstones of Indian law.

As a practical application, some examples may be helpful. Respecting tribal sovereignty means that tribes should not be required to submit to the state's licensing authority in order to receive federal funding for health programs. The government-to-government relationship means that tribes should be able to receive money and administer programs in the same manner as states and county governments. Agreements can be reached between the state government and tribal governments that are different from the state's relationships with vendors and other types of contractors.

The federal trust responsibility means that every agency of the federal government should exercise oversight as states administer federally funded programs to assure that tribes are consulted in the development of those programs, that states are responsive to tribal concerns, and that tribes receive a proportional share of the funding. The federal trust relationship means that the federal government has a duty to act in the best interest of tribes.

The concept of trust responsibility is not limited to health care. It is embedded in many concepts of Indian law and Indian programs, such as land that is taken into trust on behalf of tribes and Indian individuals. The federal trust responsibility to provide health care derives from the U.S. removal of Indians from their tribal lands in the 1800s, thus limiting tribal choices, creating a dependency on the federal government similar to other wards of the state, and then having a responsibility to take care of those who have been rendered dependent. At various times in history, the U.S. has tried to terminate this trust responsibility, however, the U.S. cannot undo the first part of the equation in which they have placed restrictions on tribes that reduce their choices and their independence. The concept of "dependent sovereign nation" continues and there is no possibility that tribes will once again be completely sovereign. This creates a "love–hate" relationship between tribes and the federal government. On the one hand, tribes want to exercise complete sovereignty and chaff at restrictions placed on them, such as gaming laws that require them to negotiate compacts with states and to pay a percentage of their profits to states. On the other hand, tribes feel that the limits on their sovereignty create a federal trust responsibility that must be honored. They want the federal government to fulfill its trust responsibility by fully funding federal programs that are designed to assist tribes and AI/AN people.

There are other important principles related to these three foundations of Indian law. These principles include tribal consultation, protecting and enhancing Indian health facilities and services, assuring that AI/AN have a choice of providers, setting reimbursement rates at a level that covers the cost of delivering services, eliminating barriers to AI/AN participation in other federal and state health programs, and simplifying the bureaucracy so that more resources are spent directly on health care.

CONSULTATION WITH TRIBES

Tribal consultation recognizes the inherent sovereignty of Indian nations by placing them in a government-to-government relationship with the federal government and individual states. Tribal consultation is a process that flows from federal laws that have created a special status and programs for American Indians, including the Indian Health Care Improvement Act (P.L. 94-437) and the Indian Self-Determination and Education Assistance Act (P.L. 93-638). In recognition of these laws, President Bill Clinton issued an Executive Order #13084 that serves to promote government-to-government consultation between the United States and tribal governments on matters affecting federal policy and budgetary concerns.

Tribal consultation is different from just holding hearings or meetings on or near AI/AN communities. Tribal consultation involves the active participation of tribal governments in setting the agenda, meeting place, and time of the meeting. Tribal governments share an equal role with the federal or state government in planning and hosting the event. The planning process establishes the climate of respect and enables all parties to take ownership for the outcomes of the meeting.

The consultation process needs to recognize the sovereignty of each tribe and not assume that one tribe can speak for another. States should issue invitations to participate in a consultation process to every tribe in the state. These invitations should be personally addressed to the tribal chairperson, governor, or chief of each respective tribal government according to sovereign protocol. Tribes may decide to let another organization represent them in discussions, but this should be done through the official tribal resolution process. Sometimes it is easier for state and federal government employees to communicate with employees of the tribe, such as the tribal health director, but all official invitations and communications should go to the elected tribal officials. If it seems too cumbersome to deal with each tribe individually, the federal and state governments can enlist the assistance of national and regional pan-tribal organizations, such as the National Indian Health Board or Area Health Boards, but they still must find a way to interact with each tribe on a government-to-government basis.

Tribal consultation should occur before decisions are made—not after. It is an opportunity to get tribal input to assure that decisions accommodate the needs and preferences of tribes. For example, states should consult with tribes in the development of their health programs and make special provisions for AI/AN consumers and Indian health system providers, particularly for Medicaid and other health programs that receive federal funding. Very few states actually invite tribal governments to consult with them on their state plans, which diminishes the capacity of health programs in meeting the needs of American Indians and Alaska Natives.

PROTECT AND ENHANCE INDIAN HEALTH FACILITIES AND SERVICES

Because there are cultural, geographic, financial, and historic barriers to accessing health care (See chapter 3), special health care delivery systems have been developed for American Indians and Alaska Natives. A fundamental value expressed by tribal leaders is maintaining a separate health care delivery system for AI/AN (Dixon, Bush, et al 1998). Both the federal and state governments must recognize the unique role of tribes in the delivery of health services (See chapter 2).

While Congress has not fully funded the Indian Health Service through direct appropriations, it has been the intent of Congress to use Medicaid, Medicare and other federal program funding to support Indian health care. To carry out this intent, both federal and state agencies should think creatively about how they can direct resources to protect and enhance Indian health facilities and services.

Thinking creatively means taking away some of the boundaries that usually creep into program designs. For example, if states are to design their Medicaid programs to protect and enhance Indian health facilities and services, they should think about providing the highest possible level of care to people both when they are Medicaid beneficiaries and when they are not receiving Medicaid. Knowing that people move on and off of Medicaid as their income and resources change, states should be concerned about continuity of care for AI/AN patients over the long term, not just providing care when they are eligible for Medicaid. That continuity is maintained when Indian health providers are also Medicaid providers for AI/AN. Also, states should be careful to avoid subsidizing non-Indian health care with federal resources intended for AI/AN.[2]

By providing 100 percent federal funding for AI/AN Medicaid recipients who are served in IHS and tribal facilities, HCFA has now given the states a great deal of opportunity to be flexible in designing Medicaid programs for AI/AN. Tribal consultation provides further opportunity for states to design Medicaid programs that meet the unique needs of AI/AN consumers. At minimum, Indian health facilities should be paid by Medicaid for every visit in which Medicaid-covered services are provided to a Medicaid beneficiary. This applies to the Indian Health Service (IHS) direct service facilities, tribally operated facilities, and urban Indian clinics, collectively known as "the I/T/U."

ASSURE THAT AMERICAN INDIANS/ALASKA NATIVES HAVE A CHOICE OF PROVIDERS

While the federal and state governments need to deal with tribes in the policy arena, their relationship with individuals who are American Indian or Alaska Native must recognize multiple citizenship. An AI/AN individual is a citizen of their tribe, a citizen of their state, and a citizen of the United States. As U. S. citizens, they need to be given the choices available to other U.S. citizens; as state citizens, they need to be given the choices available to other state citizens; and, in addition to the choices available to them as U.S. and state citizens, they should have choices to access to Indian health providers.

For example, American Indian and Alaska Native individuals who are Medicaid beneficiaries should have access to their customary Indian health providers, as well as providers that are available to other Medicaid beneficiaries. In a state with managed care Medicaid programs, AI/AN should not have to choose between the Indian health service and a managed care plan. If they choose a managed care plan, they should be able to go "off-plan" to seek care at an Indian health facility and that facility should be paid for the services provided as well.

AI/AN individuals who have alternate resources should have the opportunity to select the health care providers that will best meet their needs. Studies of AI/AN consumer behavior show that they are most likely to choose Indian

---

[2] This can happen when dollars provided under the 100 percent Federal Medical Assistance Percentage (FMAP) for AI/AN are used to pay premiums for a Medicaid managed care plan that is underutilized by AI/AN Medicaid recipients who go off plan for I/T/U services that are not reimbursed by Medicaid.

health providers for primary care, but they may prefer a private sector provider when they want a second opinion, have a serious problem, or consider their problem embarrassing and want to have more confidentiality (Dixon, Lasky, et al 1998).

SET PAYMENT RATES TO COVER THE COST OF DELIVERING SERVICES

The I/T/U should be reimbursed by Medicaid, Medicare, and other public financing programs at rates that cover the cost of delivering services, considering that there is little opportunity to shift costs to other third-party payers. Although the Federally Qualified Health Center (FQHC) payment approach recognized the need for payment rates that are fair and reasonable to community health centers and Indian health clinics, the Balanced Budget Act of 1997 phases out the FQHC rates. While tribes are protected to some extent by the Indian Health Service/Health Care Financing Administration Memorandum of Understanding (See chapter 4) that permits the IHS rate to be applied to tribes, this MOA does not apply to urban Indian clinics. Furthermore, the IHS flat daily rate does not take into account many regional variations in the cost of delivering services, nor does it include the cost of facilities depreciation and financing. Also, there is no IHS rate for outpatient surgery, which is considerably more costly than the current reimbursement rate for an outpatient visit. Despite the impact of rate setting on their operations, the tribes and urban Indian clinics are not represented in the negotiations that establish the IHS rate.

The elimination of the FQHC rate is part of an overall trend to roll Medicaid patients into large managed care plans that will absorb the cost of serving them. However, these managed care plans do not always provide accessible or culturally responsive services for AI/AN Medicaid recipients. While it may cost more to serve AI/AN Medicaid recipients in I/T/U facilities, the total cost of their care is a tiny fraction of the total Medicaid budget and providing revenues to the I/T/U may be the most cost-effective approach in the long run.

Few people in Indian Country are advocating for a return to the FQHC rates, as the calculation is very cumbersome and bureaucratic. It has been suggested that a special category of Indian health facilities be identified for the purposes of rate setting for Medicaid, Medicare and other federally funded programs. The National Steering Committee on Reauthorization of the Indian Health Care Improvement Act (P.L. 94-437) recommended the establishment of a new provider-type, entitled the "Qualified Indian Health Program" (QIHP). The proposed amendments to Title IV of P.L. 94-437 would change the Social Security Act to allow IHS and tribal facilities to be reimbursed directly by the Health Care Financing Administration under the new QIHP. Furthermore, in the legislative proposal the negotiated rulemaking process used to develop regulations for the Indian Self-Determination Act (P.L. 93-638) would be used in the rate setting process to assure tribal participation.

Fair payment rates are not just an issue for the I/T/U; combined with low population density, low reimbursement rates make it difficult for private medical services to survive in the rural areas where most tribes are located. In urban areas, many private sector physicians simply refuse to see patients who are beneficiaries of publicly-financed health programs if those programs keep their rates too low. So, payment rates can affect access to care for AI/AN consumers who are exempted from managed care Medicaid programs and choose to be served in the fee-for-service system.

ELIMINATE BARRIERS TO AI/AN PARTICIPATION IN GOVERNMENT HEALTH PROGRAMS

Barriers to participation, such as premiums, deductibles, and co-pays, should be eliminated for AI/AN for health care programs that receive any public funding. Because AI/AN are eligible for services at Indian health facilities, they are unlikely to enroll in federal and state programs that charge fees. This means that the I/T/U facilities will not get reimbursed for services delivered to people who would otherwise be eligible for those programs.

Financial barriers often exist with expanded Medicaid programs and Medicare Part B. While assistance is available for the financial costs of Medicare Part B through the Selected Low Income Medicare Beneficiary (SLIMB) and Qualified Medicare Beneficiary (QMB) programs, they have not been well advertised in Indian Country. In light of the special status of American Indians, states should waive the consumer participation requirement for those programs for AI/AN who would otherwise not be eligible.

While it is not well documented, there is a concern that many elderly AI/AN do not qualify for Medicare because they have not worked in jobs with Social Security coverage for the required number of quarters (Those people who have lived subsistence lifestyles or worked in seasonal employment are not as likely to be eligible for Medicare.). A policy approach that merits further consideration is to deem all AI/AN eligible for Medicare when they meet the age requirements, regardless of their level of contributions to the Social Security system.

SIMPLIFY THE BUREAUCRACY

Recognizing the limitations in funding, resources should be used to the maximum extent for direct patient care and prevention activities while keeping administrative functions as efficient as possible. In a situation where the Indian health system must operate on a fixed budget, the burden of additional bureaucratic requirements means reductions in direct patient care. If the bureaucracy expands without resulting in greater productivity or quality of care, limited resources will be wasted on administrative costs. For example, the requirement for Indian health facilities to bill three or more Medicaid managed care organizations creates a much heavier administrative burden than billing one state office or its fiscal intermediary. When the outcome is the payment of the same IHS rate, it makes no sense to create a more complicated path to receiving that payment.

SUMMARY OF GUIDING PRINCIPLES

While it is impossible to foresee all of the policy issues relating to Indian health in the 21st century, it is possible to approach each new issue with consistent criteria for evaluation. Policy makers and planners should ask these questions:

• Is this policy or approach consistent with the basic tenants of federal Indian policy: tribal sovereignty, government-to-government relationships, and the federal trust responsibility?

• Were tribes consulted in the process of developing this policy and do they endorse it?

• Does this approach protect and enhance Indian health facilities and services?

• Does this policy protect the right of AI/AN individuals to choose whether they receive their health services from the Indian health system, or another type of provider, or both?

• Do payment rates cover the cost of delivering services and are they sufficient to assure access to care for AI/AN consumers?

• Have steps been taken to identify and eliminate barriers to AI/AN participation?

• Is the new program or policy designed to enhance health services without creating unnecessary administrative costs for the I/T/U?

If tribes are satisfied that the answer is "yes" to all of these questions, then the proposed policy or program is probably going to benefit AI/AN people.

DIRECT APPROPRIATIONS FROM CONGRESS TO THE IHS

To exercise the federal trust responsibility, the United States Congress must appropriate the funding to the Indian Health Service that enables the I/T/U to deliver health care programs on a par with the general population. The level of congressional appropriations is a key public policy issue that affects the health of American Indians and Alaska Natives.

TRIBES CALL FOR A $15.1 BILLION BUDGET FOR IHS

Under the Clinton Administration, tribes became more involved in the development of the federal Indian health care budget that was submitted to Congress. The Presidential Executive Order #13084 on Government-to-Government Consultation and the Department of Health and Human Services' Secretarial Policy on Tribal Consultation issued by Secretary Donna Shalala requires federal agencies to consult with tribes in the development of their annual budget justification documents. The preparation of the fiscal year 2001 budget for the Indian Health Service included participation by representatives of tribal governments and their health care systems from every IHS Area. The National Indian Health Board, the Tribal Self-Governance Advisory Committee, and the National Council on Urban Indian Health met collectively with the Indian Health Service and reviewed the budget recommendations developed in each of the 12 Area budget formulation meetings. This multi-layered approach to tribal consultation resulted in a consensus that the IHS budget should be at least $15.1 billion; however, the Director of the Indian Health Service only requested $3.219 billion.

Despite the unprecedented federal budget surplus, tribes recognize that there must be an incremental approach to increasing the budget for the IHS. In 1999, NCAI passed a resolution that called for the first incremental increase to be $806 million, with at least $340 million of that amount going to Contract Support Costs (See Chapter 4 for a more thorough discussion of Contract Support Costs.), considered "critically needed to ensure that tribal governments are successful in fulfilling the goals of Indian Self-Determination and Self-Governance."[3] However, Congress only increased the IHS budget by $214 million, including only a $20 million increase for Contract Support Costs.

RESULTS OF MAINTAINING THE STATUS QUO

Just to maintain the status quo, the Indian Health Service budget must increase by approximately 7 percent per year to address the mandatory Pay Act increases for federal employees and to keep pace with inflation. In fiscal year 2000, for example, the Federal Employee Pay Act resulted in a 4.4 percent pay increase that required a $40.7 million to be added to the IHS budget just to maintain the status quo. The preceding year inflation was low, but the 2.1 percent inflation rate for non-medical costs and the 3.8 percent inflation for medical costs meant that an additional $52.5 million would have to be added to the IHS budget just to maintain the status quo. Thus, a $93.2 million increase was needed to maintain the status quo. In the final deliberations on the Fiscal Year 2000 IHS Budget, the Congress agreed to a $155 million increase to the IHS budget which amounted to a 6.9 percent increase, but $93.2 million of that amount went to simply meeting inflation. Furthermore, the IHS budget was subject to an across-the-board reduction of 0.38 percent for discretionary pro-

---

[3] The National Congress of American Indians, Resolution #VAN-99-050, Indian Health Service Fiscal Year 2001 Budget, adopted at the 1999 Mid-Year Session held in Vancouver, British Columbia, Canada, July 20-23, 1999.

grams which amounted to a decrease of $6 million agreed to by the Congress. In sum, the $155 million increase in the IHS budget was only a $55.8 million increase in real spending that could be used to expand services.

From 1992 until 1999, the IHS absorbed $323 million in unfunded mandatory costs. The agency estimated that this resulted in 65 percent of Contract Health Services requests being denied. The types of problems that went untreated in children included tympanoplasty, umbilical hernia repair, and tonsillectomies, and nearly a quarter of the deferred services involved women's health, such as routine mammograms to screen for cancer. Buford L. Rolin, Chairman of NIHB, explained the system for prioritizing health care to the Senate Committee on Indians Affairs in his testimony on July 22, 1998:

> Currently, we are forced to apply Priority One in the first quarter of the fiscal year. So for the remaining nine months, we understand that pain has become the new standard for determining who can access basic surgery and other specialized care. If an Indian patient needs gall bladder surgery, he or she will likely be denied a referral for surgery, unless this patient is in terrible pain and on the verge of passing their gallstones. If an Indian elder needs to have cataract surgery to see better or requires a referral to a heart specialist to determine potential heart damage, they will likely be denied care, until a more serious health problem arises like blindness, heart attack or stroke.

He also reported that prevention services decreased, with the number of well child visits declining by 23 percent, adult physical exams reduced by 16 percent, and an 18 percent reduction in the number of people receiving dental services.

Most dramatic was the story he told about the suicides that took a terrible toll on the Standing Rock Sioux Reservation in 1998: Within a 6-month period, there were 6 suicides among children aged 12–20. At the same time, there were 18 suicide attempts requiring hospitalization and another 150 tribal members who were identified as high risk for suicide. Yet, the under funding of mental health services in the IHS meant that people had to wait up to three months for an appointment to secure psychiatric evaluation.

ELIMINATING RACIAL DISPARITIES IN HEALTH STATUS

In 1997, President Clinton formed a Blue Ribbon Commission on Race in America; but he declined to appoint an American Indian or Alaska Native to serve on the commission. The commission identified a number of issues related to the gap in health status and health services between people of color in America and the White population. As a result of the Commission findings, the President submitted to Congress a budget that included a $1.7 billion increase for six agencies in the Department of Health and Human Services (DHHS)— the IHS was not one of those agencies. Instead, the IHS was slated for an increase of less than one percent, not enough to cover the cost of inflation or the Federal Employee Pay Act increases.

The DHHS Initiative to Eliminate Racial Disparities in Health was designed to focus on the areas of HIV/AIDS, diabetes, cancer screening and management, cardiovascular disease, infant mortality, and childhood and adult immunizations. However, little of the new funding actually filtered down to Indian Country.

A cruel hoax was perpetrated on the Indian people in the fiscal year 1999 budget. There really was no new money to close the gap in health status. In a shell game, money was taken from other vital and under-funded Indian health services to fund new initiatives. Buford Rolin, Chairman of the National Indian Health Board, explained it this way in his testimony to the House Interior Appropriations Subcommittee on March 25, 1998:

> As part of President Clinton's Race Commission recommendations, $80 million in new funding is supposed to be targeted at six priority areas as part of the increases described above. New initiatives in Breast Cancer Screening and Prevention will require the IHS to dedicate $5 million toward early cancer screening within its Hospitals and Clinics line item. This is an unfunded mandate. While we support the intent, the means to this end are wrong. The cost of providing access to 60,000 women for vitally needed cancer detection is to deprive other patients of nearly 440,000 hospital and clinic patient visits. Rather than closing the gap between the races in access to health care, the President's budget widens the gap by cutting $9.9 million in the Hospitals and Clinics line item. New funding is not provided for this important life-saving effort to address cancer in Indian Country. Instead, services are being compromised.

The disparities in health status persist in AI/AN populations. According to Mr. Rolin's testimony, the 5-year survival rate for AI/AN with breast cancer is 49 percent compared to 76 percent for Whites. Cervical cancer mortality rates for AI/AN are 1.7 times the national average. Infant mortality rates are 30 percent greater for AI/AN babies than for infants in the U.S. White population.

REAUTHORIZATION OF THE INDIAN HEALTH CARE IMPROVEMENT ACT (P.L. 93-437)

After 23 years, a major overhaul is occurring in the Indian Health Care Improvement Act (P.L. 93-437) through the reauthorization process. Tribal governments have participated in the development of more than 180 pages of bill language that is being submitted to Congress to help guide the development of a new law. In the future, there will be many twists and turns in the progress of this legislation.

Tribes have taken the view that reauthorization of the Indian Health Care Improvement Act (IHCIA) provides an opportunity to reaffirm the government's commitment to sustain existing programs, to enhance new programs, and to address broad policy issues that can affect funding for the Indian health system. For example, it is necessary for IHCIA to reauthorize the Community Health Representative programs, urban Indian clinics (See chapter 5), and scholarship programs for those important programs to continue. Reauthorization of the IHCIA may provide the vehicle to finally change the Indian Health Service into an entitlement program. This would guarantee the funding needed to provide designated services to the eligible population (See chapter 4).

ELEVATION OF THE DIRECTOR OF THE IHS TO ASSISTANT SECRETARY

Many people believe that the IHS has fared poorly in the appropriations process because the Director of the IHS is situated too low in the federal bureaucracy to advocate effectively for Indian health needs; currently, the Director of the IHS reports to an Assistant Secretary in DHHS. Tribes have supported legislation that would elevate the IHS Director to the position of Assistant Secretary for Indian Health. In testimony provided July 22, 1998, on S. 1770, a bill to elevate the Director of the Indian Health Service, NIHB Chairman Buford L. Rolin told the Senate Committee on Indian Affairs:

> This under-funding arises from the lack of positive regard provided to the IHS during the entire budget formulation process, from within the Department, to the Office of Management and Budget, and on to the Congress.

As an Assistant Secretary, the head of the Indian Health Services would have a direct line of communication with the Secretary of DHHS, more organizational independence, and the capacity to advocate at a higher level with more authority.

Even with tribal contracting and compacting reducing the administrative services of the IHS to tribes, the Indian Health Service comprises about 20 percent of the DHHS workforce. In the Indian Health Design Team (IHDT) recommendations, the headquarters of IHS retains the responsibility to advocate on behalf of all tribes in improving the Indian health system (IHDT 1997). Tribes recognize that this will be accomplished more effectively if the top position in the IHS leadership is an Assistant Secretary. This desire has been endorsed by the NIHB[4] and NCAI.[5]

One of the most significant reasons to elevate the IHS Director to Assistant Secretary is to provide greater opportunity to persuade leaders of other agencies in DHHS to direct a greater portion of their resources to meet the needs of American Indians and Alaska Natives.

FUNDING FROM OTHER AGENCIES TO MEET AMERICAN INDIANS/ALASKA NATIVES HEALTH NEEDS

There is great potential for DHHS agencies to enhance the efforts of the IHS. For example, the NIHB has requested that the Centers for Disease Control and Prevention (CDC) allocate a portion of their funding for existing programs to address diabetes, tuberculosis, HIV/AIDs, sexually transmitted diseases, epidemiology, and surveillance in Indian Country. The NIHB recommended that the National Cancer Institute should be spending at least $5.4 million in new funding in the fiscal year 2000 budget on Indian issues, such as development of tumor registries, reclassifications of AI/AN in cancer data, and provisions for technical advisors and leadership development for cancer research at Area Health Boards and tribal colleges. NIHB recommends that the Agency for Healthcare Research and Quality invest $1.5 million to conduct research on quality of care in Indian health systems.

Also, the National Indian Council on Aging has called on the Health Care Financing Administration (HCFA), the Health Resources and Service Administration (HRSA), the National Institutes of Health (NIH), and the Administration on Aging (AOA) to dedicate a portion of their research and development funds for grants to help tribes and AI/AN communities plan, develop and deliver culturally-appropriate and effective long-term care services. Only at the end of the 20th century have the various agencies in DHHS begun the process of tribal consultation to find out how they can better serve Indian Country.

MEDICAID

Since Congress has not appropriated sufficient funding through the Indian Health Service budget to meet the health care needs of American Indians and Alaska Natives, there is a growing reliance on Medicaid as a source of funding. At the same time, there has been a growing trend within states to change their Medicaid programs to managed care programs. This has created problems for AI/AN consumer access to care and has created obstacles for the Indian health system to maximize its income from Medicaid (see chapters 3 & 4).

Congress created a special rule for Indian enrollment in state Medicaid managed care programs in the Balanced Budget Act of 1997 (BBA) (Section

---

[4] NIHB Resolution 96-20, Support for Senate Bill 311: The Elevation of the Director of the Indian Health Service to Assistant Secretary of the Department of Health and Human Services, adopted at a Special Meeting in Rockville, MD, October 17-18, 1996.

[5] NCAI Resolution #GRB-98-10, Support for Senate Bill 1770: The Elevation of the Director of the Indian Health Service to Assistant Secretary of the Department of Health and Human Services, adopted at the Mid-Year Session of the NCAI in Green Bay, WI, June 14-17, 1998.

1932(a)(2)(c)). The BBA prohibits a state plan from requiring AI/AN to enroll in a managed care entity unless the entity is the IHS, an Indian health program operated by an Indian tribe or tribal organization, or an urban Indian health program. However, this special rule does not apply to states that receive waivers under Section 1115 or 1915(b), which are the most common means for states to convert their Medicaid programs to managed care.

IHS and HCFA entered into a Memorandum of Agreement (IHS/HCFA MOA) on December 19, 1996, regarding a payment policy for Medicaid services to American Indian and Alaska Natives (See chapter 4), but that MOA is not binding on states and it does not apply to urban Indian clinics. Furthermore, the MOA is subject to a variety of interpretations (Dixon 1998).

In 1998, the NIHB conducted a survey of nine states with Medicaid managed care programs to learn how AI/AN consumers and Indian health providers were being affected by the change (Dixon 1998); the report was presented at a national meeting, "Indian Health, Medicaid and Managed Care: A Call to Action," held in Denver, Colorado, September 2–3, 1998. Based upon the report and the comments at that meeting, the Advisory Committee for the project developed a series of recommendations; these recommendations were presented at the NIHB Consumer Conference in Anchorage, Alaska, October 6–8, 1998. After tribal review, the NIHB adopted these recommendations in two resolutions.

Many of the protections that tribes are requesting can be made by Medicaid administrators at the state and federal levels. However, tribes recognize that as political administrations change, so do political policies. Therefore, it is recommended that changes be made by amending the Social Security Act (Title 19). These are the highest priority Medicaid recommendations from the study (Dixon 1998) that were adopted in a resolution passed by the NIHB:[6]

1. The same protections that Congress provided for American Indians in the Balanced Budget Act of 1997 should be extended to the Social Security Act. Title 19, Sections 1115 and 1915(b), should be amended to prohibit HCFA from granting waivers that allow mandatory enrollment in managed care plans unless those waivers exempt American Indians and Alaska Natives from mandatory enrollment in plans that are not operated by the I/T/U.

2. Recognizing that the I/T/U cannot refuse services to American Indian and Alaska Native beneficiaries who voluntarily enroll in a managed care plan, the law should require all state Medicaid managed care programs to have provisions to pay the I/T/U for off-plan services provided to IHS beneficiaries who are also Medicaid beneficiaries.

---

[6] National Indian Health Board Resolution 99-01, Amending the Social Security Act (Title 19) to Protect American Indians and Alaska Natives who are Medicaid Beneficiaries and to Assure Payment to Indian Health Facilities in States with Managed Care Medicaid Programs was adopted on January 29, 1999, in Denver, Colorado.

3. The provisions in the IHS/HCFA MOA for tribally-operated facilities to have the option to use the IHS payment methodology rate and for states to receive 100 percent Federal Medical Assistance Percentage (FMAP) for services delivered in these facilities should be specified in law and should be extended to urban Indian clinics.

4. The methods for calculating the IHS payment rate and the application of that rate and the 100 percent FMAP should be developed by a joint tribal-federal rulemaking committee that includes HCFA and IHS, using the negotiated rulemaking model that was used for P.L. 93-638.

5. Indian health providers should receive payment for services to IHS beneficiaries who are also Medicaid recipients from states or their fiscal intermediaries directly and not be required to bill health plans.

6. The law should define the I/T/U provider type or payment rate methodology for non-Indian Medicaid beneficiaries served in I/T/U facilities to assure that the Medicaid payments are not lower than the cost of delivering services and thereby avoid cost shifting that would result in IHS funding subsidizing health care for non-Indians.

7. Consumer cost sharing (premiums, deductibles, and co-payments) should be waived for American Indians and Alaska Natives in Medicaid programs.

Tribes also see a need for oversight of state Medicaid programs. The NIHB has recommended a Medicaid Managed Care and Indian Health Monitoring Committee with participation from tribes, urban Indian programs, the Indian Health Service, the Health Care Financing Administration, and states to prioritize evaluation and monitoring needs and provide oversight for on-going studies. Oversight activities could include an annual meeting for researchers to share their findings about managed care and Indian health, and a newsletter to communicate findings to Indian health providers and state and federal agencies. They believe the Medicaid Managed Care and Indian Health Monitoring Committee should provide an annual report to Congress on the impact of Medicaid managed care on Indian health facilities and access to care for IHS beneficiaries.

Furthermore, there is an interest among tribes in having a more direct government-to-government relationship with HCFA. Many tribes would like to be able to bill HCFA directly for Medicaid in the same way as they bill for Medicare, without dealing with states or managed care plans. The Navajo Nation has proposed to operate a Medicaid agency that would cover tribal members on the Navajo reservation, which is located in three states and now requires the tribe to negotiate with three different state Medicaid agencies. NIHB supports the idea of a research and demonstration project for tribes or tribal organizations to contract or compact with HCFA for Medicaid programs that serve their tribal members, or to waive the state agency requirement and allow tribes or tribal organizations to function as a fiscal intermediary without going through the IHS or state governments.

MEDICARE

While Medicare provides health coverage for most senior citizens in our country, there is some evidence to suggest that the AI/AN benefit from this program is less than for other ethnic groups (Kauffman, et al 1997). The federal government could increase AI/AN participation in Medicare by deeming eligible all AI/AN who meet the age criteria, even if they do not have the requisite number of quarters of contributions to the Social Security system. Also, greater outreach to AI/AN communities is needed to inform them of the opportunities for assistance with Medicare Part B premiums and co-pays through the Selected Low Income Medicare Beneficiary (SLIMB) and Qualified Medicare Beneficiary (QMB) programs. Many advocates want to increase accessibility by waiving the Medicare premiums and co-pays for AI/AN.

Medicare does cover people with end-stage renal disease, regardless of their age or social security status. Since diabetes is disproportionately high in the American Indian population, there is also a disproportionately high rate of end-stage renal disease. Medicare coverage is making it possible for private sector and tribally operated dialysis centers to locate in Indian communities. However, tribes need more technical assistance to make more of these life-sustaining services accessible for their tribal members.

Medicare also is one of the major funding sources for home health care services (See chapter 6). While tribes have a long history of delivering services at home, including Community Health Nursing and Community Health Representatives, few tribes have been certified as Medicare Home Health Agencies to enable them to receive Medicare reimbursement. Again, technical assistance is needed for tribes to develop creative ways to meet the staffing and administrative requirements of Medicare certification. Another approach would be to create more flexible rules to allow tribes to qualify for Medicare reimbursement. Laws and regulations that impede the ability of Indian health providers to obtain reimbursement from Medicare should be reviewed and changed.

STATE CHILD HEALTH INSURANCE PROGRAMS

Congress established the State Children's Health Insurance Program (SCHIP) in the Balanced Budget Act of 1997, also known as Title 21 of the Social Security Act. The Act specifically stated that Indian Health Service beneficiaries are not excluded from participation in SCHIP; however, many states did not consult with Indian tribes in the development of their SCHIP plans (Dixon 1998). Some SCHIP programs have premiums and co-pays that effectively eliminate most AI/AN participation in these programs. Furthermore, some SCHIP programs have contracted with managed care plans that do not include all Indian health facilities in their provider networks and do not pay for off-plan services. These conditions in SCHIP programs reduce the opportunities for the I/T/U to collect payments from SCHIP even though they are providing services to AI/AN who are eligible for SCHIP.

Under Title 21, states have a choice of expanding their Medicaid programs, or creating separate SCHIP programs, or both. The federal law and policies regarding AI/AN consumers and I/T/U providers for Medicaid programs are very different from those for non-Medicaid SCHIP programs. For example, the non-Medicaid programs may be located in a state agency that offers low cost insurance to small employers and restricts services to managed care plans. States that choose to expand their Medicaid programs can better serve AI/AN children, enhance collections for I/T/U facilities, and receive greater reimbursement under the IHS/HCFA MOA.

The NIHB passed a resolution with the following recommendations for amending Title 21:[7]

1. Recognizing that the I/T/U cannot refuse services to American Indian and Alaska Native beneficiaries who voluntarily enroll in a managed care plan, the law should require all SCHIP managed care programs to have provisions to pay the I/T/U for off-plan services provided to IHS beneficiaries who are also SCHIP beneficiaries.

2. The provisions in the IHS/HCFA MOA for tribally-operated facilities to have the option to use the IHS payment methodology rate and for states to receive 100 percent Federal Medical Assistance Percentage (FMAP) for services delivered in these facilities should be applied to SCHIP programs, specified in law and extended to urban Indian clinics.

3. Consumer cost sharing (premiums, deductibles and co-payments) should be waived for American Indians and Alaska Natives in SCHIP programs.

4. States that have already expanded their Medicaid to the extent provided by the State Child Health Insurance Program should be allowed to submit 1115 or 1915(b) waivers to cover the remaining uninsured children and use the federal allocation for SCHIP to accomplish this goal.

---

[7] NIHB Resolution Number 99-02, amending the Social Security Act (Title 21) to Increase Access to State Children's Health Insurance Programs for American Indians and Alaska Natives, was adopted on January 29, 1999, in Denver, Colorado.

STRENGTHENING SELF-DETERMINATION AND SELF-GOVERNANCE

The policy of self-determination and self-governance that started in 1971 with the Indian Self-Determination and Education Assistance Act has proven successful over the years (Dixon, et al 1998). However, there has never been sufficient federal funding to allow all tribes to participate to the extent that they may choose. The problem has been not only the direct funding for health care programs, but also Contract Support Costs (See chapter 4). In the fiscal year 2000 budget, Congress made a significant effort to close the gap between the tribal requests for assistance from the Indian Self-Determination (ISD) Fund and the actual appropriations for that purpose. The $60 million increase in ISD funding covered 90 percent of the negotiated requirements; however, an additional $147.6 million was still needed to assure that all tribes that want to participate could do so. The Fiscal Year 2001 budget provided $20 million toward that goal, so there is still an unmet need of $127.6 million.

CREATING HEALTHIER AI/AN COMMUNITIES

Healthy People 2010 provides health objectives for the nation as a whole that are intended to increase quality-of-life and to eliminate health disparities. The model used by *Healthy People 2010* includes factors such as individual behavior and biology, the physical and social environment, access to quality health care, and policies and interventions. It is estimated that 70 percent of all premature deaths in the U.S. are due to individual behaviors and environmental factors (DHHS 2001)

As the incidence of chronic diseases rises, the focus of prevention and control of illness should be on nutrition, physical activity, and other lifestyle factors. Often, a healthy lifestyle accompanies a resurgence of cultural pride and an acknowledgement that tribal traditions provide a way to physical, mental, and spiritual well-being.

Health is affected by community socioeconomic status (Yen and Syme 1999). Healthier communities have greater opportunities for employment, childcare, education, housing, transportation, and recreation. Improvements in education in AI/AN communities will contribute to improved health literacy. Schools that have strong math and science programs are more likely to encourage students to pursue careers in health. Too often AI/AN students who go to college do not have the confidence to take the courses that would prepare them for health professions.

These circumstances are affected not only by federal funding for a wide-range of Indian programs, but also by policies that can enable tribes to develop greater self-sufficiency through economic development. The Indian Gaming Regulatory Act of 1988 (IGRA) created opportunities for some tribes to create greater employment opportunities for their members and increased revenue has been used for health, education, job training, and community infrastructure (Kalt 1998). However, the success of tribal gaming has been over-stated. Only about one-third of tribes have any gaming operations at all. While the successes of the eight tribal programs that account for more than half of all Indian gaming revenues are well publicized, they are not typical (Kalt 1998). Because they exercise their tribal sovereignty by not entering into gaming enterprises or because they are located in areas where gaming is not a viable option, most tribes in the country need other types of economic development.

Environmental factors that also affect health include the most basic public health measures of clean water and sewage treatment facilities, yet many tribal communities lack these necessities. Federal programs have located a number of dangerous activities on or near reservations, including uranium mining, testing of atomic bombs, and storage of nuclear wastes. While some of the biggest environmental clean-up programs in the nation are currently underway on tribal lands, other tribes are just beginning the identification and elimination of harmful contaminants. Many tribes have inherited old military and Bureau of Indian Affairs (BIA) housing that is laden with asbestos and lead paint, but few tribes have the resources to identify those environmental hazards and contain them. Perhaps the most prevalent environmental risk is tobacco abuse and second-hand smoke; there is a great need for culturally sensitive tobacco cessation programs in AI/AN communities.

The high rates of morbidity and mortality from injuries require that AI/AN communities have better roads, law enforcement, criminal justice systems, domestic violence prevention programs, and substance abuse prevention and treatment programs. Alcoholism has been associated with high rates of injury, poisoning, homicide, and suicide, as well as fetal alcohol syndrome.

No discussion of the development of alcohol and drug abuse prevention and treatment among AI/AN during the past 15 years can avoid considering the role of the federal government; funding for substance abuse awareness programs comes primarily from the federal government via appropriations authorized under a number of important public laws, including P.L. 95-570 and P. L. 100-713. There continue to be challenges and remarkable accomplishments alike due to enactment of P.L. 99-570, also known as the Indian Juvenile Alcohol and Substance Abuse Prevention Act. By the end of the century, the level of funding for prevention and treatment had increased to $100 million, but tribes estimate that an additional $290 million is needed for this important activity.

American Indian and Alaska Native cultures value the wisdom of elders and their important roles in leadership, education, spiritual activities, and cultural continuity. Healthy communities have services that support elders and others with disabilities to live with dignity as independently as possible. As the number of AI/AN elders grow, the need for a full range of home and community-based services will grow; many tribes are anxious to build nursing homes so that they can keep their elders in the community, as they have requested.

However, nursing homes are only one small part of the continuum of care that is needed. A healthy community should have senior citizen centers, nutrition programs, transportation programs, adult day care, respite care, home health care, homemaker services, and assisted living.

SUMMARY

While there are 556 federally recognized tribes in our country with many different languages and cultures, all American Indians and Alaska Natives share a common belief in the interrelatedness of all things—this basic philosophy is compatible with the holistic approach of public health. Public health policy for American Indians and Alaska Natives in the 21st century should be broader than existing health services; public health policy should strive to support healthier communities and strengthen tribal self-determination.

It has often been said that the Indian health system would be an ideal model for community-based, public health-oriented health care, if only it were adequately funded. Adequate federal and state funding is needed to build upon the traditions of public health that have evolved through a long process of creative problem solving. If we have learned anything in the past 200 years, we have learned that tribes must be part of the solution. Tribes must have the opportunity to be involved in every aspect of planning and delivering services for their tribal members. But, most tribes cannot do this alone. The federal government must honor its trust responsibility by providing the necessary funding to assure that the health of American Indian and Alaska Native people is comparable to that of other citizens of our great nation.

ACKNOWLEDGEMENTS:

The authors would like to express their deepest appreciation to the Board of Directors and the staff of the National Indian Health Board, especially the current Chair H. Sally Smith and the former Chair Buford L. Rolin, for their leadership and support in the development of the ideas in this chapter. We would also like to thank the tribes, their elected leaders, and health program directors, who are on the front lines in the development of federal and state health policy.

REFERENCES

Department of Health and Human Services. *Healthy People 2010*). Available at www.health.gov. Accessed on January 7, 2000

Dixon M. *Indian Health in Nine State Medicaid Managed Care Programs.* Denver: National Indian Health Board. 1998.

Dixon M, Bush JK, Iron PE. Factors Affecting Tribal Choice of Health Care Organizations. In *A Forum on the Implications of Changes in the Health Care Environment for Native American Health Care*. Washington, DC: The Henry J. Kaiser Family Foundation. 1997.

Dixon M, Lasky PS, Iron PE, Marquez C. Factors Affecting Native American Consumer Choice of Health Care Provider Organizations. In *A forum on the Implication of Changes in the Health Care Environment for Native American Health*. Washington, DC: The Henry J. Kaiser Family Foundation; 1997.

Dixon M, Brett Lee Shelton BL, Roubideaux Y, Mather D, Smith CM. *Tribal Perspectives on Indian Self-Determination and Self-Governance in Health Care Management*. Vol 4. Denver, CO: National Indian Health Board; 1998.

Indian Health Design Team. *Design for a New IHS: Final Recommendations of the Indian Health Design Team, Report Number II*. Rockville, MD: Indian Health Service, DHHS. 1997.

Kalt JP. Statement Before the National Gambling Impact Study Commission, March 16, 1998. Cambridge, MA: Harvard Project on American Indian Economic Development, Harvard University; 1998.

Kauffman JA, Johnson E, Jacobs J. Overview: Current and Evolving Realities of Health Care to Reservation and Urban American Indians. In *A Forum on the Implications of Changes in the Health Care Environment for Native American Health Care*. Washington, D.C.: The Henry J. Kaiser Family Foundation; 1997.

Yen IH, Syme SL. The Social Environment and Health: A Discussion of the Epidemiologic Literature. In: Fielding JE, Lave LB, Starfield B, eds. *Annual Review of Public Health*. Vol 20. Palo Alto, CA: Annual Reviews; 1999.

INDEX